Recent Results in Cancer Research 132

Managing Editors
Ch. Herfarth, Heidelberg · H.-J. Senn, St. Gallen

Associate Editors
M. Baum, London · V. Diehl, Köln
F. Gutzwiller, Zürich · M. F. Rajewsky, Essen
M. Wannenmacher, Heidelberg

Founding Editor
P. Rentchnick, Geneva

S.C. Schimpff J. Klastersky (Eds.)

Infectious Complications in Bone Marrow Transplantation

With 30 Figures and 51 Tables

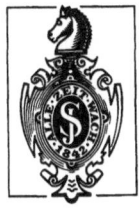

Springer-Verlag
Berlin Heidelberg New York
London Paris Tokyo
Hong Kong Barcelona
Budapest

Prof. Stephen C. Schimpff, M.D.
University of Maryland Medical System
Baltimore, MD 21201, USA

Prof. Jean Klastersky, M.D.
Institut Jules Bordet
Centre des Tumeurs de l'Université
Libre de Bruxelles
Brussels, Belgium

ISBN-13:978-3-642-84901-5   e-ISBN-13:978-3-642-84899-5
DOI: 10.1007/978-3-642-84899-5

Library of Congress Cataloging-in-Publication Data.
Infectious complications in bone marrow transplantation / Stephen C. Schimpff,
Jean Klastersky (eds.). p. cm.—(Recent results in cancer research : 132) Includes
bibliographical references and index.
ISBN-13:978-3-642-84901-5
1. Bone marrow—Transplantation—Complications—Congresses. 2. Infection—Congresses. I. Schimpff, Stephen C., 1941– . II. Klastersky, J. (Jean) III. Series.
[DNLM: 1. Bone Marrow Transplantation—adverse effects—congresses. 2. Infection—etiology—congresses. W1 RE106P v. 132 1992 / WH 380 I43 1992]
RC261.R35 no.   132 [RD123.5] 616.99'4 s—dc20 [617.4'4] DNLM/DLC
92-48504

© Springer-Verlag Berlin Heidelberg 1993
Softcover reprint of the hardcover 1st edition 1993

The use of general descriptive names, registered names, trademarks, etc. in this
publication does not imply, even in the absence of a specific statement, that such
names are exempt from the relevant protective laws and regulations and therefore
free for general use.

Product Liability: The publishers cannot guarantee the accuracy of any information
about dosage and application contained in this book. In every individual case the user
must check such information by consulting the relevant literature.

Typesetting by Best-set Typesetter Ltd., Hong Kong
19/3130/SPS-5 4 3 2 1 0 – Printed on acid-free paper

To our wives, Carol and Daisy,
and our daughters,
Elizabeth, Catherine and Sophie

Preface

As the demographics of the population shift toward an increasingly aged society, the number of individuals with cancer increases and with it the need to give the most comprehensive possible health care delivery. Although much has been written about the specific therapy best suited for the various types of cancer and about the basic and clinical research which has dramatically improved treatment, overall patient care requires attention to supportive care, which includes such items as pain management, the use of blood products, nutrition, and psychosocial needs. Yet infection remains the leading cause of death in cancer patients and is a major cause of morbidity and hospitalization, making it a major aspect of the supportive care of cancer patients. It therefore deserves a full exposition.

Bone marrow transplantation is increasingly being utilized as part of a therapeutic modality in the treatment of cancer patients. Transplantation patients are at such a particularly high risk of developing a wide variety of different types of infection, that they inevitably can serve as an excellent framework for discussion of all the types of infections that occur during the treatment of cancer. The patient undergoing allogeneic bone marrow transplantation is at particularly high risk of infection due to the major perturbations of host defenses, which include granulocytopenia, cellular immune dysfunction, humoral immune dysfunction, blood product transfusions, and vascular access devices. Each of these perturbations results in a different set of infectious disease problems. The patient with granulocytopenia tends to develop bacteremia with Gram-negative bacilli, staphylococci, and streptococci and, after receiving broad-spectrum antibiotics, is at risk for infections with *Candida* and *Aspergillus*. The patient who has dysfunction of his/her cellular immune system is at risk for viral infections, such as herpes simplex, varicella zoster, and cytomegalovirus; bacterial infections, such as reactivation of latent *Mycobacterium tuberculosis*; or infections caused by *Listeria*, *Salmonella*, or other mycobacteria, by protozoa, such as *Pneumocystis carinii* and *Toxoplasma gondii*, by the helminth, *Strongyloides stercoralis*, and by fungi, which include *Cryptococcus neoformans*; and the reactivation of latent histoplasmosis or coccidioidomycosis. The patient with humoral immune dysfunction is at risk for a totally different group of infections, most notably the encapsulated pyogenic coccus, *Streptococcus pneumoniae* and, to a lesser degree, *Haemophilus influenzae* and *Neisseria meningitidis*. Patients who have had a splenectomy or have hypoplastic splenic function are at risk for this same group of organisms causing overwhelming septicemia. Blood product transfusions have their own risk of related infection, including cytomegalovirus carried via white blood cells, hepatitis B or C, and occasionally other viruses and bacteria. Finally, the patient who has a vascular access device is at risk for an infection in connection with that device. One final set of infections are those which relate to partial obstruction of a natural passage, such as a postobstructive pneumonia and urinary tract infection, where the tumor itself creates the obstructing phenomenon.

Having now conducted three international symposia dealing with the supportive care complications of cancer and its treatment, we organized, in the summer of 1991, a workshop to look specifically at the issues of infectious disease complications and utilized as our model a patient who received an allogeneic bone marrow transplantation for acute nonlymphocytic leukemia. We invited 23 internationally recognized experts to deal with the issues, both to name areas of controversy and, concurrently, to seek consensus. This workshop, graciously funded by an educational grant from Merck Sharp & Dohme, brought forth sufficient valuable information that we felt, along with Dr. H. J. Senn, our cochairman and, likewise, organizer of supportive care symposia, that it would be useful to make this information available to a broader audience through the publication of this text. Thus, we present for your review a summary of these topics, as noted above, plus discussions of new pathogens, drug delivery systems, and, finally, some thoughts on clinical trials and clinical trial methodology.

Baltimore, MD, USA   Stephen C. Schimpff
Brussels, Belgium   Jean Klastersky

Acknowledgment

The symposium-workshop which served as the basis for this text was funded by an educational grant from Merck Sharp & Dohme. We wish to acknowledge the corporation's generosity and, equally importantly, acknowledge the personal efforts of Mr. Lawrence C. Rappaport, Executive Coordinator, Health Science Services, Infectious Diseases. In addition to the presenter/authors, the success of the symposium was due to the organizational efforts of Paula Rosen with on sight assistance from her husband, Marc. Mrs. Rosen was also responsible for all of the organizational work required to ensure the successful completion of this text. Finally, we wish to thank Professor Hans-Jörg Senn, Editor of this series and our co-chairman of the symposium-workshop, for assuring timely editing and publishing.

Contents

XIV   Contents

List of Contributors*

Anaissie, E. *137*[1]
Andriole, V. T. *117*
Aoun, M. *127*
Barrett, A. J. *185*
Bustamante, C. I. *45*
Comis, R. L. *257*
Davis, G. L. *213*
Diamond, R. D. *109*
Dick, J. D. *221*
Feld, R. *249*
Feldman, S. *175*
Flaherty, J. P. *79*
Gallagher, J. G. *89*
Gèrain, J. *127*
Hurd, D. D. *1*
Jacoby, G. A. *241*

Karp, J. E. *221*
Klastersky, J. *127, 147*
Mandell, G. L. *103*
Peters, W. P. *97*
Pinczowsky, H. *137*
Pizzo, P. A. *57*
Saral, R. *155*
Schimpff, S. C. *15, 35, 261*
Schmidt, G. M. *161*
Shenep, J. L. *67*
Tutschka, P. J. *197, 205*
Van der Auwera, P. *127*
Vogelzang, N. J. *79*
Vollmer, K. *103*
Zinner, S. H. *231*

---

* The addresses of the authors are given on the first page of each contribution.
[1] Page on which contribution begins.

I. Introduction

Bone Marrow Transplantation for Cancer: An Overview

D.D. Hurd

Comprehensive Cancer Center of Wake Forest University, Bowman Gray School of Medicine, Winston Salem, NC 27157, USA

Introduction

Although allogeneic bone marrow transplantation has been attempted for over 50 years (Bortin 1970), it was not until 1968 that the first successful transplant was achieved in a child with an immunodeficiency syndrome (Gatti et al. 1968). Since that time, allogeneic, and more recently autologous, transplantation has grown repidly as a means of treating a variety of malignant and nonmalignant disorders. In a recent survey conducted by the International Bone Marrow Transplant Registry (IBMTR), data from 342 institutions in 47 countries revealed that 14 745 patients had been treated with either allogeneic or syngeneic transplants during the years 1988–1990 (Bortin et al. 1992). Overall, it is estimated that over 32 500 allogeneic or syngeneic transplants have been performed worldwide since the first successful transplant.

Autologous transplants were first attempted in the 1950s but their usefulness was limited, and it was not until the early reports of success with allogeneic transplantation that there was a rekindling of interest in the use of high-dose therapy and autografting for the treatment of malignant diseases. It is estimated that over the past two decades more than 18 000 patients have undergone autologous bone marrow transplants (Advisory Committee of the International Autologous Bone Marrow Transplant Registry 1989; Bortin, et al. 1992). Of these, 70% have been performed since 1988 (Bortin et al. 1992).

There has also been a significant growth in the number of centers performing transplants. Of the current 342 allogeneic transplant centers, 246 were established in the last 10 years (Bortin et al. 1992). While the majority of allogeneic transplantation is still undertaken at university medical centers, there has been a rapid growth in the number of autologous transplants in larger community hospitals. With the widespread and increasing use of these treatment modalities, it is important to understand some of the basic principles

Recent Results in Cancer Research, Vol. 132
© Springer-Verlag Berlin · Heidelberg 1993

of the application of both allogeneic and autologous bone marrow transplantation to the management of patients with cancer.

Overview

There are three major principles on which bone marrow transplantation is based. The first is that bone marrow suppression is the major dose-limiting side effect of total body radiation and of many of the chemotherapeutic agents that are used to treat malignant disorders. The second is that there is a dose response for many of these agents so that higher doses of cytotoxic drugs and radiation can have greater antitumor effects (Frei and Canellos 1980). And lastly, a bone marrow transplant can protect against the lethal effects of high-dose chemotherapy and radiation.

The successful use of bone marrow transplantation requires a disease that is responsive to effective cytoreductive therapy where the dose-limiting toxicity is marrow suppression. Bone marrow transplantation is of little use if the treatment program causes major damage to other vital organs such as the liver, lungs, heart, kidneys, and central nervous system. Importantly, the transplant should be performed at a time in the course of the malignancy when there is minimal tumor burden and before the development of resistance to therapy. Patients should have a relatively normal performance status as judged by history, physical examination, and evaluation of pulmonary, cardiac, renal, and hepatic function. Patients with significant co-morbid disease are not good candidates for intensive therapy since this would increase significantly the morbidity and mortality associated with transplantation.

Finally, there must be a source of hematopoietic stem cells free of clonogenic tumor cells that can be used to rescue the patient from high-dose therapy and insure both hematopoietic and immunologic recovery. The source of these cells may be allogeneic derived from a compatible donor, syngeneic derived from an identical twin, or autologous using the patient's own bone marrow.

The most frequent diseases that are being treated with either allogeneic or autologous bone marrow transplantation are shown in Table 1.

Allogeneic Bone Marrow Transplantation

Allogeneic transplantation was originally used in the early 1970s as a "last ditch" salvage therapy for patients with end-stage leukemia and aplastic anemia (Thomas et al. 1977). Those studies indicated that even with advanced leukemia, approximately 10% of patients could be salvaged and cured with an allogeneic transplant. It was noted, however, that patients who were in better physical condition, who were not infected, and who had a low tumor burden at the time of treatment did better than those with a poorer performance status. Because of this, studies were begun in 1976 utilizing transplantation for treatment of patients with acute myeloid leukemia in first

Table 1. Diseases treated with bone marrow transplantation 1988–1990. (Modified from Bortin et al. 1992)

	Transplantations (n)	Percentage of total
Allogeneic		
Acute leukemia	6891	46.7
Chronic leukemia	3910	26.5
Lymphoma	698	4.7
Other malignancy	780	5.3
Aplastic anemia	1258	8.5
Thalassemia major	339	2.3
Congenital immunodeficiency	386	2.6
Genetic/metabolic disorders	243	1.6
Other	240	1.6
Autologous		
Acute leukemia	3616	27.5
Chronic leukemia	286	2.2
Lymphoma	5306	40.4
Breast cancer	1017	7.7
Neuroblastoma	721	5.5
Other solid tumors	2193	16.7

complete remission (Thomas et al. 1979). By adapting this strategy, it was demonstrated that approximately 60% of young patients could be cured by the use of allogeneic transplantation earlier in the course of the disease.

Initially, the focus was on diseases that affected the bone marrow with the intent being to destroy the diseased marrow and replace it with a normally functioning marrow. However, it was quickly determined that the effectiveness of intensive therapy with bone marrow rescue could be applied to other malignancies, such as Hodgkin's disease, where the bone marrow is infrequently involved by tumor cells. In these instances, the high-dose therapy is directed at treating the specific malignancy and rendering the patient disease free. During the high-dose therapy, however, other rapidly growing cells are injured. Of these, the hematopoietic stem cells are the most important and the transplant is necessary to rescue the patient from the irreversible damage to the normal bone marrow. For other disorders, the transplant is done to replace defective enzyme production (e.g., the in-born errors of metabolism) or to replace abnormal red blood cell production for patients with hemoglobinopathies (e.g., thalassemia).

Allogeneic bone marrow transplantation is the use of marrow derived from an HLA/MLC histocompatible donor. The HLA complex is located on chromosome 6 and is comprised of more than 30 class I and class II genes (Hansen et al. 1990). Class I comprises the HLA-A, -B, and -C genes which have been traditionally characterized by the use of alloantisera. While additional class I genes exist, their relevance to clinical bone marrow transplantation is unclear at this time.

Class II alloantigens are encoded by the DR, DQ, and DP genes that make up the HLA-D region of chromosome 6. DR, DQ, and DP can be serologically defined, and the reactivity of the D-region overall can be measured by the mixed lymphocyte culture (MLC). Since one chromosome 6 is inherited from each parent, there is a 25% chance that any two siblings will inherit the same HLA genes and be compatible for an allogeneic transplant. The ideal donor for an allogeneic transplant has a six-antigen match (two each A, B, and DR loci) and is nonreactive in MLC with the recipient.

While the vast majority of allogeneic transplants have utilized matched family (usually siblings) donors, only 25%–30% of patients needing an allogeneic transplant have a six-antigen matched family donor. Transplants have been done between one-, two-, and three-antigen mismatched family donors; however, the complications arising from the increasing disparity generally limits the successful use of this approach to the no more than one-antigen mismatched donor–recipient pairs (Ash et al. 1991).

Based on the assumption that there are a limited number of A, B, and DR antigens, it has been postulated that there are a finite number of HLA haplotypes. This would mean that, by chance alone, there should be individuals in the general population that would share the same HLA phenotype and would be compatible to serve as unrelated bone marrow donors for patients needing an allogeneic transplant. In 1987, the National Marrow Donor Program was established in the United States to recruit volunteer bone marrow donors. In addition, there are several other donor registries throughout the world (e.g., Canadian Donor Registry, the Anthony Nolan Registry in Great Britain) which can be searched to help find a compatible donor. Over the last few years the use of matched unrelated donors has accounted for nearly 8% of all allogeneic transplants and this percentage continues to increase (Bortin et al. 1992).

In allogeneic transplantation, the goals are twofold. The first is to eliminate the disease process and prepare the marrow space to accept the transplanted marrow; and the second is to suppress the immune system of the recipient to allow the donor marrow to engraft. This requires the use of high-dose chemotherapy with or without total body irradiation. Examples of preparative regimens for allogeneic transplantation are shown in Table 2.

The successful use of allogeneic bone marrow transplantation is limited by several factors. These include age of the patient, graft-versus-host disease (GVHD), toxicities of the preparative regimens, infections, graft failure and graft rejection, and recurrence of the disease for which the transplantation was performed. Despite improvements is the prevention and treatment of GVHD, it remains the major factor in the outcome of allogeneic transplantation. GVHD is caused by immunocompetent lymphocytes of donor origin being able to recognize important transplantation isoantigens in the

Table 2. Seclected examples of preparative regimens for allogeneic transplantation

Regimen	Dosage
Cylcophosphamide,	60 mg/kg per day × 2 days
total body irradiation	200 cGy b.i.d. × 3 days
Cyclophosphamide,	60 mg/kg per day × 2 days
total body irradiation	165 cGy b.i.d. × 4 days
Cyclophosphamide,	50 mg/kg per day × 5 days
total lymphoid irradiation	750 cGy × 1 day
Busulfan,	1 mg/kg every 6 h × 16 doses
cyclophosphamide	50 mg/kg per day × 4 days
Busulfan,	1 mg/kg every 6 h × 16 doses
cyclophosphamide	60 mg/kg per day × 2 days

recipient that are lacking in the donor so that the recipient appears foreign to the donor marrow (Ferrara and Deeg 1991). GVHD is generally divided into two phases: acute and chronic. While historically acute GVHD was a disease that occurred prior to day 100 post transplant and chronic GVHD was disease that occurred after day 100, GVHD can be better defined by its manifestations and target organs. Acute GVHD generally affects the skin, gastrointestinal tract, and liver and is manifested by rash, diarrhea, and bilirubin elevations. The severity (grades 1–4) of acute GVHD is based on the extent and characteristics of the rash, the volume of diarrhea, and the degree of elevation of the bilirubin. Using the grade of GVHD for each organ involved, a staging system (stages I–IV) can be derived to describe the significance of the acute GVHD (Table 3).

Despite the increased morbidity associated with GVHD, some acute GVHD (stages 1 and 2) may be beneficial to the patient. The phenomenon of graft-versus-leukemia (GVL) was first noted in patients transplanted for acute lymphoblastic leukemia (Weiden et al. 1981). Patients with GVHD who survived had a lower relapse rate following transplantation than those patients who never developed GVHD. It was postulated that the immune reaction of the donor lymphocytes against the host associated with GVHD would also impart an immune response against any residual leukemia cells (GVL) that had not been destroyed by the high-dose cyclophosphamide and total body irradiation. This graft-versus-disease effect has been subsequently demonstrated by other investigators for some but not all cancers treated with allogeneic transplants.

Manifestations of chronic GVHD are similar to those seen in patients with a variety of autoimmune disorders and can involve nearly every organ in the body. Limited chronic GVHD (skin or liver) has a better prognosis than patients with more extensive disease (Ferrara and Deeg 1991). Infections are the major complication of both acute and chronic GVHD leading to increased morbidity and mortality.

Table 3. Grading and staging of acute graft-versus-host disease

Grade	Skin	Liver	Gastrointestinal
1	Rash <25%	Bili 2–3.5 mg/dl	Diarrhea 500–1000 ml/day 10–15 ml/kg per day
2	Rash 25%–50%	Bili 3.5–8 mg/dl	Diarrhea 1000–1500 ml/day 16–20 ml/kg per day
3	Erythroderma	Bili 8–15 mg/dl	Diarrhea 1500–2500 ml/day 21–25 ml/kg per day
4	Bullae, desquamation	Bili >15 mg/dl	Diarrhea >2500 ml/day ≥26 ml/kg per day
Stage			
I	Skin 1–2	Liver 0	Gastrointestinal 0
II	Skin 1–3	Liver 1	Gastrointestinal 1
III	Skin 2–3	Liver 2–3	Gastrointestinal 2–4
IV	Skin 2–4	Liver 2–4	Gastrointestinal 2–4

Factors associated with GVHD include age of the donor and recipient (older is worse than younger), sex mismatch donor–recipient pairs (especially a parous female donor for a male recipient), and prior infections with herpes group viruses (especially cytomegalovirus, CMV). Because of the age-associated GVHD morbidity and mortality, allogeneic transplants are usually restricted to patients under the age of 45 although newer methods of prevention and treatment of GVHD, including T cell depletion, may allow allogeneic transplants to be performed in older individuals (up to 55 years of age).

Despite these limitations, allogeneic bone marrow transplantation has proven beneficial in a variety of disorders (Table 1). It is now generally accepted that allogeneic transplantation is the treatment of choice for aplastic anemia, thalassemia major, chronic myelogenous leukemia, immunodeficiency disorders (other than acquired immunodeficiency disorder, AIDS), and certain subsets of patients with acute lymphocytic leukemia (ALL) and acute myelogenous leukemia (AML) who have poor prognostic features associated with their disease. For ALL and AML these would include patients who have experienced a relapse, unfavorable cytogenetics in the leukemic clone, high white blood cell count at diagnosis, mixed lineage phenotype, and leukemias arising from an antecedent hematologic disorder. However, it has become increasingly clear since the report by Thomas et al. (1979) that newer treatment approaches for selected younger patients with AML who have favorable prognostic features may lead to long-term disease-free survival and cure without having to undergo an allogeneic transplant in first remission (Hurd 1987). For this small subset of AML patients, transplantation should be undertaken only if they relapse.

Autologous Bone Marrow Transplantation

Patients who do not have a donor identified within the family or from one of the donor registries, but for whom bone marrow transplantation would be the treatment of choice, may benefit from the use of autologous bone marrow as the source of stem cells after dose-intensive therapy. Currently the only application of autologous bone marrow transplantation is in the management of patients with malignant disorders (Table 1). As has been noted (Frei and Canellos 1980), dose-intense therapy may lead to greater tumor cell kill and improvement in disease survival over standard chemo-therapeutic regimens. There is increasing clinical evidence that this may be true for the leukemias and a variety of "sensitive" solid tumors (e.g., non-Hodgkin's lymphoma, Hodgkin's disease, germ cell neoplasms, ovarian car-cinoma, breast carcinoma); however, for the vast majority of malignancies including gastrointestinal malignancies (stomach, pancreas, colon, rectum), non-small cell lung cancer, bladder cancer, prostate cancer, kidney cancer, etc., there is no evidence that autologous transplantation has any role in the management of these diseases with the currently available chemotherapeutic agents or intensive radiation therapy programs.

Many of the same principles applied to allogeneic transplantation are equally important in autologous transplantation, but there are some major differences. Since GVHD is not a significant factor in autologous bone marrow transplantation, one can apply autologous transplantation to an older age group (usually up to age 60–65 years). One can focus the preparative regimens for transplantation on combinations of cytotoxic agents that may be disease specific rather than having to be concerned about selecting therapies that are immunosuppressive as well as cytotoxic. Indeed, the degree of immunosuppression that is usually seen following an autologous transplant is generally not as severe nor does it last as long as the immunosuppression seen in patients undergoing an allogeneic transplant for the same disorder.

On the other hand, since the patient being considered for an autograft has a malignancy, there are two additional factors that must be considered. The first is the concern that the hematopoietic stem cell may have been depleted or damaged by prior cytotoxic therapy and may not be an optimal product to use to consistently insure recovery of hematologic and immunologic function. Also, one must be able to obtain and viably store sufficient numbers of autologous stem cells that are free of clonogenic tumor cells; or, alterna-tively, there must be a way of removing the abnormal cells in vitro prior to cryopreservation and storage so that they will not be reinfused along with the normal hematopoietic stem cells. For tumors that rarely affect the bone marrow (e.g., germ cell neoplasms), this is not an important issue; however, for those diseases that involve the marrow (e.g., acute leukemia) or that frequently metastasize to the bone marrow (e.g., non-Hodgkin's lymphoma, advanced breast cancer, etc.), some form of marrow purging may be necessary to rid the marrow of overt or occult disease.

Table 4. In vitro purging techniques

Negative selection
  Chemotherapy
    4-Hydroperoxycyclophosphamide (4HC)
    Mafosfamide (Asta-Z)
    Deoxycorformycin (DCF)
    Etoposide (VP-16)
  Monoclonal antibodies plus complement
  Antibody-toxin immunoconjugates
    Pokeweed antiviral protein (PAP)
    Ricin
  Antibody-magnetic microspheres
  Phototherapy – Merocyanine-540

Positive selection
  Long-term bone marrow cultures
  Stem cell-specific selection
    Avidin-biotin immunoabsorption columns
    Cell sorter
    Panning

There have been a variety of techniques investigated to attempt to purge the marrow of contaminating tumor cells (Gulati et al. 1992). Some of the more commonly applied approaches are shown in Table 4. While attempting to purge the marrow of the malignant cells would appear to be a reasonable approach (Gorin et al. 1990), to date there have been no randomized studies comparing purged to nonpurged autologous marrow transplantation to convincingly demonstrate the value of purging. An alternative approach to purging (negative selection) of the malignant cells is the isolation and purification of the pluripotential stem cell (positive selection). While this technology appears promising (Berenson et al. 1991), few studies have been done to demonstrate the utility of this approach.

An increasingly popular alternative to the use of bone marrow for autografting is the collection and use of peripheral blood progenitor cells (PBPC). It has been known for many years that committed and pluripotential stem cells can be isolated from the mononuclear cell fraction in the peripheral circulation. For patients whose marrow is involved by tumor, or who have had prior pelvic radiation that would make it impossible to harvest bone marrow, these PBPC can be collected by multiple leukapheresis procedures. More recently, it has been demonstrated that the numbers of circulating PBPC can be increased by the use of hematopoietic growth factors (granulocyte-macrophage colony-stimulating factor, GM-CSF, or granulocyte colony-stimulating factor, G-CSF) or collection of PBPC during the regrowth phase after cytotoxic (e.g., cyclophosphamide) chemotherapy. PBPC have most commonly been applied in autologous transplantation for breast cancer, Hodgkin's disease, and the non-Hodgkin's lymphomas. While

PBPC appear to be a reasonable alternative to marrow in autologous transplantation, there are currently no data that would support the use of PBPC in allogeneic transplantation.

Transplant Procedure

Once it has been determined that a patient has a disease that might benefit from intensive therapy with marrow support, they undergo extensive evaluation. This will include pulmonary function studies, cardiac studies, liver and renal function studies, and evaluation of the extent of disease prior to transplant. All patients should also be evaluated for prior illnesses that might affect their post transplant care. Routinely hepatitis A, B, and C serologies are obtained. Cytomegalovirus (CMV) serology and screening urine for CMV culture are done since this one infection has been a significant cause of morbidity and mortality following allogeneic transplantation. Frequently Epstein Barr, herpes simplex, varicella zoster, and toxoplasmosis immune status are determined. In allogeneic transplantation, many of these same serologic studies are also determined for the donor.

Bone marrow is collected under general or spinal anesthesia in an operating room. For autologous transplantation, this is usually done several days to several months before the patient is actually admitted for transplant. Once the autologous marrow has been collected, it is processed to isolate the nucleated cell fraction. This cellular product contains the pluripotential and committed stem cell pool needed for repopulation of the hematopoietic and immunologic functions. If purging is not being done, this product is mixed with an appropriate cryoprotectant agent (dimethylsulfoxide, DMSO, in most transplant centers) and undergoes controlled rate freezing in a liquid nitrogen freezing chamber. Care must be taken to prevent damage to the cells during the freezing process. Once the temperature of the temperature of the eproduct reaches about $-80°C$, it is transferred to a liquid nitrogen storage container at $-190°$ C where it may be kept for future use. While some studies have demonstrated that marrow remains viable for several years, the practice of most centers is to not use any marrow that has been stored for more than 5 years.

For allogeneic transplantation, the donor marrow is usually harvested on the same day as the transplant. For both allogeneic and autologous transplants, marrow is obtained by multiple aspirations from the posterior iliac crests. Through a quarter-inch incision in the skin, the marrow harvest needle is guided into the iliac crest beginning at the posterior superior iliac spine and working laterally along the crest until a sufficient amount of marrow has been obtained. It is estimated that 10 ml/kg body weight of the recipient should provide enough marrow for the transplant procedure, but most centers will also obtain nucleated cell counts on the product to insure that an adequate amount of marrow has been harvested. This volume of marrow represents approximately 5%–10% of total bone marrow, and for the allogeneic donor it will be regenerated over a period of several weeks.

Once the patient has been prepared for transplant with high-dose chemo-therapy or chemotherapy and total body irradiation, the marrow can then be infused. If the donor and the recipient are the same ABO blood type, the marrow product can be taken directly from the operating room to the bedside where it is infused through a central venous catheter just like any other blood product. If the blood types are different, the marrow must be first depleted of red cells, plasma, or both depending on the ABO incompatibility.

For the autologous reinfusion, the marrow is brought to the bedside where it is rapidly thawed and, as soon as it is in a liquid state (about 4°C), it is drawn up in a syringe and given by rapid intravenous bolus infusion. Side effects of infusion of this product may include fevers, chills, shortness of breath, chest pain, headaches, nausea, vomiting, and hemoglobinuria (Stroncek et al. 1991).

The duration of hospitalization following transplantation is quite variable depending on the disease being treated, the type of transplant being done, the cellular product being used to support the patient, the preparative regimen used for transplant, the application of hematopoietic growth factors, and complications that develop. While many uncomplicated autologous patients may be discharged 2–3 weeks following marrow infusion, the more typical patient will require 4–5 weeks of hospital care. Allogeneic patients frequently spend 6–8 weeks in the hospital. During this time, patients are monitored closely for complications and transfused on a regular basis to maintain an adequate platelet count and hemoglobin. Patients should be in a dedicated nursing unit that is equipped with an appropriate air-handling systmen to help decrease the acquisition of *Aspergillus* and other opportunistic fungal infections.

During the early post-transplant period, prior to marrow recovery, patients are highly susceptible to bacterial, fungal, and viral infections. This is secondary to profound neutropenia and injury to the mucosal barriers from the preparative regimen for transplant. While prophylactic antibiotics, antifungal and antiviral agents appear to be of some value, the majority of patients will require treatment for neutropenic febrile episodes. The allogeneic patients also receive immunosuppressive therapy to help prevent acute GVHD. This adds to the potential for infectious complications, es-pecially reactivation of CMV. The major risk factor associated with CMV disease in allogeneic transplantation is a positive serology in either the donor or recipient. Since the degree of immunosuppression experienced by autologous transplant patients is significantly less than that seen in the allogeneic patient, the risk of developing CMV disease in these patients is quite low, even if they have a positive serology pre-transplant.

With the recent availability of recombinant hematopoietic growth factors, the duration of neutropenia following marrow reinfusion has been significantly decreased (Nemunaitis et al. 1991). Both G- and GM-CSF will hasten white blood cell recovery. This may lead to a decrease in the morbidity associated with transplantation by decreasing the duration of neutropenia and the number of infections associated with prolonged marrow suppression. Since G- and GM-CSF are lineage specific, their use is of little value for red cell and platelet recovery. Other cytokines, such as interleukin 3 (IL-3), or stem cell factor (SCF), may effect earlier progenitor cells and may be useful in promoting recovery of all three cell lines. Clinical investigations are beginning into IL-3 and combinations of IL-3 with GM-CSF.

Late complications of bone marrow transplantation include delayed toxicities from the preparative regimens for transplantation, poor marrow graft function, and recurrence of disease for both allogeneic and autologous transplants. In addition, late complications of allogeneic transplantation include chronic GVHD requiring prolonged immunosuppressive therapy. Chronic GVHD is associated with mucosal damage and prolonged deficits in both humoral and cellular immunity that predispose to infectious complications. The more common bacterial infections associated with chronic GVHD are streptococcal and staphylococcal infections causing recurring pneumonias, sinusitis, and soft tissue infections. With the prolonged use of steroids to manage chronic GVHD, recurring Candida infections are seen.

Results of Transplantation

The expected results of transplant programs are dependent on the stage of the disease being treated, the type of transplant (autologous versus allogeneic), and the selection of patients for these therapies. As an example, leukemia-free survival of allogeneic transplants for AML, ALL, and CML based on the status of the leukemia at transplant and the age of the recipient are shown in Table 5.

Complications of GVHD and infections associated with GVHD remain the major factors that limit the successful outcome of allogeneic transplants for most diseases. Relapse of the underlying disease also limits the benefits of allogeneic transplantation with higher relapse rates being seen with more advanced disease at the time of transplantation.

The major cause of failure in autologous transplantation is recurrence of disease despite the aggressive treatment programs. Since these patients frequently receive identical therapy that is used in the allogeneic preparative regimens for transplantation, two possible explanations have been proposed for the excess relapse rate. The first is that the marrow cell inoculum harbors occult tumor cells that are reinfused along with the normal cells. The second hypothesis suggests that the immune response associated with GVHD in allogeneic transplantation is responsible for the low relapse rate (see above), and, since it is rare to have GVHD with an autologous transplant, there will be a higher relapse of disease.

Table 5. Results of allogeneic transplantation for leukemia: 4-year probability of leukemia-free survival. (From International Bone Marrow Transplant Registry 1992)

	ALL		AML		CML	
	Patients (n)	Probability[a]	Patients (n)	Probability[a]	Patients (n)	Probability[a]
Leukemia status at Transplant						
Early	514	50 ± 5	1122	51 ± 4	1227	45 ± 4
Intermediate	600	33 ± 5	230	31 ± 7	370	32 ± 6
Advanced	284	18 ± 5	424	21 ± 5	150	9 ± 6
Age at transplant (years)						
≤19	195	58 ± 8	316	59 ± 7	120	63 ± 11
10–29	175	49 ± 9	345	49 ± 6	309	47 ± 8
≥30	140	36 ± 11	460	47 ± 6	795	41 ± 5

[a] Actuarial probability of leukemia-free survival ±95% confidence interval.
ALL, acute lymphocytic leukemia; AML, acute myelogenous leukemia; CML, chronic myelogenous leukemia.

Still, for the diseases listed in Table 1, autologous transplantation would offer the best opportunity for curative therapy and would be the treatment of choice in appropriately selected patients. For the majority of patients with these diseases, age alone would preclude them from consideration of an allogeneic transplant; for others, it would be the lack of a suitably matched donor. To date, there have been no truly randomized comparative studies between autologous and allogeneic transplantation. For some diseases such as breast cancer, lymphoma, and other solid tumors, the number of autologous transplants far exceeds allogeneic transplantation. In other diseases, such as the chronic leukemias and the nonmalignant marrow disorders, allogeneic transplantation predominates.

Future Directions

Bone marrow transplantation is an evolving technology. Clearly transplantation is safer and more effective than it was 20 years ago. This has been achieved by improvements in supportive care, improvements in the prevention and treatment of GVHD, improvements in cancer chemotherapy and radiation therapy techniques, and through a better understanding of the biology of the diseases treated with transplantation. This latter fact has allowed a more rational application of these treatment modalities to the management of the patient with cancer.

The goal of transplantation is the achievement of long-term, disease-free survival and cure in a significant fraction of patients treated. This is an important principle since transplantation is an expensive therapy and should not be undertaken merely as a palliative treatment.

Despite the significant advances that have been made in transplantation in the last 2 decades there are many areas that will still need improvement to make transplantation safer, more effective, and less costly. Some of these areas include the development of more effective preparative regimens for the prevention of recurrent disease, the development of better ways of preventing GVHD without jeopardizing the potential benefits of the immune response against residual disease, the development of better means of preventing and treating infections, and the development of better overall treatment programs to prevent both acute and delayed adverse effects.

As with any therapeutic modality, the benefits and risks of transplantation must be continually evaluated in the light of advances being made in other areas. There have been significant strides made in the understanding and treatment of many cancers. Those malignancies that have benefited from transplantation are among the same ones for which newer, more effective treatment programs, without transplantation, now exist.

References

Advisory Committee of the International Autologous Bone Marrow Transplant Registry (1989) Autologous bone marrow transplants: different indications in Europe and America. Lancet ii:317–318

Ash R, Horowitz MM, Gale RP, van Bekkum DW, Casper JY, Gordon-Smith EC, Henslee-Downey PJ, Kolb JH, Lowenberg B, Masaoka T, McGlave PB, Rimm AA, Ringdén O, van Rood JJ, Sondel PM, Vowels Mr, Bortin MM (1991) Bone marrow transplantation from related donors other than HLA-identical siblings: effect of T-cell depletion. Bone Marrow Transplant 7:443–452

Berenson RJ, Bensinger WI, Hill RS, Andrews RG, Garcia-Lopez J, Kalamasz DF, Still BJ, Spitzer G, Buckner CD, Bernstein ID, Thomas ED (1991) Engraftment after infusion of CD34+ marrow cells in patients with breast cancer or neuroblastoma. Blood 77:1717–1722

Bortin MM (1970) A compendium of reported human bone marrow transplants. Transplantation 9:571–587

Bortin MM, Horowitz MM, Rimm AA (1992) Increasing utilization of allogeneic bone marrow transplantation. Results of the 1988–1990 survey. Ann Intern Med 116:505–512

Ferrara JLM, Deeg HJ (1991) Mechanisms of disease: graft versus host disease. N Engl J Med 324:667–674

Frei E III, Canellos GP (1980) Dose: a critical factor in cancer chemotherapy. Am J Med 69:585–594

Gatti RA, Allen HD, Meuwissen HJ, Hong R, Good RA (1968) Immunological reconstitution of sex-linked lymphopenic immunological deficiency. Lancet ii:1366–1369

Gorin NC, Aegerter P, Auvert B, Meloini G, Goldstone AH, Burnett A, Carella A, Korbling M, Herve P, Maraninchi D, Löwenberg R, Verdonck LF, de Planque M, Hermans J, Helbig W, Porcellini A, Rizzoli V, Alesandrino EP, Franklin IM, Reifiers J, Collesslli P, Goldman JM (1990) Autologous bone marrow transplantation for acute myelocytic leukemia in first remission: a European survey of the role of marrow purging. Blood 75:1606–1614

Gulati SC, Lemoli RM, Acaba L, Igaraeshi T, Wasserheit C, Fraig M (1992) Purging in autologous and allogeneic bone marrow transplantation. Curr Op in Oncol 4:264–278

Hansen JA, Choo YS, Geraghty DE, Mickelson E (1990) The HLA system in clinical marrow transplantation. Hematol Oncol Clin North Am 4:507–515

Hurd DD (1987) Allogeneic and autologous bone marrow transplantation for acute nonlymphocytic leukemia. Semin Oncol 14:407–415

Nemunaitis J, Rabinowe SN, Singer Jw, Bierman Pj, Vose Jm, Freedman AS, Onetto N, Gillis S, Oette D, Gold M, Duckner CD, Hansen JA, Ritz J, Applebaum FR, Armitage JO, Nadler LM (1991) Recombinant granulocyte-macrophage colony-stimulating factor after autologous bone marrow transplantation for lymphoid cancer. N Engl J Med 324:1773–1778

Stroncek DF, Fautsch S, Lasky L, Hurd DD, Ramsay N, McCullough JJ (1991) Adverse reactions in patients transfused with cryopreserved marrow. Transfusion 31:521–526

Thomas ED, Buckner CD, Banaji M, Clift RA, Fefer A, Flournoy N, Goodell BW, Hickman HO, Lerner KG, Neiman PE, Sale GE, Sanders JE, Singer J, Stevens M, Storb R, Weiden PL (1977) One hundred patients with acute leukemia treated by chemotherapy, total body irradiation, and allogeneic marrow transplantation. Blood 49:511–533

Thomas ED, Buckner CD, Clift RA, Fefer A, Johnson LF, Neiman PE, Sale GE, Sanders JE, Singer J, Shulman H, Storb R, Weiden PL (1979) Marrow transplantation for acute nonlymphoblastic leukemia in first remission. N Engl J Med 301:597–599

Weiden PL, Sullivan KM, Flournoy N, Storb R, Thomas ED, Seattle Marrow Transplant Team (1981) Antileukemic effect of graft-versus-host disease: contribution to improved survival after allogeneic marrow transplantation. N Engl J Med 304:1529–1533

Infection in Bone Marrow Transplantation: A Model for Examining Predisposing Factors to Infection in Cancer Patients

S.C. Schimpff

University of Maryland School of Medicine, 22 South Greene Street, Baltimore, MD 21201, USA

Infection is recognized as not only a common complication of cancer and its therapy but also the most common call upon the physician to provide supportive care to the hospitalized cancer patient. Despite dramatic improvements in therapeutics over the past 20 years, infection remains the most frequent cause of death for patients with leukemia, lymphoma, and many forms of advanced metastatic cancer.

The patient who undergoes bone marrow transplantation, especially allogeneic bone marrow transplantation, usually develops multiple infections. As increasing numbers of these procedures are being done, it is a relevant time to consider the associated infectious disease complications. Further, the bone marrow transplant patient provides a unique model to examine the factors which predispose to infection.

Figure 1 details the infections which occur in relation to time after the transplant. One can "lump" these infections into one of several categories based upon the major factor(s) predisposing to each infection. It is important to recognize that this requires some oversimplification and that all of the elements leading to infection are undoubtedly not known. Nevertheless, this division of infections based upon predisposing factors can be very useful in the diagnostic evaluation of a patient in that it will direct the clinician to the most immediately useful approaches. Further, it can greatly aid therapy, especially initial empiric therapy before definitive microbiologic data have been returned. Finally, recognition of the infection patterns associated with each predisposing factor will assist in the design of rational prevention strategies.

The basic groupings of predisposing factors include: obstruction of natural passages, granulocytopenia – disruption of normal anatomic barriers and shifts of normal microbial flora, cellular immune dysfunction, humoral immune dysfunction, vascular access devices, and transfusions and infusions.

Recent Results in Cancer Research, Vol. 132
© Springer-Verlag Berlin · Heidelberg 1993

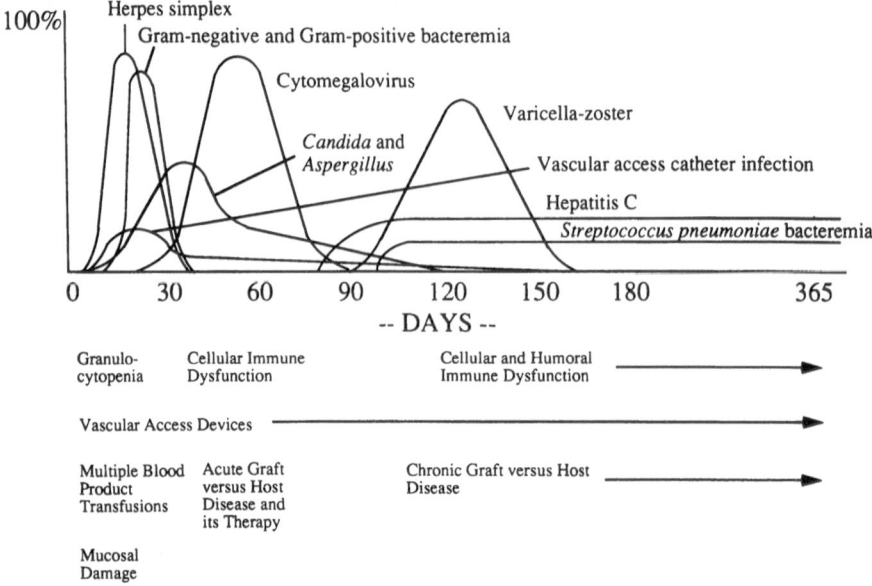

Fig. 1. Infection in marrow transplantation: time frames and relative frequency

Obstruction

The old pathology adage "obstruction leads to infection" is very relevant with the cancer patient. A primary or secondary lung tumor partially obstructing a bronchus leads to postobstructive pneumonia. The etiologic organisms will be oral flora, a flora which may have been altered by disease or antibiotics. Prostate cancer may lead to cystitis from local bowel flora such as *Escherichia coli*, ovarian or colon cancer obstruction of a ureter to unilateral pyelonephritis. Lymphoma obstructing the common bile duct will be associated with ascending colangitis caused by flora in the small bowel and obstruction of the eustachian tube by large nodes in a child with acute lymphocytic leukemia will lead to otitis. Although antibiotics may be appropriate in each situation, infection will not be resolved unless the obstruction can be relieved, usually through some form of anticancer therapy. Without relief of obstruction, the antibiotics will probably encourage a shift of flora toward more resistant bacteria or fungi.

Local flora, especially oral flora, changes in relation to underlying illness. Normal individuals have "normal" oral flora but with moderate to serious underlying illness (trauma, cardiac disease, or cancer) or with advancing age, the oral flora shifts toward Gram-negative bacilli. This apparently relates to changes in fibronectin on the surface of the epithelial cells such that Gram-negative rods now avidly bind to the oral mucosa. These then become the organisms responsible not only for oral infections such as pharyngitis but also pneumonia and esophagitis.

The mucosa of not only the mouth but most of the alimentary canal is populated, normally, with high numbers of anaerobes. These bind tightly to the epithelial cells, and their presence deters transient organisms from gaining a "foothold" and locally colonizing. Natural changes in binding, as noted above, occur with disease states, but antibiotics which suppress these anaerobes reduce their ability to protect against colonization by transient organisms, a mechanism termed "colonization resistance." Colonization resistance is markedly reduced by many antibiotics including most of the broad-spectrum penicillins and many of the newer cephalosporins in addition to tetracyclines and others.

Granulocytopenia

Granulocytopenia by itself is usually not a major cause of infection but rather a condition that allows what might have been a minor infection to progress rapidly to bacteremia and death. In most instances, other factors interact in the presence of granulocytopenia to increase the risk of infection at a specific location. Damage to anatomic barriers, particularly the skin, mucosal membranes of the alimentary canal, and the lining of the respiratory tract, are such factors which increase infection risk. However, shifting patterns of microbial colonization secondary to the disease state and the acquisition of potential pathogens from the hospital environment are important.

Granulocytopenia is a major predisposing factor in the bone marrow transplant patient because the process of intensive therapy with cytotoxic drugs with or without total body radiation renders the bone marrow aplastic, and hence these patients will have no circulating granulocytes until the marrow engrafts and becomes functional.

Although granulocyte counts of less than $1000/\mu l$ usually define the "granulocytopenic state," a substantial increased risk of infection really does not begin until the granulocyte count has dropped below $500/\mu l$, and essentially Gram-negative bacteremia or disseminated candidiasis occurs when the granulocyte count is less than $100/\mu l$ (Fig. 2). This has substantial import in decision making for both infection prevention and infection therapy (Bodey et al. 1966).

Sites

The sites (Fig. 3) of infection are localized to regions of damaged anatomic barriers, which allow for easy entry of otherwise relatively nonpathogenic organisms (Table 1) (Schimpff et al. 1972b). The alimentary canal is the

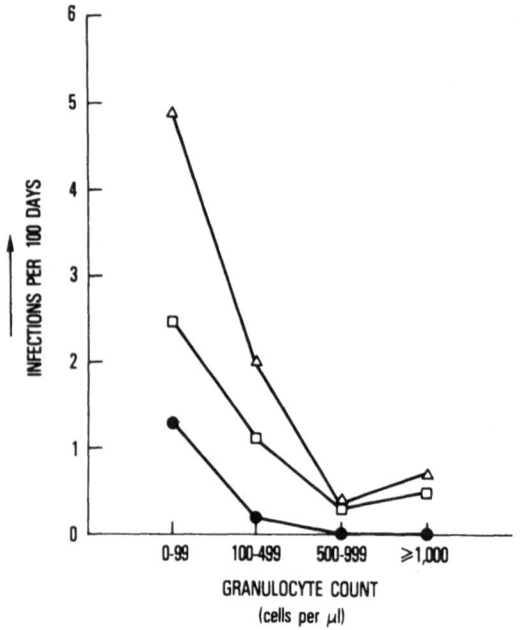

Fig. 2. Incidence of infection in acute nonlymphocytic leukemia during induction therapy. *Triangles*, all infections; *squares*, severe infections; *circles*, bacteremias. (From Joshi and Schimpff 1984)

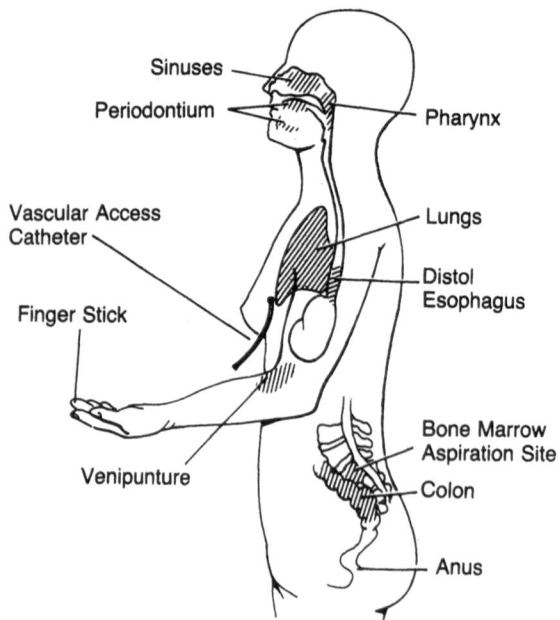

Fig. 3. Sites of infection among granulocytopenic cancer patients. (From Schimpff 1991)

Table 1. Infection granulocytopenic patients[a]

Sites	Pathogens
Alimentary canal	Gram-negative bacilli
Periodontitis	*Escherichia coli*
Pharyngitis	*Pseudomonas aeruginosa*
Esophagitis	*Klebsiella pneumoniae*
Colitis	
Perianal lesions	Gram-positive cocci
	Streptococcus species
Respiratory tract	*Staphylococcus aureus*
Sinusitis	*Staphylococcus epidermidis*
Pneumonitis	
	Yeasts/fungi
Skin	*Candida* species
Local trauma	*Aspergillus fumigatus/flavus*
Vascular access	
	Anaerobes
	Clostridium difficile

[a] These patients can become infected at any site and by any potential pathogen, but the sites and pathogens listed here represent more than 85% of acute infections.

principal site of infection and includes exacerbation of previously chronic subacute periodontitis, pharyngitis, esophagitis localized to the distal third of the esophagus, colitis, and perianal lesions. Infections along the respiratory tract are limited essentially to sinusitis and pneumonia, whereas infections of the skin occur in the axillae, groin, or at areas of direct damage due to venipuncture, bone marrow aspiration, fingersticks, or vascular access devices. In addition, there are bacteremias of unknown origin, some of which are presumed to relate to bacterial translocation along the intestinal wall. A group of infections will be infusion related and occur secondary to the placement of intravascular catheters or infusion of products which are contaminated with bacterial or viral (hepatitis; cytomegalovirus, CMV) pathogens.

These predominating infection sites are readily explainable: acute periodontitis, which at some centers has been recognized to cause approximately 20% of febrile episodes, occurs as a result of acute exacerbation of previously unrecognized chronic periodontal disease. Esophagitis occurs in the distal esophagus because of mucosal damage due to chemotherapeutic agents exacerbated by acid reflux from the stomach, which is secondary to chemotherapy-induced vomiting. Perianal lesions occur particularly in patients with acute monocytic or myelomonocytic leukemia (for reasons which are unclear) and can reach an incidence of 33% among patients who do not receive alimentary tract decontamination. Patients with a history of hemorrhoids are most frequently affected because of the development of small mucosal tears at the base of the hemorrhoid at the anal opening (Schimpff et al. 1972a). The high pressures developed in the process of defecation exacerbate this process. Sinusitis seems to develop in patients with a previous history of sinus infections, perhaps suggesting a tendency toward obstruction to the ostia. Pneumonia results from damaged ciliary function with consequent reduced tracheobronchial clearance of mucous. These alterations in the normal clearance mechanisms allow the organisms normally aspirated during sleep to establish local infection which is then unchecked by either granulocytes or pulmonary macrophages. The axillae are common sites of infection because of the warm, moist environment which allows for the growth of organisms in an area that has been damaged by shaving or in an area where hair follicles have been occluded by anti-perspirants. Infection at areas of direct damage to the skin, such as bone marrow aspiration sites and fingersticks, occurs because healing is slow after chemotherapy and because the number of organisms necessary to induce infection in the individual who is granulocytopenic is substantially less than in the normal host.

"Bacterial translocation" is a term used to define the movement of bacteria across the intact intestinal epithelium into the mesenteric lymph nodes and possibly beyond to cause systemic infection. This process is well recognized with *Salmonella typhi* in the production of typhoid fever. However, data are now accumulating from animal experimentation to show that certain aerobic Gram-negative organisms, principally *E. coli*, *Klebsiella pneumoniae*, and *Pseudomonas aeruginosa* can also translocate across the normal alimentary canal mucosa under at least the following conditions: suppression of the anaerobic flora of the intestinal tract or suppression of cellular immune function. It is therefore possible that many episodes of so-called bacteremia of unknown origin have their origin in the intestinal tract as a result of bacterial translocation in the absence of specific mucosal epithelial damage.

Pathogens

The most common causes of infection in the granulocytopenic patient are the aerobic Gram-positive cocci *Staphylococcus epidermidis* and alpha *Streptococcus* spp. and the aerobic Gram-negative rods, especially *E. coli*, *K. pneumoniae*, and *P. aeruginosa*. At most cancer centers, 80% or more of the Gram-negative bacteremias are caused by the three organisms noted. Despite colonization with other aerobic Gram-negative bacilli, patients who are granulocytopenic rarely develop infection or bacteremia with such organisms (Schimpff et al. 1972b). *Bacteroides fragilis*, an anaerobic Gram-negative rod which is known to cause infection in many other settings, and other anaerobes are also uncommon causes of infection during granulo-cytopenia. Gram-positive aerobic organisms such as *S. epidermidis*, alpha

Streptococcus spp., and *Staphylococcus aureus* cause most of the Gram-positive infections, and each commonly causes bacteremias. The principal yeasts and fungi are *Candida* spp. (especially *Candida albicans* and *Candida tropicalis*), and *Aspergillus* (especially *Aspergillus flavus* and *Aspergillus fumigatus*).

Inflammatory Response

The absence or near absence of granulocytes substantially limits the inflammatory response which in turn affects both diagnosis and prognosis. There are very few early signs and symptoms except for fever (Sickles et al. 1975). It is this ability of an otherwise minor-appearing and localized infection to rapidly progress to a systemic bacteremia which makes the need for early diagnosis and prompt empiric therapy critical. The patient with a Gram-negative bacteremia who is not treated promptly will usually die within 24–48 h unless antimicrobial therapy is initiated within the first few hours.

Therapy

Empiric therapy for the febrile, neutropenic patient must be: (a) prompt; (b) empiric; (c) bactericidal; and (d) broad in spectrum.

The need for prompt institution of therapy is due to the rapid and high mortality rate of patients with Gram-negative bacteremia and, occasionally, the bacteremias caused by *Streptococcus* spp. The need for prompt therapy makes the use of empiric antibacterial regimens clear. It should be emphasized that an antibiotic regimen must be chosen which is most appropriate for the specific patient in a specific institution. It is necessary to know what organisms are or are likely colonizing the patient and what the likely susceptibility patterns will be. It is critical to have continually updated information on the susceptibility patterns of organisms frequently recovered from the area of the hospital where the patient is being treated.

It is obvious that bactericidal rather than bacteriostatic antibiotics are important since, in the absence of granulocytes, this is a battle of "bugs versus drugs" without help from host defenses. The agents should have a broad spectrum so as to "cover" the great majority of hospital pathogens. In the past, this required the combination of two or more antibiotics to ensure coverage of most Gram-negative rods, especially *P. aeruginosa, K. pneumoniae*, and *E. coli* plus *S. aureus* and other Gram-positive cocci (Schimpff et al. 1971). The use of antibiotic combinations may also slow the emergence of resistant bacterial strains. Many neutropenic patients will be adequately treated with monotherapy; however, combination therapy is advantageous for those with <100 polymorphonuclear neutrophils (PMN)/µl and suspected Gram-negative bacteremia.

Therapy of Persistent Fever and Persistent Granulocytopenia

A major concern for the clinician dealing with the febrile, granulocytopenic patient is what to do with the patient who has persistence of fever following the administration of empiric antibiotic therapy with persistence of granulocytopenia (Pizzo et al. 1982). The questions relate to whether the initial antibiotic should be continued or discontinued, whether an additional antibacterial antibiotic should be added, whether an antifungal agent such as amphotericin B or an antiviral such as acyclovir should be added, or whether polymorphonuclear leukocyte transfusions should be administered. Clearly, there is no single correct answer applicable to all patients. The first step should be to carefully repeat the history and physical examination, to repeat the chest X-ray, and to review the results of the original cultures with the microbiology laboratory. More often than not, such a careful review will reveal an infection site, if in fact one exists. However, other causes of fever must be considered: blood product transfusions, a history of fever with the underlying tumor, and drug fever from compounds such as cytosine arabinoside or from the empiric antibiotics themselves.

Therapy of Persistent Granulocytopenia with Febrile Response

Some patients who have persistent granulocytopenia and have no specific evidence of infection on history or physical examination, have a "febrile response," i.e., the fever abates promptly after institution of antibiotics. This raises the question as to whether the patient was infected and, if so, should antibiotics be continued? The critical step is to repeat the history and physical examination, review all cultural data, and repeat the chest X-ray. If no specific evidence of infection can be determined, yet it would appear that the patient has had a febrile response secondary to antibiotic therapy, it would seem reasonable to continue the antibiotics for a total of about 10 days. If at that time the granulocyte count remains very low, one would have to decide whether to continue antibiotic therapy. I usually discontinue antibiotics at this time, but there is evidence to suggest that continuing antibiotic therapy is appropriate. However, continuation must be balanced against the potential risk of predisposing toward fungal infection; continuation may demand the addition of amphotericin B or other antifungal agents (EORTC International Antimicrobial Therapy Cooperative Group 1989).

Therapy of Fungal Infections

The fungal infections that occur during granulocytopenia can be divided into those caused by yeasts, principally as *C. albicans* and *C. tropicalis*, and those caused by filamentous fungi, especially *A. flavus* and *A. fumigatus*.

Candidiasis begins as a localized mucosal infection usually in the pharyngeal region or in the distal esophagus. When localized, it can perhaps be treated topically, but systemic therapy is usually indicated because the infection is not only on the mucosal surface but is also locally invasive. Until recently, the only clearly effective agent was amphotericin B, today fluconazole also appears effective. The disadvantages of amphotericin B, of course, are its multitude of side effects, including fever, shaking chills, nausea, anorexia, and nephrotoxicity. Disseminated candidiasis is a life-threatening, rapidly fatal disease which usually originates from the distal esophagus or alimentary canal but which is exceedingly difficult to detect in its earliest stages. Blood cultures are usually nonrevealing, because the absolute numbers of circulating yeasts in the blood are usually very low, yet autopsy will demonstrate involvement of liver, spleen, kidneys, adrenals, lungs, and other organs despite repeatedly negative blood cultures. Any positive blood culture for *Candida* in a granulocytopenic patient should be considered adequate evidence of disseminated candidiasis, and the patient should be treated with amphotericin B or fluconazole at full dosage immediately. Additional clues to suggest dissemination in the absence of positive blood cultures would be evidence of esophagitis, presence of *Candida* at multiple surveillance culture sites, persistent fever despite antibacterial antibiotics, the occasional development of biopsy-positive skin lesions, or the rare development of endophthalmitis. Amphotericin B has been the drug of choice to which 5-fluorocytosine or rifampin may be added because of their proven synergistic activity in animal models. Ketoconazole or miconazole may be useful for localized mucosal infection but are not adequate for disseminated candidiasis. The new agent fluconazole appears to be a satisfactory substitute for amphotericin B.

The filamentous fungi that cause the greatest percentage of infections in neutropenic patients are *A. flavus* and *A. fumigatus*. The most common site of *Aspergillus* infection is the lung with the upper respiratory passages, especially nasal turbinates or sinuses, frequently involved. From the respiratory sites, essentially any organ can become involved, especially the gastrointestinal tract and the central nervous system. Factors predisposing to infection with *Aspergillus* species include prolonged granulocytopenia with associated broad-spectrum antimicrobial administration (Aisner et al. 1979). Antibiotics apparently have their effect by suppressing the normal flora of the upper airways thus allowing colonization by environmentally present airborne spores of *Aspergillus* species. As a result, an early diagnostic clue is the presence of pathogenic species of *Aspergillus* in cultures of the anterior nares or by observation of necrotic lesions high on the nasal turbinates. Biopsy of these lesions will usually reveal the characteristic branched septated hyphae of *Aspergillus*. This finding in the presence of an otherwise unexplained pulmonary infiltrate should lead to initiation of therapy with amphotericin B.

Pulmonary infiltrates caused by *Aspergillus* may be single or, more commonly, multiple and may involve multiple lobes. A common pattern of pulmonary infiltration is a wedge-shaped infiltrate that results from the propensity of *A. fumigatus* and *A. flavus* to invade large vessels leading to thrombosis and distal infarction. The infection can progress slowly or rapidly, and death is usually due to either respiratory insufficiency or massive hemoptysis.

Treatment is with amphotericin B at a dose of about 0.6–1.2 mg/kg per day. There are no data that 5-fluorocytosine, although active in vitro, is useful in these patients. Miconazole and ketoconazole are not active against these organisms. Fluconazole is likewise not effective for aspergillosis. There is evidence from animal models that either 5-fluorocytosine or rifampin combined with amphotericin B are synergistic. Combination therapy could therefore be recommended for treating invasive aspergillosis, but no clinical data are available. There are no data on the use of granulocyte transfusions but, if available in sufficient numbers, should be useful because it is known that, in vitro, polymorphonuclear leukocytes destroy the hyphae of *Aspergillus* by encirclement and direct damage by lysosomal enzymes and because this infection tends to occur in patients with aplastic marrows with little chance of prompt marrow recovery.

Prevention and Infection During Granulocytopenia

The information presented regarding granulocytopenia offers some approaches for prevention of infection. These fall into the following categories: reducing acquisition of new potential pathogens, suppressing potential pathogens already colonizing the patient, and improving host defense factors (Pizzo and Schimpff 1983).

Acquisition can be reduced by placing the patient in a "sterile" environment such as a laminar air flow room, but much can be accomplished with less aggressive measures. The major routes of acquisition are contact, food, water, and air. Contact acquisition can be reduced dramatically by careful handwashing procedures. Serve the patient a low microbial content diet (i.e., avoid salads, tomatoes, uncooked vegetables, unpasteurized fruit juices, etc.) and be sure that water supplies are satisfactory (Remington and Schimpff 1981). The major added value of the LAF room (i.e., sterile air) is to reduce acquisition of *Aspergillus* spores, a not inconsequential issue for bone marrow transplant patients.

Organisms which are potential pathogens can be suppressed with a variety of antimicrobials. Recall that the key offenders are aerobic Gram-negative bacilli in the oral cavity and rectal-perianal area, aerobic Gram-positive cocci in the oral cavity, yeasts in the oral cavity, esophagus, and intestines, *Aspergillus* in the upper and lower airways, and herpes simplex lying latent to reinfect the oral or genital regions, and anaerobes which produce chronic periodontal infection.

Gram-negative bacilli can be suppressed with oral nonabsorbable anti-biotics (aminoglycosides, polymyxins) or oral absorbable agents (quinolones, trimethoprim-sulfamethoxazole). In my opinion, based upon review of the literature, these approaches should be limited to the patient who will experience profound ($<100\,\text{PMN}/\mu l$) prolonged (>14 days) granulo-cytopenia, i.e., the marrow transplant patient.

Gram-positives can be suppressed with nonabsorbables (vancomycin, aminoglycosides), or absorbable agents (some, but not all, quinolones).

Yeasts can be suppressed to a limited degree with nonabsorbable polyenes (nystatin), but it appears useful to also use an absorbable agent (such as ketoconazole or fluconazole). Attempts at nasal sprays with amphotericin B have not been proven successful to reduce aspergillosis. Acyclovir, however, clearly is efficacious in preventing recrudescence of herpes simplex during the risk period. Finally, a good dental prophylaxis done before induction of granulocytopenia will reduce the frequency of acute exacerbations of periodontitis.

As to improving host defense mechanisms, the key is to obtain return of circulating granulocytes. White cell transfusions have been shown useful in preventing bacteremia but are expensive, difficult to obtain, create problems for donors, and may lead to other infections, notably CMV. The current interest is to determine whether granulocyte colony-stimulating factor (G-CSF) or granulocyte-macrophage CSF (GM-CSF) (Table 3) will sub-stantially shorten the granulocytopenic period such that infections will be reduced. Early data from Peters (this volume, pp. 97–101) are suggestive.

Cellular Immune Dysfunction and Infection

Infections associated with cellular immune dysfunction are considered by Klastersky (this volume). In effect, this is an issue of inadequate T cell function, although T cells are also relevant in abnormal humoral (B cell) immune function. Methods for evaluating T and B cell function are shown in Table 2. Table 3 reviews the major recognized cytokines and their currently appreciated functions. An appreciation of the cytokines is particularly appropriate given the use of GM-CSF and G-CSF in attempts to speed engraftment and return of granulocyte function after transplantation, inter-ferons for some types of hepatitis, and possibly others to reduce the possibility of graft-versus-host disease. This is a new field but one rapidly evolving in relevance for both prevention and treatment of infection.

Humoral Immune Dysfunction and Infection

There is yet another group of infections associated with humoral immune dysfunction. Patients who have defects in humoral immunity (multiple

Table 2. Laboratory tests for evaluating immune function. (From American College of Physicians Medical Knowledge Self-Assessment Program 1991)

Screening tests
B cell studies
  Serum immunoglobulin studies: IgG, IgA, IgM, IgE
  Natural antibody titers: isohemagglutinins, antibodies to previous immunizations
    or infections
T cell studies
  Lymphocyte count
  Delayed-type hypersensitivity testing to recall antigens

Second-level tests
B cell studies
  Tests of in vivo production
    IgG subclasses: IgG_1, IgG_2, IgG_3, IgG_4
    Antibody response to antigen challenge: protein and carbohydrate antigens
  In vitro assays
    B cell enumeration: surface immunoglobulin and B cell-specific antigens
    Immunoglobulin production assays: polyclonal and antigen-specific activation
T cell studies
  T cell enumeration: T cell-specific antigens
  T cell function: T cell proliferation (mitogens, antigens, allogeneic cells), T cell
    help, T cell suppression, T cell cytotoxicity
Natural immunity studies
  Natural killer cell (NK cell) enumeration: NK cell markers
  NK cell function (with and without cytokines)
  Antibody-dependent cellular cytotoxicity

---

myeloma, chronic lymphocytic leukemia, chronic graft-versus-host disease) tend to have infections for which opsonizing antibody is the major means of infection prevention, i.e., *Streptococcus pneumoniae*, *Hemophilus influenzae*, and (rarely) *Neisseria meningitidis*.

The absence of normal production of immune serum globulins impairs the phagocytic activity not only of granulocytes but also of monocytes and macrophages. In multiple myeloma, there is both a decrease in synthesis and an increase in catabolism of normal immunoglobulins. The degree of impairment increases with increased tumor burden. Apparently, suppressor macrophages, as an exaggerated expression of the natural control mechanisms, suppress the remaining normal B lymphocytes and plasma cells. Also, patients with a heavy tumor burden may be deficient in C3 activation. The net result is an increased incidence and severity of *S. pneumoniae* infections. *H. influenzae*, *N. meningitidis*, and *E. coli* infect less commonly in these patients but host resistance for each depends upon complement and, for the Gram-positive cocci, opsonizing antibody (Jacobson and Zolla-Pazner 1986).

In chronic lymphocytic leukemia, infections with these same organisms may occur. The degree of hypogammaglobulinemia accelerates with tumor

Table 3. Selected cytokines and their major biologic functions. (From American College of Physicians Medical Knowledge Self-Assessment Program 1991)

Cytokine	Cell source	Biologic effects
Interleukin 1 (IL-1)	Mononuclear leukocytes and endothelial cells	Acute-phase reaction; activates resting T cells; cofactor for B cell, T cell, bone marrow cell proliferation; activates macrophages and endothelial cells; was known as endogenous pyrogen
Interleukin 2 (IL-2)	T cells	Growth factor for B cells and T cells, activates cytotoxic lymphocytes, promotes synthesis of other cytokines, enhances NK cell function
Interleukin 3 (IL-3)	T cells, stromal cells	Promotes proliferation of pluripotent marrow stem cells; growth factor for mast cells, basophils, eosinophils, and macrophages
Interleukin 4 (IL-4)	T cells	Induces IgE synthesis, up-regulates Fc_ε receptors and MHC class II molecules, growth factor for T cells
Interleukin 5 (IL-5)	T cells	Eosinophil growth and differentiation factor
Interleukin 6 (IL-6)	Mononuclear leukocytes, fibroblasts	Induces differentiation of activated B cells
Interleukin 7 (IL-7)	T cells, bone marrow stromal cells	Induces growth of immature B cells and T cells
Interleukin 8 (IL-8)	Monocytes, macrophages	Activates neutrophils
Interferon-alpha	Mononuclear leukocytes	Interferes with viral replication, decreases cell replication, increases MHC class I expression
Interferon-beta	Fibroblasts, endothelial cells	Increases NK cell function, induces fever
Interferon-gamma	T cells, NK cells	Interferes with viral replication, decreases cell replication, increases expression of MHC class I and II, enhances macrophage function, down-regulates IgE synthesis

Table 3. *Continued*

Cytokine	Cell source	Biologic effects
Tumor necrosis factor-alpha	Mononuclear leukocytes, mast cells	Acute-phase reaction, antitumor and antiviral activity, increases endothelial cell adherence and MHC class I expression, enhances PMN adherence and cidal activity
Tumor necrosis factor-beta	T cells	Induces production of tumor necrosis, IL-1, and colony-stimulating factors
Transforming-growth factor (TGF)-beta	Platelets, endothelial cells, mononuclear leukocytes, mast cells, stromal cells	Suppresses lymphocyte proliferation; regulates antibody production; suppresses generation of cytotoxic T cells; promotes tissue repair, chondrogenesis, and osteogenesis
Granulocyte-macrophage colony-stimulating factor (GM-CSF)	T cells, endothelial cells, monocytes, macrophages, fibroblasts, stromal cells	Promotes proliferation of neutrophil, macrophage, eosinophil precursors; enhances function of macrophages, eosinophils, and neutrophils; inhibits mast cell differentiation
Macrophage colony-stimulating factor (M-CSF)	Monocytes, macrophages, fibroblasts, endothelial cells, stromal cells	Promotes proliferation of monocytes, enhances function of macrophages
Granulocyte colony-stimulating factor (G-CSF)	Monocytes, macrophages, fibroblasts, endothelial cells	Promotes proliferation of granulocytes, enhances function of granulocytes
Stem cell factor	Fibroblasts, stromal cells	Promotes expansion of precursor cells

burden (stage) but, unlike myeloma, does not generally revert following chemotherapy.

Antibody production against *S. pneumoniae* is depressed following bone marrow transplantation, and these patients tend to have an increased risk of pneumococcal infection. Patients who have had a splenectomy for any cause, including trauma or as a diagnostic procedure (e.g., staging laparotomy for Hodgkin's disease) are at an increased risk of infection with the encapsulated pyogenic cocci. Although pneumococcal bacteremia appears to be quite unusual even in the splenectomized patient with Hodgkin's disease, it is important to recall that a very small but real percentage of patients may develop the "overwhelming pneumococcal sepsis syndrome" (Bisno 1971). This has been reported sporadically in adults in whom an overwhelming septicemia without apparent origin of infection leads to the patient's demise in a matter of a day or less. The syndrome mimicks in many ways the Waterhouse-Friderichsen syndrome described with meningococcal sepsis and which has also been seen occasionally as a result of *Hemophilus* sepsis in splenectomized patients. Therefore, patients who have had a splenectomy (e.g., Hodgkin's disease, hairy cell leukemia) should be advised that the sudden onset of fever and chills should prompt immediate medical attention, and physicians should be aware that immediate hospitalization with institution of i.v. ampicillin (to cover *S. pneumoniae*, *H. influenzae*, and *N. meningitidis*) is appropriate except in those settings where ampicillin-resistant *H. influenzae* are prevalent (in which case cefotaxime or other third-generation cephalosporins with good penetration of the blood–brain barrier should be effective).

The severity of humoral immune deficiencies depends on maturation of B cells through a complex process along with their interaction with multiple other cell populations and cytokines. Defects in the complement system can have some similar effects as to infection development and progression. When complement (C3) binds to a bacterium, it makes it more readily phagocytized by granulocytes or attacked by splenic macrophages or hepatic Kupffer cells. If splenic function is reduced, as in chronic graft-versus-host disease following bone marrow transplantation, or absent, as in traumatic splenectomy, bacteria are not cleared from the bloodstream effectively and septic death may result. Alternatively, reduced antibody production makes splenic clearance much less effective. Thus, the patient who has had a bone marrow transplant is at risk of infection due to the combined effect of reduced antibody production, impaired splenic function, and, perhaps, less than optimal complement activity. Pneumococcal infections, especially during chronic graft-versus-host disease, are encountered commonly in these patients. Elsewhere, Tutschka (this volume, "Late Bacterial Infections in Humoral Immune Deficiency") explores the use of intravenous immune serum globulin to reduce these infections and reduce the severity of chronic graft-versus-host disease.

Infections Associated with Vascular Access Devices

Implanted vascular access catheters are in common usage and in many patients, especially leukemia and transplant patients, may be left in place for many months or even years. Three types of infection occur: exit site infections, tunnel infections, and catheter-related bacteremia/fungemia. Using Hickman catheters as an example (Fig. 4), about one-quarter will develop

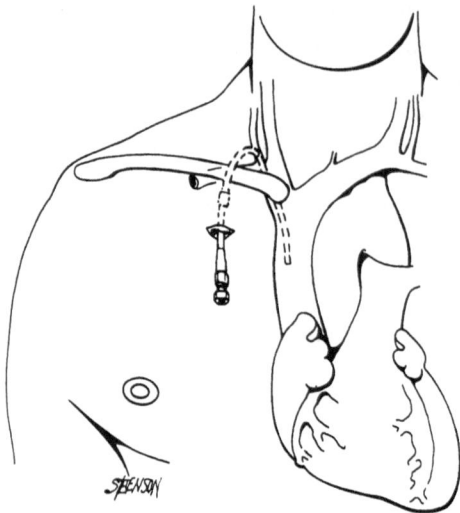

Fig. 4. Central venous catheter placement. The catheter is placed into the external jugular vein. Note the Dacron cuff in the subcutaneous portion of catheter approximately 2 cm from the exit site in the skin. (From Schimpff 1990)

an exit site infection, usually caused by *S. epidermidis*. Generally, these can be treated with vancomycin or other antibiotics without the need to remove the catheter. Tunnel infections are much less common (about 5% of patients) but are very serious, fulminant infections usually requiring prompt catheter removal in addition to antibiotic therapy. Catheter-associated bacteremias/ fungemias appear to be relatively uncommon provided meticulous attention is paid to initial insertion and daily maintenance. Bacteremias caused by *S. epidermidis*, the most common etiology, can usually be resolved by vancomycin given via the catheter without catheter removal. Those caused by Gram-negative bacilli or yeasts generally require removal of the catheter in addition to antimicrobials. Most catheters will develop a biofilm (glycocalyx) produced by *S. epidermidis* along the inner lumen (Tenney et al. 1986). Scanning electron microscopy will detect the bacteria and biofilm along most catheters within 6 weeks after placement; surprisingly few patients develop a catheter-associated bacteremia however.

Infections Associated with Infusions

One of the most common iatrogenic causes of infection is related to blood and blood product administration, with resultant non-A/non-B hepatitis (hepatitis C) and, less frequently, infections caused by CMV, Epstein-Barr virus, or *Toxoplasma gondii*. Less common are infections associated with contamination of physiological fluids, such as the nationwide epidemic of *Enterobacter* bacteremia in the United States about 20 years ago, which was related to contamination during manufacture of intravenous fluids. Rarely, Gram-negative bacteria can contaminate platelets or other blood products. Vigilence will be necessary as new approaches to drug delivery systems become widespread.

For the present, *hepatitis C virus* infection is the major cause of hepatitis among multiply transfused individuals. Characteristically, hepatitis occurs in the third, or later, month after transplantation and may present as a difficult diagnostic challenge as the same presentation may herald acute or chronic graft-versus-host disease, venoocclusive disease, CMV or other infection (Davis, this volume, pp. 213–220).

New Pathogens and Resistance Patterns

Not only are Gram-positive organisms more common, but a host of organisms are now recognized more frequently than just a few years ago. Included among them are bacteria such as *Streptococcus mitis*, *Xanthomonas maltophilia*, and *Leuconostoc* spp.; fungi such as *Trichosporon*, *Rhodotorula rubra* and viruses such as herpesvirus type 6 (McWhinney et al. 1992; Oren and Sobel 1992). Resistance remains a notable problem, from Gram-negative bacillary resistance to gentamicin to broad resistance to many beta-lactams. Resistance to vancomycin and amphotericin B, although rare, is being reported.

Specifics of Infection in Marrow Transplant Patients

The first major predisposing factor is absolute granulocytopenia, generally lasting 18–23 days after allogeneic transplantation (Fig. 1). These patients also have significant mucosal damage and shifts of oral microbial flora toward Gram-negative bacilli, and may have acquired resistant organisms from the hospital environment. Hence, they are subject to Gram-negative (especially *E. coli*, *K. pneumoniae*, or *P. aeruginosa*) infection and bacteremia, Gram-positive (especially *S. epidermidis*, *S. mitis*) infection and bacteremia, as well as possibly fungal infection caused by *Candida* or *Aspergillus*. This is also the same time frame when herpes simplex is reactivated, especially orocutaneous lesions.

Table 4 outlines the impairments in host defenses after engraftment. As the marrow engrafts, acute graft-versus-host disease and its therapy predispose to CMV infection, most notably CMV pneumonia. *Candida* and *Aspergillus* infection can also occur in this setting, now one of cellular immune dysfunction. Somewhat later, varicella zoster virus infections, either zoster with possible dissemination or a variant form of varicella occur in nearly two thirds of patients.

Table 4. Host defenses associated with marrow transplant patients after engraftment (From Donowitz 1992)

Host defense system	Defect	Time of recovery[a]
Cell mediated immunity	↓ Numbers and function of nonspecific cytotoxic cells (NK cells, ADCC)	30 Days
	↓ T cell numbers	120 Days
	↓ CD_4 (helper-inducer cells)	4–6 Months to 1 year
	↑ CD_8 cells (cytotoxic suppressor cells) (↓ CD_4–CD_8 ratio)	1–6 Months
	↓ Interleukin-2 production	100 Days–1 year
	↓ Blastogenic response in CD_4 cells	2 Years
	↓ Response to recall antigen	4 Years
Humoral immunity	↓ IgG, IgM levels	30–160 Days
	↓ IgA response to antigenic stimuli	180 Days
	↓ Response to pneumococcal polysaccharide	180 Days
Phagocytic defense		
– Neutrophil function	↓ Chemotaxis	4 Months
– Alveolar macrophage function	↓ Chemotaxis	>1 Year
	↓ Phagocytosis	
	↓ Bactericidal, fungicidal activity	

[a] In the absence of graft-versus-host disease.
From Donowitz GR (1992) Infections in bone marrow transplant recipients. In: Mandell GL, Douglas RG Jr, Bennett JE (eds) Principles and practice of infectious diseases, quarterly update 12, Churchilll Livingstone, 1992.

As the acute graft-versus-host disease wanes and is replaced by chronic graft-versus-host disease, the infections associated with humoral immune dysfunction and splenic dysfunction predominate, especially pneumococcal bacteremia and cutaneous lesions.

Enough time has now passed so that this multiply transfused patient may develop *hepatitis C virus* infection.

At any time over the course of recovery, implanted vascular access catheters may have associated infections at the exit site, along the tunnel, or as a lumen-associated bacteremia.

The clinician must be cognizant of local hospital/center resistance patterns, of endemic patterns of colonization and of possible clusters of special problem organisms. Finally, in patients with solid tumors with potential for natural passage obstruction, it is necessary to recall that any partial obstruction will usually lead to postobstructive infection.

References

Aisner J, Murillo J, Schimpff SC, Steere AC (1979) Invasive aspergillosis in acute leukemia: correlation with nose cultures and antibiotic usage. Ann Intern Med 90:4–9

American College of Physicians Medical Knowledge Self-Assessment Program (MKSAP IX) (1991) part A, book 2, Allergy and Immunology. American College of Physicians, Philadelphia

Bisno AL (1971) Hyposplenism and overwhelming pneumococcal infection: a reappraisal. Am J Med Sci 262:101–107

Bodey GP, Buckley M, Sathe YS, Freireich EJ (1966) Quantitative relationships between circulating leukocytes and infection in patients with acute leukemia. Ann Intern Med 64:328–340

Donowitz GR (1992) Infections in bone marrow transplant recipients. In: Mandell GL, Douglas RG Jr, Bennett JE (eds) Principles and practice of infectious diseases. Quarterly update 12, pp 3–12

EORTC International Antimicrobial Therapy Cooperative Group (1989) Empiric antifungal therapy in febrile granulocytopenic patients. Am J Med 86:668–672

Jacobson DR, Zolla-Pazner S (1986) Immunosuppression and infection in multiple myeloma. Semin Oncol 13:282–290

Joshi JH, Schimpff SC (1984) Infections in the compromised host. In: Mandell GL, Douglas RG, Bennett JE (eds) Principles and practice of infectious diseases, 2nd edn. Wiley, New York, p 1664

McWhinney PHM, Kibbler CC, Gillespie SH, Prentice HG (1992) Stomatococcus mucilaginosus: an emerging pathogen in neutropenic patients. Clin Infect Dis 14:641–646

Oren H, Sobel JD (1992) Human herpesvirus type 6: review. Clin Infect Dis 14: 741–746

Pizzo PA, Robichaud KJ, Wesley R et al. (1982) Fever in the pediatric and young adult patient with cancer. A prospective study of 1001 episodes. Medicine 61:153

Pizzo PA, Schimpff SC (1983) Strategies for the prevention of infection in the myelosuppressed or immunosuppressed cancer patient. Cancer Treat Rep 67: 223–234

Remington JS, Schimpff SC (1981) Please don't eat the salads. N Engl J Med 304:443–435

Schimpff SC (1990) Infection in the leukemia patient: diagnosis, therapy and prevention. In: Henderson ES, Lister TA (eds) Leukemia, 5th edn. Saunders, Philadelphia, p 702

Schimpff SC (1991) Infections in cancer patients: overview and epidemiology. In: Moossa AR, Schimpff SC, Robson MC (eds) Comprehensive textbook of oncology, 2nd edn. Williams and Wilkins, Baltimore, p 1721

Schimpff S, Satterlee W, Young VM, Serpick A (1971) Empiric therapy with carbenicillin and gentamicin for febrile patients with cancer and granulocytopenia. N Engl J Med 284:1061–1065

Schimpff SC, Wiernik PH, Block JB (1972a) Rectal abscesses in cancer patients. Lancet ii:844–847

Schimpff S, Young V, Greene W, Vermeulen G, Moody M, Wiernik P (1972b) Origin of infection in acute nonlymphocytic leukemia – significance of hospital acquisition of potential pathogens. Ann Intern Med 77:707–714

Sickles EA, Greene WH, Wiernik PH (1975) Clinical presentation in granulocytopenic patients. Arch Intern Med 135:715–719

Tenney JH, Moody MR, Newman KA, Schimpff SC, Wade JC, Costerton JW, Reed WH (1986) Adherent microorganisms on lumenal surfaces of long-term intravenous catheters: importance of Staphylococcus epidermidis in patients with cancer. Arch Intern Med 146:1949–1954

Further Reading

Hughes WT, Armstrong D, Bodey GP, Feld R, Mandell GL, Meyers JD, Pizzo PA, Schimpff SC, Shenep JL, Wade JC, Young LS, Yow MD (1990) Guidelines for the use of antimicrobial agents in neutropenic patients with unexplained fever. J Inf Dis 161:381–396
  The consensus report of a group of experts in the empiric treatment of infections during granulocytopenia. The major issues and controversies are reviewed.
Lum LG (1987) The kinetics of immune reconstitution after human bone marrow transplantation. Blood 69:369
  A thorough review of immune function in relation to marrow transplantation.
Pizzo PA (1989) Evaluation of fever in the patient with cancer. Eur J Cancer Clin Oncol 25[Suppl]:S9–S16
  A good overview of the treatment of infection in cancer patients.
Rubin M, Hathorn JW, Marshall D et al. (1988) Gram-positive infections and the use of vancomycin in 550 episodes of fever and neutropenia. Ann Intern Med 108:30–35
  A discussion of the increased frequency of S. epidermidis infections and the authors' approach to early use of vancomycin.
Schimpff SC (1991) Infections in patients with cancer: overview and epidemiology. In: Moossa AR, Schimpff SC, Robson MC (eds) Comprehensive textbook of oncology, 2nd edn. Williams and Wilkins, Baltimore, pp 1720–1732
  A general discussion of infection in cancer patients.
Schimpff S, Young V, Greene W, Vermeulen G, Moody M, Wiernik P (1972) Origin of infection in acute nonlymphocytic leukemia – significance of hospital acquisition of potential pathogens. Ann Intern Med 77:707–714
  A study which demonstrated the importance of acquired organisms in infection during granulocytopenia and the relative invasive potential of the various Gram-positive and Gram-negative bacteria during granulocytopenia.

II. Case Presentation

Introduction to Case Presentation

S.C. Schimpff

University of Maryland School of Medicine, 22 South Greene Street,
Baltimore, MD 21201, USA

The following case presentation was used at The Greenbrier Conference in August 1991 as a stimulus to the invited experts. The questions were prepared to be consistent with the type of problems commonly encountered by clinicians caring for patients who have undergone a bone marrow transplant. The questions were designed to be straightforward yet raise issues for which the answer is frequently controversial. There was lively discussion regarding most answers, a summary of which is given at the end of this monograph.

Case Presentation

A 33-year-old previously healthy male is found to have acute myelocytic (monocytic) leukemia. He is treated with cytotoxic combination chemotherapy, and a complete remission is achieved following a stormy course. He goes home for 2 months and then is readmitted for bone marrow transplantation. The donor is to be his HLA-identical sister. In advance preparation, he has a Hickman catheter placed into his venous system.

Three days before the transplantation, he receives total body irradiation and 3 consecutive days of high-dose cyclophosphamide. The bone marrow material is infused intravenously without incident. Within 4 days, he has no circulating granulocytes, and his platelets are being supported by every-other-day platelet transfusions.

On day 9 following transplantation, without concurrent symptomatology, he develops a fever of 102°F (38.9°C) with a shaking chill. Complete history and physical examination are unremarkable. Chest X-ray is negative, and urinalysis is negative.

1. In the absence of any other detectable historical, physical, or X-ray finding should this patient be treated empirically with broad-spectrum antibiotic(s)?

Recent Results in Cancer Research, Vol. 132
© Springer-Verlag Berlin · Heidelberg 1993

A. Yes
B. No

2. Assuming the decision was to begin a combination of antibiotics, which one of the following combinations would not be appropriate?
A. Cephalothin plus gentamicin
B. Ceftazidime plus gentamicin
C. Imipenem plus gentamicin
D. Piperacillin plus gentamicin

3. The hospital microbiology laboratory reports that approximately 20% of Gram-negative rod isolates in recent months have been resistant to gentamicin. In that situation, which one of the following would be an appropriate aminoglycoside to utilize?
A. Gentamicin
B. Tobramycin
C. Netilmicin
D. Amikacin

4. Under what circumstances would a "double beta lactam" combination (e.g., piperacillin plus ceftazidime) be utilized?
A. Never
B. Patient with pre-existing renal dysfunction
C. Patient with aminoglycoside ototoxicity
D. Hospital with high incidence of gentamicin resistance

5. Which of the following (choose one or more) have an adequate spectrum of coverage when using monotherapy as an initial empiric regimen?
A. Piperacillin
B. Ticarcillin plus clavulanate
C. Imipenem
D. Ceftazidime

6. Monotherapy is appropriate initial therapy when the initial granulocyte count is (choose one or more):
A. 0–99/μl
B. 100–499/μl
C. 500–999/μl
D. ≥1000/μl

7. Some institutions have noted a particularly high frequency of *Staphylococcus epidermidis*, streptococcal species bacteremias and a near absence of Gram-negative rod infections among their patients who develop fever during neutropenia. Given that setting, which of the following might be appropriate regimens for empiric therapy in the febrile neutropenic cancer patient? (Choose one or more.)
A. Piperacillin plus gentamicin plus vancomycin
B. Piperacillin plus vancomycin

   C. Ceftazidime plus vancomycin
   D. Imipenem plus vancomycin
   E. Vancomycin

8. The changing epidemiology of infections in neutropenic patients continues. Which Gram-positive cocci are most likely to cause bacteremia in this patient?
   A. *Staphylococcus aureus*
   B. *Staphylococcus epidermidis*
   C. *Viridans* streptococci
   D. *Streptococcus pneumoniae*

9. Repeat history and examination on a daily basis demonstrates a site of infection 48 h after initial fever documentation. Which of the following are the five most likely sites for infection in this patient?
   A. Acute exacerbation of chronic periodontitis
   B. Sinusitis
   C. Pharyngitis
   D. Otitis media
   E. Pneumonitis
   F. Esophagitis
   G. Perianal lesion
   H. Urinary tract infection
   I. Prostatitis
   J. Hickman catheter exit site infection
   K. Hickman catheter tunnel infection
   L. Hickman catheter-related bacteremia

10. Blood cultures drawn when fever first began are reported negative. However, which of the following organisms are likely causes of bacteremia in patients such as this one? (Choose one or more.)
   A. *Pseudomonas aeruginosa*
   B. *Xanthomonas (Pseudomonas) maltophilia*
   C. *Escherichia coli*
   D. *Enterobacter cloacae*
   E. *Staphylococcus epidermidis*
   F. *Clostridium difficile*
   G. *Candida albicans*
   H. *Streptococcus mitis*

11. What novel bacteria are emerging as agents of bacteremia in neutropenic patients?
   A. *Corynebacterium jikeium*
   B. *Leuconostoc* species
   C. *Xanthomonas maltophilia*
   D. *Pseudomonas putrefaciens*
   E. *Leptotrichia buccalis*
   F. *Rhodococcus equi*

12. Fever resolves over a 3-day period as do symptoms and signs of perianal cellulitis (recognized the day after fever occurred) by day 5. How long should the empiric antibiotic regimen be continued? (Choose one.)
    A. Discontinue when fever/symptoms and signs resolve
    B. For a total course of 7–10 days
    C. Until resolution of granulocytopenia

13. If fever had persisted, but the signs and symptoms of local infection had resolved, which course of action would be appropriate? (Assume daily repeat examinations are negative, chest X-rays every 2–3 days are unrevealing, and the empiric regimen was a beta lactam or carbapenem plus gentamicin.) (Choose one or more.)
    A. Add amphotericin B (i.v.)
    B. Add acyclovir (i.v.)
    C. Replace gentamicin with amikacin
    D. Add vancomycin
    E. Replace beta lactam/carbapenem with a different class (e.g., substitute carbapenem for cephalosporin or vice versa)
    F. Removal of indwelling catheter

14. Should this patient have been the recipient of granulocyte–macrophage colony-stimulating factor (GM-CSF) to hasten marrow engraftment and return of circulating granulocytes?
    A. Yes
    B. No

15. Should this patient have been the recipient of granulocyte transfusions?
    A. Yes
    B. No

16. What about other growth factors or growth factor antagonists? (Choose one or more.)
    A. Granulocyte CSF (G-CSF)
    B. Macrophage CSF (M-CSF)
    C. Tumor necrosis factor (TNF)
    D. Anti-TNF compound
    E. Interleukin 1 (IL-1)
    F. IL-6
    G. None of above

17. Are granulocytes that are released "early" due to GM-CSF (or other growth factors) functionally normal?
    A. Yes
    B. No

18. Granulocyte transfusions have fallen from use largely due to limited yields with current technology even following donor priming with corticos-

teroids. Would the priming of donors with GM-CSF be of potential value in collecting adequate numbers of granulocytes for transfusion?

A. Yes
B. No

19. The patient is treated as above; however, by day 18, with still no circulating granulocytes, he develops new fever and chest X-ray shows a left upper lobe pulmonary infiltrate. Bronchoscopy with biopsy is done, and appropriate stains might show which of the following organisms? (Pick the two most likely.)

A. Gram-negative bacilli
B. Branching septated hyphae
C. *Pneumocystis carinii*
D. *Toxoplasma gondii*

20. The biopsy shows branching septated hyphae. You would now treat with (choose all correct answers):

A. Amphotericin B
B. Amphotericin B plus rifampin
C. Fluconazole
D. Ketoconazole

21. Amphotericin B should be at what dosage? (Choose one best answer.)

A. 0.3 mg/kg per day
B. 0.6 mg/kg per day
C. 1.2–1.5 mg/kg per day
D. 1.2–1.5 mg/kg q.o.d.

22. Should amphotericin B be given as a liposomal preparation?

A. Yes
B. No

23. Assume that the biopsy in Q16 had demonstrated a nonfungal origin for the pulmonary infiltrate and that a few days later the patient developed difficulty swallowing. Esophagoscopy was performed and demonstrated invasive candidiasis. Which of the following would be appropriate therapy? (Choose one or more.)

A. Amphotericin B
B. Amphotericin B plus flucytosine
C. Fluconazole
D. Nystatin
E. Ketoconazole
F. Amphotericin B plus acyclovir

24. How often is *Candida* esophagitis preceded by herpetic infection? (Choose one.)

A. Frequently
B. Occasionally
C. Rarely

25. Which species of *Candida* is more invasive?
   A.   *Candida albicans*
   B.   *Candida tropicalis*

26. Which species of *Candida* is more frequently found to cause infection in this setting?
   A.   *Candida albicans*
   B.   *Candida tropicalis*

27. Which fungi are emerging as new pathogens in the immunocompromised patient with cancer?
   A.   *Pseudallescheria boydii*
   B.   *Trichosporon* spp.
   C.   *Fusarium* spp.
   D.   Drechslera spp.
   E.   *Encephalitozoon cuniculi*

28. This patient was antibody positive for herpes simplex virus at the time of initial admission. Given that such patients have a very high incidence of reactivation of the latent herpes simplex virus, which of the following agents should have been used, beginning on day 0, as prophylaxis?
   A.   Ganciclovir
   B.   AZT
   C.   Acyclovir
   D.   Foscarnet

29. Would the same prophylactic approach have been appropriate for this patient when he was receiving his initial remission induction chemotherapy?
   A.   Yes
   B.   No

30. Again, the patient improves, and by day 23, the granulocyte count begins to return toward normal. Antibacterial therapy is given for 14 days and antifungal therapy is planned for 6 weeks. On day 40, new fever develops and chest X-ray now shows bilateral pulmonary infiltrates with an interstitial pattern. Bronchoscopy and biopsy are done again, avoiding the original area of infiltrate known to be fungal in origin. The findings are most likely which one of the following?
   A.   *Pseudomonas aeruginosa*
   B.   Cytomegalovirus (CMV)
   C.   *Toxoplasma gondii*
   D.   *Streptococcus pneumoniae*
   E.   *Aspergillus flavus*
   F.   *Pneumocystis carinii*
   G.   Herpes simplex virus
   H.   Idiopathic IP (regimen-related toxicity)

31. The appropriate therapy for this patient would be:
   A. Acyclovir
   B. Piperacillin plus gentamicin
   C. Pyrimethamine plus sulfadiazine
   D. Ganciclovir plus immune serum globulin

32. If this patient had been CMV seronegative prior to bone marrow transplantation and also received his graft from a CMV-negative donor,
   A. the patient should have received CMV-negative blood component support exclusively
   B. filtered blood component support is equivalent
   C. Unscreened blood support is adequate

33. The patient improves and is discharged to home. On day 63, he develops an erythematous painful rash at the level of T4 on the right side. By the next day, a number of vesicles have appeared which are filled with a clear, slightly straw-colored fluid. The diagnosis is herpes zoster caused by the latent varicella zoster virus. The physician prescribes codeine for pain, careful washing with an antiseptic soap, and a skin cream. In addition, this patient should be treated with:
   A. Nothing
   B. Ganciclovir
   C. Acyclovir
   D. Adenine arabinoside

34. About day 70 following transplantation, the patient develops myalgia, abdominal pain, nausea, and malaise. He is afebrile. White blood count and platelet count are normal with no evidence of recurrence of primary disease. Serum ALT is 1330 IU/l, AST is 890 IU/l (nl ALT and AST < 40), alkaline phosphatase is 115 IU/l (nl < 120), bilirubin is 2.1 mg/dl (1.3 mg/dl direct). Differential diagnosis includes viral hepatitis (A, B, C, D, CMV), drug-induced hepatitis, hepatic recurrence, veno-occlusive disease and hepatic graft-versus-host disease. Initial serologic evaluation include negative IgG anti-HAV, HBsAg, anti-HBc, and anti-HCV. Blood and urine cultures for CMV are negative. The most effective means of establishing the diagnosis is:
   A. CT scan
   B. Wedged hepatic venogram
   C. Percutaneous liver biopsy
   D. Laparoscopic liver biopsy

35. The most likely diagnosis is:
   A. CMV hepatitis
   B. Hepatitis C
   C. Veno-occlusive disease

36. The patient is observed. Although the liver tests decline slightly over the next week, the patient becomes jaundiced. A liver biopsy is performed

which shows acute hepatitis without viral inclusions. Terminal hepatic venules are normal (no veno-occlusive disease). The presumptive diagnosis is seronegative hepatitis C (post-transfusion). Appropriate treatment is:

A. Recombinant interferon alfa-2b
B. Ribavirin
C. Decrease immunosuppression
D. Observation

37. About day 90 the patient is driving in his car and is obliged to make a sudden stop; his shoulder seat belt strap forcibly restrains him. He notices some discomfort along the Hickman catheter tunnel site for the next week and then begins to have low-grade fever and increased discomfort along the tunnel. Within 2 more days the overlying skin is erythematous and examination demonstrates fluctuance; temperature is now 100.4°F (38°C). Gram stain of an aspirate shows Gram-positive cocci. The treatment approach should be (choose one):

A. Vancomycin (i.v.)
B. Nafcillin (i.v.)
C. Cloxacillin (p.o.)
D. Vancomycin plus remove catheter
E. Nafcillin plus remove catheter

38. The patient is well until he calls his physician at 10 p.m. on the evening of the 97th day. He indicates that he has been well except for a minor sore throat for the past day or two. However, 1 h ago, he had the sudden onset of fever to 103°F (39.4°C) with very intense shaking chills. He has no other particular symptomatology. His physician had seen him in the office a few days before for routine follow up, and, at that time, he had been in complete remission of leukemia, white blood cell count was normal with a normal differential, and the platelet count was normal. The physical examination was entirely normal. Given the high fever and shaking chills, the patient is instructed to meet his physician in the emergency room immediately. The physician is concerned about the possibility of an overwhelming bacteremia, in its very earliest stages, caused by which (choose the single best answer) of the following organisms?

A. *Pseudomonas aeruginosa*
B. *Staphylococcus epidermidis*
C. *Streptococcus pneumoniae*
D. *Staphylococcus aureus*

39. Should this patient have received any of the following vaccines following transplantation? (Circle correct choices.)

A. *Haemophilus influenzae B*
B. *Streptococcus pneumoniae*
C. *Neisseria meningiditis*
D. Varicella zoster
E. Measles – mumps – rubella

40. Should this patient have received serum immune globulin (i.v.) prophy-lactically on a regular basis after transplantation?
   A. Yes
   B. No

41. Should this patient have received trimethoprim-sulfamethoxazole (TMP-SMX) as prophylaxis for pneumocystis pneumonia?
   A. Yes
   B. No

42. Would TMP-SMX therapy have prevented this febrile illness?
   A. Yes
   B. No

43. Should the patient have received prophylaxis with another antibiotic, e.g., amoxacillin?
   A. Yes
   B. No

44. On day 120 after bone marrow transplant on a routine review, he complains of an unusual sensation which he described as "not being able to take a complete breath." Examination of the chest is unremarkable, blood count shows a fall in neutrophils from $2.4 \times 10^9/l$ to $1.3 \times 10^9/l$, the platelet count also fell from 110 to $92 \times 10^9/l$. A chest radiograph showed no abnormalities, but lung function showed a restrictive-obstructive pattern with a decreased KCO and a prolonged FEV1. He was given a bronchodilator inhaler, and a DEAFF test for CMV was carried out on blood and urine. What possible diagnosis should be considered?
   A. CMV pneumonitis
   B. Chronic graft-versus-host disease (GVHD) affecting the lungs
   C. Pneumocystis pneumonia
   D. Bacterial pneumonia
   E. *Aspergillus* pneumonia

45. Three days later, he reports that the tightness in the chest has improved but he is nevertheless more dyspneic and has developed an unproductive cough. On examination, there are a few scattered crepitations to be heard on auscultation of the chest, and the chest radiograph now shows a widespread diffuse increase in density particularly around the midzones. On further examination, he is noted to be mildly icteric and has a generalized fine erythema. Liver function results taken 3 days previously show a rise in alkaline phosphatase and raised bilirubin. The DEAFF test for CMV early antigens taken 3 days previously is negative. What would you do next?
   A. Bronchoscopy and examination of bronchial washings
   B. Open lung biopsy
   C. Empiric high-dose intravenous cotrimoxazole
   D. Repeat DEAFF test

E. Empiric intravenous ceftazidime

F. Empiric intravenous amphotericin

46. Bronchial washings were shown to be positive for CMV. How would you treat the patient?

A. CMV-specific immunoglobulin and ganciclovir

B. Prednisolone and cyclosporine to treat chronic graft-versus-host disease

C. Add antibacterial prophylaxis with seprin, and antifungal prophylaxis with ketaconazole

D. Give high-dose intravenous methyl prednisolone to improve lung function

47. He was admitted to the hospital and treated with ganciclovir and anti-CMV immunoglobulin. After 4 weeks of treatment, his lung function had improved and the DEAFF test was negative. He is discharged from the hospital. What prophylactic treatment should he continue with and for how long?

A. Alternate-day prednisolone and cyclosporine

B. Regular cotrimoxazole

C. Penicillin daily

D. Repeated monthly infusions of anti-CMV immunoglobulin

III. Infection and Granulocytopenia

Initial Empiric Therapy for Fever in Neutropenia

C.I. Bustamante

Private Practice of Infectious Diseases, 16800 NW 2nd Avenue, Suite 606,
N. Miami Beach, FL 33169, USA

Despite significant improvements in supportive care, infection remains a significant cause of morbidity and mortality for patients with cancer undergoing intensive chemotherapy. This is particularly important for patients with hematologic malignancies receiving induction-chemotherapy or bone marrow transplantation. Neutropenia (<1000 granulocytes/μl) is the most significant risk factor with the majority of the infections developing at a granulocyte count $<500/\mu$l and almost all the bacteremias at <100 granulocytes/μl (Bodey et al. 1966).

The lack of adequate cellular inflammatory response during neutropenia leaves fever, invariably present, as the earliest sign of infection. Approximately 60% of febrile episodes in neutropenic patients are associated with infection, one third of these are bacteremias. Prompt empiric initiation of intravenous therapy with broad-spectrum antibiotics with the development of fever has been the standard of care for neutropenic patients for almost 3 decades. With the currently available antibiotic regimens, response rates of 60%–80% for neutropenic patients with documented infection should be expected. Patients with Gram-negative rod bacteremia have lower response rates and, if they present with septic shock or antibiotics are not initiated promptly, experience the highest morbidity and mortality (Schimpff 1990).

The search for more effective and less toxic antibiotic regimens has intensified in recent years with the availability of new classes of antibiotics (carbapenems, quinolones) and the development of new treatment strategies (monotherapy, oral therapy). Some critical issues remain regarding the ideal choice of agents for initial therapy: number of agents, need for Gram-positive coverage, need for double Gram-negative coverage, adequacy of monotherapy, etc. (Schiffer and Wade 1987; Wade et al. 1985, Wade 1986).

I will review the patterns of infection, the complicating underlying risk factors and the various therapeutic alternatives available for the initial antibiotic management of the neutropenic cancer patient with fever.

Recent Results in Cancer Research, Vol. 132
© Springer-Verlag Berlin · Heidelberg 1993

Sites of Infection and Organisms

The most common sites of infection are within the alimentary tract (pharynx, esophagus, rectum), the respiratory tract (sinuses, lung), and the skin (bone marrow site, catheter related). Infections of the urinary tract are uncommon in this patient population. The bacterial pathogens responsible for the initial infection are relatively few. *Escherichia coli*, *Klebsiella pneumoniae*, and *Pseudomonas aeruginosa* are the most common Gram-negative organisms and account for almost 50% of the initial infections. Coagulase-negative staphylococci today represent the most frequently recovered Gram-positive cocci, although *Staphylococcus aureus* continues to be a frequent isolate. Other important Gram-positive pathogens are *Streptococcus* species, diphtheroids, and *Bacillus* species. Anaerobes are infrequently recovered from blood cultures, but they may play a significant role as components of polymicrobial infections of the gastrointestinal tract (i.e., necrotizing gingivitis, perirectal cellulitis) (Schimpff 1990).

Patterns of Infection During Neutropenia

The initial infections are usually caused by bacterial pathogens originating from the colonizing flora already present in the patient when first admitted to the hospital or at the time chemotherapy is initiated. Subsequent infections, in contrast, are often caused by antibiotic-resistant bacteria, yeasts, filamentous fungi, and viruses (e.g., cytomegalovirus, CMV). These infections constitute a major diagnostic and therapeutic challenge for the management of the neutropenic patient.

Approximately 15%–20% of the initial febrile episodes are bacteremias, half of which are caused by Gram-negative bacilli; 20% are microbiologically documented infections without bacteremia; and 20% are clinical infections. Confounding factors in the assessment of febrile neutropenic patients are other causes of fever (underlying cancer, drug reactions, blood products).

Clinical Evaluation

Clinical assessment must include history and physical examination with special attention to the skin, the mucous membranes, periodontal tissues, the sinuses and lungs, and the perianal and rectal areas. Blood and urine cultures should be obtained and intravenous broad-spectrum antibiotics started immediately. Radiographic studies of the sinuses and lungs can be postponed after antibiotics have begun and the patient has been monitored for the onset of untoward reactions (chills, hypotension).

Risk Assessment

A careful analysis of specific risk factors may help anticipate the potential source of infection as well as the likelihood of infection with certain pathogens. The most significant risk factors include:

– Type of underlying disease
– Intensity of chemotherapy
– Degree of neutropenia
– Duration of neutropenia
– Prior infection history
– Colonization data if available
– Presence of a long-term intravenous catheter
– Use of prophylactic antibiotics

Patients with acute leukemia with profound ($<100\,PMN/\mu l$) and prolonged neutropenia (>14 days) who are colonized with *P. aeruginosa* are considered as being in the highest risk category. In contrast, patients with solid tumors with moderate neutropenia ($500-1000\,PMN/\mu l$) for a short duration of time (<7 days) are considered within a low-risk category. Patients with oropharyngeal mucositis or with indwelling intravenous catheters may be at greater risk to present with a Gram-positive infection (*Streptococcus* species or coagulase-negative staphylococci).

Likewise, the use of prophylactic antibiotics with activity predominantly against Gram-negative bacilli (TMP/SMX, quinolone antibiotic) may place patients at increased risk of infection by antibiotic-resistant bacteria or by Gram-positive pathogens. This has been the case in some centers, particularly in Europe, where these agents are routinely used for prophylaxis (i.e., increased incidence of streptococcal infection in patients receiving ciprofloxacin prophylaxis).

A serologic evaluation for herpes simplex virus (HSV) is important to determine the need for prophylactic acyclovir to prevent HSV reactivation, which could increase the morbidity associated with chemotherapy-induced mucositis and facilitate bacterial superinfection. A study by Baglin et al. (1989) showed that patients with febrile episodes associated with HSV infection were less likely to respond to empiric antibacterial therapy alone. The high incidence of antibiotic-resistant fever in neutropenic patients underscores the importance of recognizing those patients at risk for HSV infection so that prophylaxis or early antiviral therapy can be instituted promptly.

Another important factor is the prior history of infection and type of clinical response to antibiotics. Some patients have a tendency to suffer recurrent infections at the same site with the same organism. History of drug allergies, presence of renal dysfunction, colonization with certain organisms, and clinical response to previous or concomitant infections are also important. Physicians should be aware of the often worldwide changes in the epidemiology of infections in neutropenic cancer patients and of the trends in antibiotic susceptibilities in their local communities.

Initial Empiric Antibiotic Therapy in Neutropenia

Optimal Antibiotic Regimen

The ideal empiric regimen should have some essential attributes:

- Broad spectrum of activity
- High bactericidal levels
- Effective in absence of neutrophils
- Low potential of emergence of resistance

The spectrum of activity should naturally include the organisms previously discussed. This is, of course, difficult to achieve with only one antimicrobial agent. Over the past 3 decades, a large number of studies has underscored the importance of utilizing combination therapy with at least two agents active against Gram-negative bacilli (Klastersky et al. 1988). Double Gram-negative coverage, preferably with demonstrable synergism against the infecting pathogen, has been the cornerstone of empiric therapy (Love et al. 1980; Klastersky et al. 1977). Synergism appears to be important for patients with Gram-negative bacteremia and profound and persistent neutropenia. An analysis of 75 neutropenic patients with Gram-negative rod bacteremia demonstrated a significantly better response rate for patients with profound and persistent bacteremia if treated with a synergistic combination (de Jongh et al. 1986) (Table 1). Patients with recovering neutrophil counts did not benefit from the presence of synergism. The standard of care in the community has, by large, conformed to such types of regimens, the most acceptable of which have included an aminoglycoside (e.g., gentamicin, tobramycin, or amikacin) in combination with an antipseudomonal β-lactam antibiotic (a ureidopenicillin or a third-generation cephalosporin). The addition of a third agent with antistaphylococcal activity has been recommended by some investigators.

Therapeutic Alternatives

Over the past 10 years, numerous studies have been performed with non-aminoglycoside-containing regimens in search of less toxic but equally efficacious alternatives. The various regimens available today or under investigation include:

1. Aminoglycoside-containing combination regimens:
   - Aminoglycoside + antipseudomonal penicillin

Table 1. Seventy-five patients with Gram-negative bacteremia and initial granulocyte count $<100/\mu l$: response, antibiotic susceptibility, and in vitro synergism. (From de Jongh et al. 1986)

Antibiotic susceptibility and synergism	Granulocyte Count			
	Remained $<100/\mu l$		Increased to $>100/\mu l$	
	(n)	(%)	(n)	(%)
Two antibiotics	11/26	42	22/26	85
Synergy	7/11	64	9/12	75
No synergy	0/6		7/8	88
Not evaluable	4/9	44	6/6	100

     – Aminoglycoside + third-generation cephalosporin (including "front-loading" approach)
     – Aminoglycoside + carbapenem
2. Nonaminoglycoside combination regimens:
     – Double β-lactam combinations
     – β-Lactam + quinolone antibiotic
     – β-Lactam + carbapenem
     – Carbapenem + quinolone
3. Monotherapy
     – Third-generation cephalosporin (ceftazidime)
     – Carbapenem (imipenem)
     – Quinolone (?)

The aminoglycoside-containing regimens have given the most predictable response rates, particularly for patients with Gram-negative rod bacteremia. Synergism is seen frequently, whereas emergence of resistance is rare. These attributes have made the aminogly-coside-containing regimen the gold standard for empiric therapy of the febrile neutropenic patient; however, their potential toxicities and the need for close monitoring of blood levels make them somewhat impractical.

Selected double β-lactam regimens have been as successful as the aminoglycoside-containing regimens. In some centers like the University of Maryland Cancer Center (UMCC), the combination of ceftazidime plus piperacillin has been routinely used for a number of years. The in vitro activity of the double β-lactam regimens against Gram-negative bacilli is characterized by additiveness or indifference, with synergism seen infrequently. Concern, however, has been raised over the years regarding the potential for drug antagonism and the possibility of emergence of resistance among Gram-negative bacilli.

The azlocillin-ciprofloxacin combination, a β-lactam–quinolone regimen, is currently under study at the UMCC. This regimen would obviate the disadvantages of the aminoglycoside and the double β-lactam regimens, and yet provide double (sometimes synergistic) coverage against Gram-negative pathogens (Bustamante et al. 1990).

In vitro studies have shown that imipenem, a potent inducer of β-lactamases, antagonizes the bactericidal activity of several β-lactams (Bustamante et al. 1986). Imipenem-induced antagonism is most obvious at low imipenem concentrations and disappears as the imipenem concentration increases. The significance of these findings is unknown, but at the present time the use of imipenem–β-lactam combinations is not recommended. Whether such combinations can be used effectively, in vivo, without the induction of antagonism, has yet to be investigated.

The carbapenem–quinolone approach has yet to be studied in vivo, but in vitro data would suggest the potential for synergism against *P. aeruginosa* and possibly increased Gram-positive activity as well (Bustamante et al. 1987). Concern exists, however, regarding the possibility of added neurotoxicity for this combination.

Monotherapy Controversy

Is monotherapy adequate? When is it a safe and ethical approach? Which antibiotics, if any, are best suited for monotherapy in profoundly neutropenic patients with single Gram-negative bacillary bacteremia?

A number of studies utilizing a host of agents as monotherapy have now been published. Criticisms and reservations have been raised by many investigators and infectious disease practitioners. However, this concept has gained strength in some sectors of the medical community, and practitioners are presently utilizing this approach and deciding which patients to treat with monotherapy on the basis of the underlying risk factors of their individual patients. Patients with solid tumors and moderate neutropenia are frequently treated with single agents.

Ceftazidime has been extensively studied, and a fairly definitive study by Pizzo et al. (1986) from the National Cancer Institute showed that this agent was adequate as initial empiric therapy for neutropenia. Multiple antibiotic modifications, however, became necessary to maintain a favorable clinical response and achieve patient survival through the episode of neutropenia (Table 2). Those antibiotic modifications are clearly critical for patients with profound neutropenia and Gram-negative bacteremia and must be made promptly before the patient deteriorates clinically. Ceftazidime, as expected, was suboptimal therapy for the treatment of severe Gram-positive and anaerobic infections.

More recently, neutropenic patients treated with imipenem as a single agent have demonstrated good clinical response, similar to that of piperacillin plus amikacin, even when single Gram-negative rod bacteremia developed in the presence of profound neutropenia (Wade et al. 1987) (Tables 3, 4). The response of Gram-positive infections to imipenem is marginal at best,

Table 2. Response to ceftazidime versus carbenicillin plus cephalothin and gentamicin. (From Pizzo et al. 1986)

Evaluable episodes	Triple-antibiotic combination		Monotherapy – ceftazidime	
	(n)	(%)	(n)	(%)
Fever of undetermined origin	204		190	
Documented infection	64		92	
Success without modification	20	31	28	30
Success with modification	38	60	54	59
Added antibiotic	24	38	46	50
Added antifungal	12	19	11	12
Added antiviral	1		2	
Crossover or change	20	31	12	13
Failure	6	9	10	11

Table 3. University of Maryland Cancer Center: response to imipenem versus piperacillin plus amikacin. (From Wade et al. 1987)

	Imipenem		Piperacillin + amikacin	
	(n)	(%)	(n)	(%)
Microbiologically documented				
With bacteremia	20/35	57	27/45	60
Without bacteremia	28/36	77	35/39	89
Clinically documented	64/71	90	53/71	75
Total	112/142	78	116/155	75

Table 4. University of Maryland Cancer Center: response to monotherapy in patients with single organism Gram-negative bacteremia. (From Wade et al. 1987)

Initial granulocyte count	Subsequent	Imipenem	Piperacillin + amikacin
<100/μl	<100/μl		
Pseudomonas aeruginosa		3/5	–
Escherichia coli		1/1	3/5
Klebsiella pneumoniae		–	1/3
Other		1/2	0/1
<100/μl	>100/μl		
Pseudomonas aeruginosa		2/2	2/2
Escherichia coli		4/5	9/12
Klebsiella pneumoniae		2/2	2/4
Other		1/1	0/2
Total		14/18	17/29

and the addition of specific antistaphylococcal therapy is usually the norm. Similar observations have been made in studies comparing ceftazidime to imipenem with fewer antibiotic modifications for patients treated with imipenem. Modifications to the initial regimen are, however, unavoidable. Depending on the specific study criteria, modifications include addition or subtractions of antibiotics and the institution of antiviral and/or antifungal therapy. The latter, however, should not be construed as failure of the initial empiric antibacterial therapy, since the concept of empiric therapy has traditionally been directed toward the therapy of bacterial sepsis. Changes in these criteria have now been introduced by many investigators (Pizzo et al. 1990).

Finally, the eventual emergence of resistance to ceftazidime and imipenem will probably limit their future use as monotherapy in the years to come. Resistance to ceftazidime is being increasingly reported for *P. aeruginosa* and *Enterobacter* species. Imipenem-resistant *Bacteroides fragilis* have been reported. *Streptococcus faecium* and *Xanthomonas maltophilia* are emerging as significant pathogens in patients treated with imipenem. Methicillin-resistant *Staphylococcus aureus* is a problematic organism for the antibiotics presently being used as monotherapy.

An approach evaluated by the EORTC is not strange to many infectious disease and oncology practitioners. This approach consists of "front loading" with an aminoglycoside-containing regimen and withdrawing the amino-glycoside once the patient stabilizes, particularly if the patient does not have a Gram-negative bacteremia. For patients with Gram-negative bacteremia studied by the EORTC (trial IV), this approach was inferior to continuing therapy with the aminoglycoside regimen (ceftazidime plus amikacin) (EORTC International Antimicrobial Therapy Cooperative Group 1987) (Table 5). This study suggested that combination therapy was necessary for the successful outcome of patients with neutropenia and Gram-negative bacteremia. Such findings are similar to those reported previously by the UMCC (de Jongh et al. 1986; Love et al. 1980).

Table 5. Response to treatment in 129 patients with single organism Gram-negative bacteremia. (Modified from EORTC International Antimicrobial Therapy Cooperative Group 1987)

	Ceftazidime–short amikacin		Ceftazidime–long amikacin	
	(n)	($\%^a$)	(n)	($\%^a$)
Escherichia coli	10/21	48	18/24	75
Pseudomonas aeruginosa	5/13	38	8/9	89
Klebsiella pneumoniae	0/1		4/5	80
Other	5/7	71	8/9	81

[a] Patients with response/patients with bacteremia.

Vancomycin Controversy

Should vancomycin be included in the initial empiric antibiotic regimen? If so, which patients might benefit from this approach?

Staphylococcus epidermidis and other coagulase-negative staphylococci have become the most frequent pathogens causing infection in neutropenic cancer patients (Rubin et al. 1988). *Streptococcus* species (*S. mitis*, *S. viridans*) have been increasingly reported in patients receiving high-dose cytosine arabinoside and in those on prophylaxis with quinolone antibiotics (norfloxacin, ciprofloxacin). These streptococci cause significant morbidity (prolonged fevers; acute respiratory distress syndrome, ARDS) and mortality. This is in contrast to the general consensus that the more common Gram-positive infections, caused by coagulase-negative cocci, are not associated with significant mortality.

A number of studies have concluded that the initiation of specific antistaphylococcal therapy (usually vancomycin) can be delayed and should only be instituted if staphylococci or other Gram-positive organisms are recovered from blood cultures (Rubin et al. 1988). Vancomycin is also added empirically in patients with persistent fevers despite optimal "Gram-negative coverage." In centers where the incidence of Gram-positive infections is high, the opposite approach might make sense: start with vancomycin as part of the initial regimen and stop it if blood cultures are negative for Gram-positive pathogens (Table 6 Shenep et al. 1988; Karp et al. 1986). The latter approach, however, does not appear to be justified in most medical centers. If there are signs of infection along the subcutaneous tunnel of an intravenous catheter, vancomycin should probably be included as initial therapy. This would not be considered empiric therapy in the true sense of the word but rather "directed" antimicrobial therapy.

A recent position paper by a consensus panel of the Infectious Diseases Society of America (IDSA) proposed using vancomycin as part of the initial

Table 6. Clinical outcome of antibiotic therapy in 101 febrile patients with neutropenia. (From Shenep et al. 1988)

Outcome	Vancomycin, ticarcillin, and amikacin ($n = 53$)		Ticarcillin-clavulanate and amikacin ($n = 48$)	
	(n)	(%)	(n)	(%)
Treatment success	45	85	30	62
Treatment failure	8	15	18	38
Persistence of fever	8	15	11	23
Fatal breakthrough bacteremia	0		5	10
Nonfatal breakthrough bacteremia	0		1	2
Other reasons	0		1	2

therapy in patients with suspected staphylococcal or intravenous catheter-related infection. This consensus panel suggested that certain criteria need to be met before considering the use of nonaminoglycoside regimens. For example, double β-lactam regimens may be acceptable in patients without profound (<100 PMN/μl) neutropenia or with previous or impending renal dysfunction. Likewise, monotherapy may be utilized, according to the IDSA, in patients in low-risk categories. For patients with profound neutropenia, the IDSA Consensus Panel recommended the use of an aminoglycoside-containing regimen, particularly if *P. aeruginosa* infection is expected (Hughes et al. 1990).

Conclusions

In my opinion, the empiric therapy of the febrile neutropenic patient is moving away from the "cookbook" stereotype to a more individualized patient-directed approach. Clearly, there is room for all the above-mentioned therapeutic alternatives, and continued understanding of the epidemiology of these infections will open this arena for even more novel approaches. Regardless of the initial empiric antibiotic regimen, the physician has to be ready to make modifications (additions or subtractions) as the clinical picture changes.

References

Baglin TP, Gray JJ, Marcus RE, Wreghitt TG (1989) Antibiotic resistant fever associated with herpes simplex virus infection in neutropenic patients with haematological malignancy. J Clin Pathol 42:1255–1258

Bodey GP, Buckley M, Sathe YS et al. (1966) Quantitative relationships between circulating leukocytes and infection in patients with acute leukemia. Ann Intern Med 64:328–340

Bustamante CI, Wharton RC, Moody MA, Novak M, Talley E, Saba G, Wade JC (1986) Imipenem induced concentration dependent antagonism when combined with β-lactams. American Society of Microbiology, Washington, D.C., abstract #A95

Bustamante CI, Drusano GL, Wharton RC, Wade JC (1987) Synergism of the combinations of imipenem plus ciprofloxacin and imipenem plus amikacin against Pseudomonas aeruginosa and other bacterial pathogens. Antimicrob Agents Chemother 31:632–634

Bustamante CI, Wharton RC, Wade JC (1990) In vitro activity of ciprofloxacin with ceftazidime, aztreonam and azlocillin against multiresistant isolates of Pseudomonas aeruginosa. Antimicrob Agents Chemother 34:1814–1815

de Jongh CA, Joshi JH, Newman KA, Moody MR, Wharton R, Standiford HC, Schimpff SC (1986) Antibiotic synergism and response in Gram-negative bacteremia in granulocytopenic cancer patients. Am J Med 80:96–100

EORTC International Antimicrobial Therapy Cooperative Group (1987) Ceftazidime combined with a short or long course of amikacin for empiric therapy of Gram-negative bacteremia in cancer patients with granulocytopenia. N Engl J Med 317:1692–1698

Hughes WT, Armstrong D, Bodey GP, Feld R, Mandell GL, Meyers JD, Pizzo PA, Schimpff SC, Shenep JL, Wade JC, Young LS, Yow MD (1990) Guidelines for the use of antimicrobial agents in neutropenic patients with unexplained fever. J Infect Dis 161:381–396

Karp JE, Dick JD, Angelopulos C et al. (1986) Empiric use of vancomycin during prolonged treatment-induced granulocytopenia. Am J Med 81:237–242

Klastersky J, Meunier-Carpentier F, Prevost J-M (1977) Significance of antimicrobial synergism for the outcome of Gram-negative sepsis. Am J Med Sci 273:157–167

Klastersky J, Zinner SH, Calandra T et al. (1988) Empiric antimicrobial therapy for febrile granulocytopenic patients: lessons from four EORTC trials. Eur J Cancer Clin Oncol 24[Suppl]:S35–S45

Love LJ, Schimpff SC, Schiffer, CA, Wiernik PH (1980) Improved prognosis for granulocytopenic patients with Gram-negative bacteremia. Am J Med 68:643–648

Pizzo PA, Hathorn JW, Hiemenz J et al. (1986) A randomized trial comparing ceftazidime alone with combination antibiotic therapy in cancer patients with fever and neutropenia. N Engl J Med 315:552–558

Pizzo PA, Armstrong D, Bodey G et al. (1990) The design, analysis and reporting of clinical trials on the empiric antibiotic management of the neutropenic patient. J Infect Dis 161:397–401

Rubin M, Hathorn JW, Marshall D et al. (1988) Gram-positive infections and the use of vancomycin in 550 episodes of fever and neutropenia. Ann Inter Med 108:30–35

Schiffer CA, Wade JC (1987) Supportive care: issues in the use of blood products and treatment of infection. Semin Oncol 14:454–467

Schimpff SC (1990) Infections in the compromised host – an overview. In: Mandell GL, Douglas RG JR, Bennett JE (eds) Principles and practice of infectious diseases, 3rd edn. Churchill Livingstone, New York, pp 2258–2265

Shenep JL, Hughes WT, Roberson PK, Blankenship KR, Baker DK Jr, Meyer WH, Gigliotti F, Sixbey JW, Santana VM, Feldman S et al. (1988) Vancomycin, ticarcillin, and amikacin compared with ticarcillin-clavulanate and amikacin in the empirical treatment of febrile, neutropenic children with cancer. N Engl J Med 319:1053–1058

Wade JC, Standiford HC, Drusano GL, Johnson DE, Moody MR, Bustamante CI, Joshi JH, de Jongh CA, Schimpff SC (1985) Potential of imipenem as single-agent empiric antibiotic therapy of febrile neutropenic patients with cancer. Am J Med 78:62–72

Wade JC, Johnson DE, Bustamante CI (1986) Monotherapy for empiric treatment for fever in granulocytopenic cancer patients. Am J Med 80[Suppl 5C]:85–95

Wade JC, Bustamante CI, Devlin A, Finley R, Drusano G, Thompson B (1987) Imipenem versus piperacillin plus amikacin as empiric therapy for febrile neutropenic patients: a double blind trial. Proceedings of the 27th Interscience Conference on Antimicrobial Agents and Chemotherapy. American Society for Microbiology, Washington (abstr) 1251

Further Reading

Hughes WT, Armstrong D, Bodey GP, Feld R, Mandell GL, Meyers JD, Pizzo PA, Schimpff SC, Shenep JL, Wade JC, Young LS, Yow MD (1990) Guidelines for the use of antimicrobial agents in neutropenic patients with unexplained fever. J Infect Dis 161:381–396

A concerted effort by leading members of the Infectious Diseases Society of America to design guidelines for the use of antimicrobial agents in neutropenic patients with fever.

Pizzo PA, Armstrong D, Bodey G et al. (1990) The design, analysis and reporting of clinical trials on the empiric antibiotic management of the neutropenic patient. J Infect Dis 161:397–401
  The results of a consensus panel of the Immunocompromised Host Society to facilitate the implementation of uniform designs and analysis of empiric antibiotic trials in neutropenic cancer patients worldwide.
Schiffer CA, Wade JC (1987) Supportive care: issues in the use of blood products and treatment of infection. Semin Oncol 14:454–467
  Comprehensive review on the supportive care of the neutropenic cancer patient with emphasis on the management of empiric antibiotic therapy.

Approach to the Patient with Prolonged Granulocytopenia

P.A. Pizzo

Pediatric Branch, National Cancer Institute, National Institutes of Health, Bethesda, MD 20892, USA

The optimal management of the neutropenic cancer patient should include a prompt evaluation and the initiation of broad-spectrum antibiotic therapy when fever occurs. However, the survival of the patient depends not only on the infectious agent(s) responsible for the initial fever and the antibiotics chosen for the primary empiric therapy, but also on the duration of the neutropenia, the secondary infections that arise, and the adjustments or modifications employed to treat them.

During the past two decades, a number of changes have occurred in the spectrum of infectious complications in the cancer patient. Of particular importance has been the fact that the incidence of infections with Gram-negative organisms, especially *Pseudomonas aeruginosa*, have declined in most cancer centers in the United States and Europe. The reasons for this are not clearly understood, but the decreased frequency of *P. aeruginosa* has had a significant impact on therapeutic programs for the management of neutropenic patients and presumably on patient survival as well. At the same time, infections due to Gram-positive bacteria (especially the coagulase-positive and -negative staphylococci) have increased. Some of these infections are associated with the widening use of indwelling Silastic catheters in cancer patients. As patients have survived their initial infectious event more successfully and as the periods of neutropenia have become more prolonged as a consequence of more intensive chemotherapy regimens, secondary infections due to invasive mycoses (especially *Candida* and *Aspergillus*) have increased and constitute a major therapeutic stumbling block to the effective management of the cancer patient with prolonged granulocytopenia. Further, in addition to infections caused by bacteria and fungi, it is also important to underscore that viral and protozoal pathogens can be important at various stages of the neutropenic patient's clinical course and that combined or mixed infections can also occur. Thus, awareness of the fact that the patient with prolonged neutropenia is subject to infection by a wide range of pathogens and that multiple sequential infections or mixed infectious com-

Recent Results in Cancer Research, Vol. 132
© Springer-Verlag Berlin · Heidelberg 1993

plications can occur during a single episode of neutropenia highlights the importance of planning for the additions or modifications of the patient's antimicrobial armamentarium as new clinical or microbiological events emerge. Indeed, it is best to consider these modifications or additions to the antimicrobial regimen (i.e., antibiotic additions or changes and/or addition of antiviral, antifungal, antiparasitic agents) as important to the overall outcome as was the initiation of antibiotics when the patient first became febrile. Some of the common reasons for antibiotic modifications that are likely to arise in the management of the patient with prolonged granulo-cytopenia are listed in Table 1. The importance of including such modifications of therapy in the evaluation and management plans of the patient with fever and neutropenia has been highlighted by two recent consensus conferences (Pizzo et al. 1990; Hughes et al. 1990).

In tandem with changes in the patterns of infections has been the intro-duction of a variety of new potent antimicrobial agents that have offered new therapeutic options to cancer patients. Included are the third-generation

Table 1. Modifications of therapy during the course of granulocytopenia

Clinical event	Possible modifications of therapy
Breakthrough bacteremia	If Gram-positive isolates (e.g., *S. epidermidis*), add vancomycin
	If Gram-negative isolate (i.e., presumably resistant), switch to regimen containing non-cross-resistant antibiotics (e.g., aminoglycoside plus a carbapenem or extended-spectrum penicillin)
Catheter-associated infection	Add vancomycin (as well as Gram-negative coverage if not already being given)
Severe oral mucositis or necrotizing gingivitis	Add specific antianaerobic agent (e.g., clindamycin or metronidazole)
Esophagitis	Trial of oral clotrimazole, ketoconazole, intravenous amphotericin B, or acyclovir
Pneumonitis, diffuse or interstitial	Trial of trimethoprim-sulfamethoxazole and erythromycin (plus broad-spectrum antibiotics if the patient is granulocytopenic)
New infiltrate in a granulocytopenic patient also receiving antibiotics	If granulocyte count is rising, watch and wait
	If granulocyte count is not recovering, biopsy to establish diagnosis; if biopsy cannot be done, add amphotericin B empirically
Perianal tenderness	If patient is already receiving broad-spectrum antibiotics, add a specific antianaerobic agent
	If patient is not on antibiotics, begin broad-spectrum therapy with anaerobic coverage
Persistent fever and neutropenia	Continue antibiotics after 1 week of persistent fever and neutropenia, add systemic antifungal therapy empirically

cephalosporins, carbapenems, extended-spectrum penicillins, monobactams and the fluoroquinolones. Some of these agents (e.g., selected third-generation cephalosporins or carbapenems) possess such broad antibiotic activity and achieve such high serum bactericidal levels that they can be used for initial monotherapy. This permits the use of more simple, less toxic, and more cost-effective therapy when the patient first becomes febrile (Pizzo et al. 1986). But it necessitates that patients be closely monitored and that other antibiotics be added or modified depending on the patient's clinical course (Pizzo 1987).

In addition to new antibiotics, some progress has also been made in the development of newer antifungal and antiviral agents. Notable, for example, has been the introduction of imidazole and triazole antifungal agents. Although promising, however, none yet has the spectrum of amphotericin B, and accordingly this agent still remains the standard when treating most serious invasive mycoses in neutropenic cancer patients. Newer antiviral agents have mainly been directed at the herpes viruses. Acyclovir has become the standard for the treatment of herpes simplex and varicella zoster, and ganciclovir and foscarnet have activity against cytomegalovirus. Newer antiviral agents are likely to become available, stimulated in part by the problems these viruses pose to patients with human immunodeficiency virus (HIV) infection.

One of the most notable advances during the past several years has been the development and increasing availability of hematopoietic cytokines that can accelerate bone marrow recovery or bolster the immune systems. Since most of the serious infections that threaten the cancer patient are associated with prolonged periods of neutropenia, the prospect for shortening the duration of neutropenia has enormous implications. Already agents such as granulocyte–macrophage colony-stimulating factor (GM-CSF) and granu-locyte CSF (G-CSF) have been studied in patients being treated with myelosuppressive chemotherapy or who are undergoing bone marrow trans-plantation, and have been demonstrated to shorten the periods of neutropenia (Pizzo et al. 1992). By themselves, these agents do not eliminate the nadir of the neutrophil count, but they do appear to abbreviate the duration of the neutropenia. Thus, although patients may still become febrile and require antibiotics, the duration of therapy and the need for antimicrobial modifications may be decreased.

At present, therefore, the management of the patient at risk for prolonged neutropenia includes the initiation of broad-spectrum antibiotics with the onset of fever. Depending on the spectrum of pathogens and the antibiotic patterns at the hospital where the patient is being treated, it may be possible to commence with a single antibiotic and then modify therapy as necessary. This process might be further simplified by the concurrent use of cytokines that might shorten the duration of neutropenia. However, it is important to underscore that the experience with cytokines is still relatively nascent, and it remains to be determined whether their putative beneficial effects will extend to more intensive chemotherapy regimens or whether their benefits will decrease in patients requiring multiple courses of chemotherapy.

The question of how long to continue empiric antibiotic therapy in persistently neutropenic patients is also a matter of practical significance (Pizzo et al. 1979, 1984). Generally, this can be approached by placing patients in one of two categories: those whose initial evaluation (at the time of presentation with fever and neutropenia) did not reveal a source of infection (i.e., unexplained fever), and those whose initial studies revealed a documented infection to account for the fever [i.e., a positive culture, or clinically infected site, or both (Fig. 1)]. At most centers, the majority of patients fall into the unexplained fever category, although this will vary with the institution, the therapy, and the patient population (Pizzo et al. 1982b).

Patients with Unexplained Fever. For patients who have a short duration of granulocytopenia (e.g., <1 week), stopping antibiotics after recovery of the white blood cell (WBC) counts is practical and effective (Pizzo et al. 1979, 1984). However, a dilemma arises in the population with more prolonged granulocytopenia. In a study from the National Cancer Institute (NCI), patients with unexplained fever and persistent granulocytopenia were randomized either to discontinue antibiotics on day 7 of therapy, or to continue them until the resolution of the neutropenia (Pizzo et al. 1979). Nearly 40% of afebrile patients who stopped antibiotic therapy developed recurrent fever, and 38% of febrile patients whose antibiotics were discontinued developed hypotensive episodes. It was concluded that day 7 was too early to discontinue antibiotic treatment in this group.

A subsequent study conducted at the NCI randomized persistently neutropenic, afebrile patients to continue or discontinue antibiotics on day 14 (Pizzo et al. 1984). Analysis showed no difference between the two groups: approximately one third of patients became febrile again regardless of whether they stopped or continued treatment with antibiotics. However, those whose fevers recurred following discontinuation of antibiotics responded to a reinstitution of their initial regimens, whereas those remaining on antibiotics required addition of amphotericin B. On this basis, it seems reasonable to discontinue antibiotics on day 14 in patients who have remained consistently afebrile and neutropenic on empirical therapy, recognizing that when the antibiotics are stopped, these patients must be closely monitored for recurrent fever or infection until the resolution of their granulocytopenia (Fig. 1). The question of whether antibiotic therapy could be delivered orally for these patients is presently being explored by a study at the Pediatric Branch of the NCI, in which patients expected to remain neutropenic but who have defervesced within the first 5 days of empirical broad-spectrum intravenous antibiotic therapy are being randomized either to continue the intravenous antibiotic (ceftazidime) or receive oral ciprofloxacin. The results of the study will help to define both the safety of ciprofloxacin in children (see above) as well as its utility for simplifying continuation of therapy for patients with

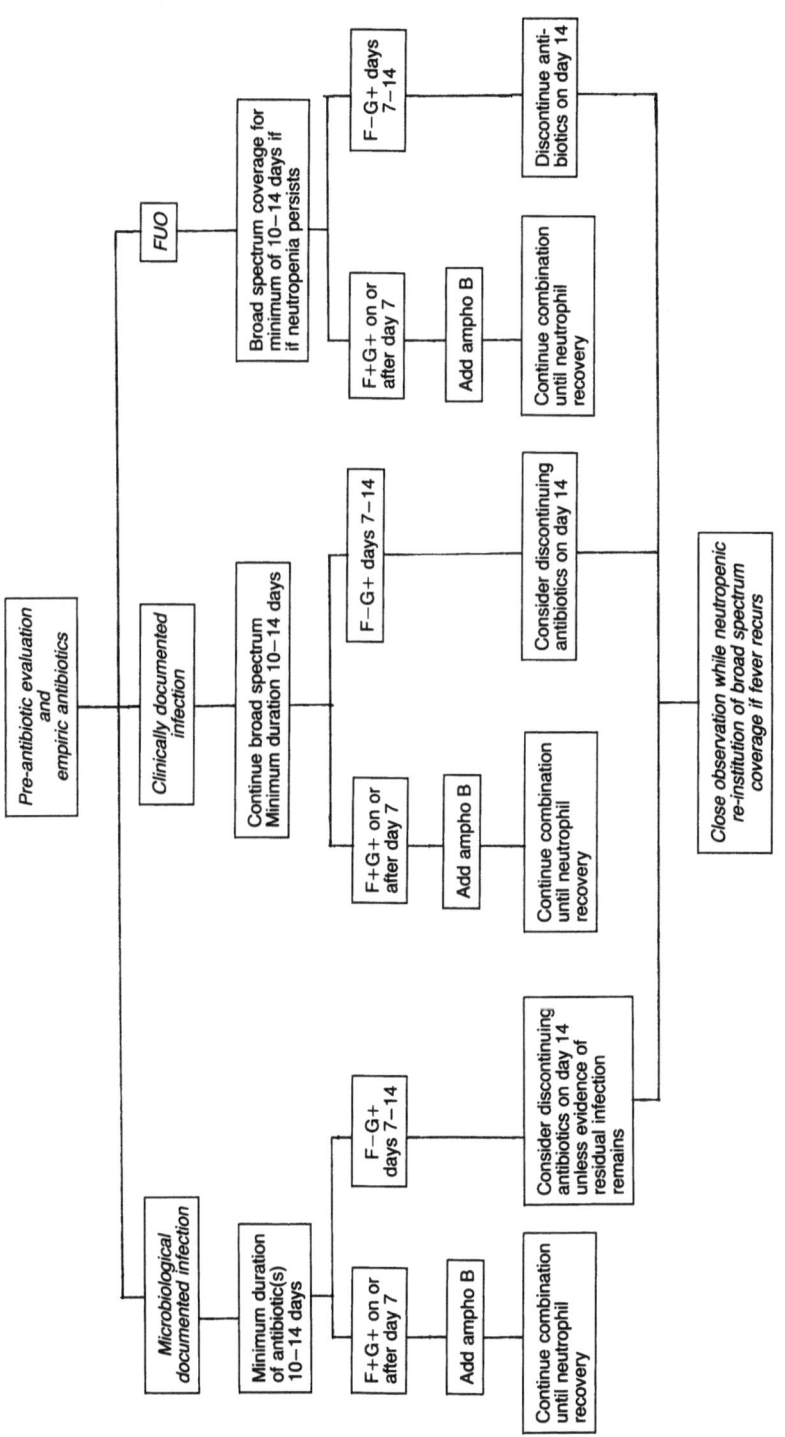

Fig. 1. Management of fever and neutropenia. *F+G+*, febrile, granulocytopenic; *F−G+*, afebrile, granulocytopenic; *FUO*, no source for fever on preantibiotic evaluation; *AMPHO B*, amphotericin B

prolonged neutropenia. This strategy may be advanced if the duration of neutropenia can be shortened with the use of cytokines.

Patients showing signs of bone marrow recovery, even though still neutropenic, can also have their antibiotics discontinued as long as they are being monitored closely.

Patients Presenting with Documented Infections. For persistently neutropenic patients who have had clinical and microbiological resolution of their infection and who are afebrile at day 14 (for a minimum of 7 days), antibiotics may be discontinued. The ultimate decision of whether to continue or discontinue antibiotics rests on a number of clinical considerations, including potential antibiotic toxicity, the predicted duration of neutropenia, the seriousness of the initial infection, and the presence or absence of other factors predisposing to subsequent infection. In general, antibiotics are usually administered for 10–14 days of treatment unless there is a residual site of infection [e.g., perianal cellulitis (Glenn et al. 1988) and the patient remains neutropenic (Fig. 1)]. In such cases, the antibiotics should be continued either until the resolution of the signs of infection and/or the recovery from neutropenia.

The question of whether the spectrum of antibiotics can be narrowed when a specific isolate is determined is also of practical relevance. Although a primary infection caused by an identified organism can be treated successfully with either a broad-spectrum or pathogen-specific antibiotic, the risk for second (or breakthrough) infections is increased in patients with prolonged neutropenia (>7 days) who received a narrow-spectrum antibiotic (Pizzo et al. 1980, 1984).

Empiric Antifungal Therapy

Patients who experience prolonged periods of profound neutropenia following intensive cytotoxic chemotherapy or ablative radiation are at increased risk of acquiring invasive fungal infections. The early diagnosis of invasive fungal infections in granulocytopenic children can be difficult, and fever may be the only manifestation of infection. Moreover, withholding antifungal therapy until infection is proven by culture or histologic examination increases the likelihood for disseminated infection. This has led to the concept of employing empiric antifungal therapy to prevent the fungal overgrowth in patients with prolonged granulocytopenia and to provide early treatment of clinically occult infection (Pizzo et al. 1982b; Walsh et al. 1991b; EORTC International Antimicrobial Therapy Cooperative Group 1989). The value of empiric antifungal therapy has been documented by the results of two randomized clinical trials (Pizzo et al. 1982b; EORTC International Antimicrobial Therapy Cooperative Group 1989). These studies demonstrated that the use of empirically administered amphotericin B in persistently or recurrently febrile granulocytopenic patients decreased the frequency, morbidity and mortality of invasive fungal infections, especially in patients who are profoundly granulocytopenic and not receiving antifungal prophylaxis. The morbidity and mortality of untreated or under-treated invasive fungal infections in granulocytopenic patients usually supersede the toxicity of amphotericin B, which is usually reversible. Thus, treatment with amphotericin B, 0.5 mg/kg per day, should be instituted in granulocytopenic patients who remain persistently or recurrently febrile after 7 days. Nonetheless, because of the side effects associated with amphotericin administration, less toxic alternatives are highly desirable. We explored the use of oral ketoconazole in comparison to amphotericin B (Walsh et al. 1991b). Although comparable to amphotericin B in preventing the onset of a fungal disease, when infection did arise it invariably progressed unless the patient was switched to amphotericin B. Fluconazole, a new antifungal triazole with significant activity against *Candida* is currently being evaluated for empiric antifungal therapy in children (Walsh et al. 1990). However, the absence of activity against *Aspergillus* and break through infections with nail resistant organisms such as *C. Kruzei* are likely to limit the value of fluconazole, underscoring the need for newer antifungal agents with broader profiles.

Indeed, even empiric amphotericin B therapy does not completely prevent the development of invasive fungal infections since invasive fungal infection with organisms more resistant to amphotericin (e.g., *Aspergillus*, *Pseudoallescheria*, *Trichosporon*, *Fusarium*) has been reported in patients who were receiving amphotericin at dosages of 0.5–0.6 mg/kg per day (Navarro et al. 1990). Such patients might benefit from either higher doses of amphotericin B (e.g., 1–1.5 mg/kg per day) or from liposomal amphotericin B (which is still not widely available in the United States) or newer agents. Again, the cytokines might also play a beneficial role if they can accelerate bone marrow recovery or improve the host's residual phagocytic defenses. The use of combinations of biologicals with antimicrobial agents also needs to be studied for patients with already established infections.

Summary

In most centers treating cancer patients, significant progress has been made in permitting patients to survive even prolonged courses of neutropenia. This has resulted from a better understanding of the epidemiology of infection and the points during the clinical course when they pose a risk for the patient with prolonged neutropenia. Considerable benefit has been derived from the availability of more potent broad-spectrum antimicrobial agents and from organized strategies for when they should be initiated, how and when they should be modified, and for how long they should be continued. The possibility that the duration of neutropenia might be attenuated in patients receiving chemotherapy now seems real with the ever-expanding repertoire of cytokines and other biologic agents that augment the hematopoietic and immune systems. Coupled with the use of peripheral stem cell reconstitution or the insertion of genes into hematopoietic stem cells that might render them resistant to the cytocidal effects of certain chemo-therapeutic agents, it now seems possible to envision regimens that might alter the consequences of neutropenia as we have come to know them. It is likely, therefore, as additional experience is garnered and as chemotherapy regimens are devised, that the optimal approach to the management of the patient with prolonged neutropenia will include the rational use of antibiotics together with cytokines and other biologicals. Hopefully, such regimens will permit the delivery of chemotherapy in a manner that might enhance its tumorical activity and improve the outcome of patients with cancer.

References

EORTC International Antimicrobial Therapy Cooperative Group (1989) Empiric antifungal therapy in febrile granulocytopenic patients. Am J Med 86:668–672

Glenn J, Cotton D, Wesley R, Pizzo PA (1988) Anorectal infections in patients with malignant diseases. Rev Infect Dis 10:42–52

Hughes WT, Armstrong D, Bodey GP, Feld R, Mandell GL, Meyers JD, Pizzo PA, Shenep JL, Schimpff SC, Wade JC, Young LS, Yow MD (1990) Guidelines for the use of antimicrobial agents in neutropenic patients with unexplained fever. A statement by the Infectious Diseases Society of America. J Infect Dis 161:381–396

Navarro E, Lecciones J, Witebsky F et al. (1990) Invasive aspergillosis developing during antifungal therapy. Proceedings of the 90th Am Soc Microbiol, Anaheim, p 420 (abstr)

Pizzo PA (1987) After empiric therapy. What to do until the granulocyte comes back. Rev Infect Dis 9:214–219

Pizzo PA, Robichaud KJ, Gill FA, Witebsky FG, Levine AS, Deisseroth AB, Glaubiger DL, MacLowery JD, Magrath IT, Poplack DA, Siman RM (1979) Duration of empiric antibiotic therapy in granulocytopenic cancer patients. Am J Med 67:194–200

Pizzo PA, Ladisch S, Robichaud K (1980) Treatment of Gram-positive septicemia in cancer patients. Cancer 45:206–207

Pizzo PA, Robichaud KJ, Gill FA, Witebsky FG (1982a) Empiric antibiotic and antifungal therapy for cancer patients with prolonged fever and granulocytopenia. Am J Med 72:101–111

Pizzo PA, Robichaud KJ, Wesley R, Commers J (1982b) Fever in the pediatric and young adult patient with cancer: a prospective study of 1001 episodes. Medicine (Baltimore) 161:153–165

Pizzo PA, Conners J, Cotton D et al. (1984) Approaching the controversies in the antibacterial management of cancer patients. Am J Med 76:436–449

Pizzo PA, Hathorn J, Hiemenz J, Browne M, Commers J, Cotton D, Gress J, Longo D, Marshall D, McKnight J, Rubin M, Skelton J, Thaler M, Wesley R (1986) A randomized trial comparing ceftazidime alone with combination antibiotic therapy in cancer patients with fever and neutropenia. N Engl J Med 315:552–558

Pizzo PA, Armstrong D, Bodey G, de Pauw B, Feld R, Glauser M, Gaya H, Karp J, Klastersky J, Todeschini G, Verhoef J, Wade J, Young LS, Remington J (1990) The design, analysis and reporting of clinical trials on the empirical antibiotic management of the neutropenic patient: report of a consensus panel for the Immunocompromised Host Society. J Infect Dis 161:397–401

Pizzo PA, Rubin M, Freifeld A, Walsh T (1992) The child with cancer and infection: I. Practical issues in the empirical therapy and preventive strategies of fever and neutropenia. J Pediatr 119:679–694

Walsh TJ, Lee J, Aoki S, Mechinaud F, Bacher J, Lecciones J, Thomas V, Rubin M, Pizzo PA (1990) Experimental basis for usage of fluconazole for preventive or early treatment of disseminated candidiasis in granulocytopenic hosts. Rev Infect Dis 12:S307–S317

Walsh TJ, Lee JW, Lecciones J et al. (1991a) Empirical amphotericin B in febrile granulocytopenic patients. Rev Infect Dis 13:496–503

Walsh TJ, Rubin M, Hathorn J et al. (1991b) Amphotericin B versus high-dose ketoconazole for empirical antifungal therapy among febrile granulocytopenic cancer patients: a prospective randomized study. Arch Intern Med 151:765–770

Simplification of Empiric Therapy for the Febrile, Neutropenic Oncology Patient

J.L. Shenep

Department of Infectious Diseases, St. Jude Children's Research Hospital,
332 North Lauderdale, Memphis, TN 38105-2794, USA, and Department of
Pediatrics, University of Tennessee College of Medicine, Memphis, TN, USA

Empiric therapy for the neutropenic oncology patient with unexplained fever appears quite complicated to the uninitiated. However, as is the case with the game of chess, once a few basic rules are learned, a handful of principles are comprehended and a set of opening moves that have passed extensive field testing are adopted, empiric therapy of febrile, neutropenic cancer patients can be surprisingly straightforward in many respects. Management strategy is virtually independent of the patient's age. The variety of organisms that commonly infect the neutropenic host is limited (Table 1). The usual sites of infection are few: the periorbital tissues, sinuses, oral and gastrointestinal mucosa, pharynx, cervical nodes, lungs, liver, spleen, kidneys, perirectal tissues, and skin, particularly at catheter exit sites and biopsy sites. The most daunting aspect of the management of the neutropenic cancer patient is, ironically, selecting empiric therapies from the large array of available antimicrobial agents and adjuvant therapies. The other common pitfall in treating infectious complications in neutropenic cancer patients is failure to recognize that management of these patients is a unique aspect of the practice of infectious diseases.

Driven by efforts to maximize efficacy, empiric therapy has been steadily expanding in recent years. With the advent of new antibiotics and antifungals, growth factors, cytokines, immunomodulators and monoclonal antibodies, emphasis is increasingly directed to complex management strategies. For certain high-risk patient cohorts with manifest susceptibility to infection, expanded therapy is clearly warranted. However, in quest of therapeutic optimization, the clinician must balance expanded therapy aimed at maximizing efficacy against simplified therapy aimed at minimizing toxicity and cost (Fig. 1).

Despite inherent advantages, streamlined management of febrile neutropenic episodes is seldom stressed in the medical literature. Simplification of empiric therapy for the febrile, neutropenic oncology patient facilitates management of increasingly complex patients, education of the medical

Recent Results in Cancer Research, Vol. 132
© Springer-Verlag Berlin · Heidelberg 1993

Table 1. Common infections in neutropenic cancer patients

Microorganisms	Initial infection	Secondary infection
Bacteria		
Escherichia coli	Yes	Yes
Klebsiella species	Yes	Yes
Pseudomonas aeruginosa	Yes	Yes
Enterobacter species	Yes	Yes
Coagulase-negative staphylococci	Yes	Yes
Staphylococcus aureus	Yes	Yes
Viridans streptococci	Yes	Yes
Streptococcus pneumoniae	Yes	Rare
Fungi		
Histoplasma capsulatum	Yes	Rare
Coccidioides immitis	Yes	Rare
Cryptococci neoformans	Yes	Rare
Candida species	Uncommon	Yes
Aspergillus species	Uncommon	Yes
Mucor species	Uncommon	Yes
Rhizopus species	Uncommon	Yes
Protozoa		
Pneumocystis carinii	Yes	Uncommon
Viruses		
Cytomegalovirus	Yes	Yes
Herpes simplex	Yes	Yes
Varicella zoster	Yes	Yes

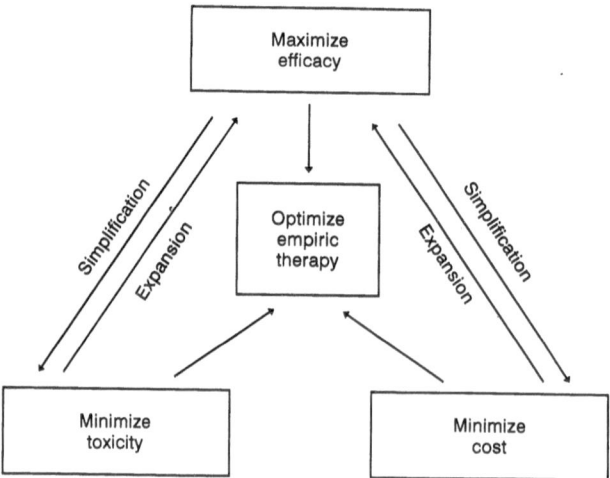

Fig. 1. Relation of simplification and expansion of empiric therapy to therapeutic optimization. Simplification of therapy reduces toxicity and cost, but eventually at the expense of efficacy

staff, and monitoring for therapeutic shortfalls; streamlined therapy also avoids unnecessary drug toxicity and reduces medical costs. Only if the clinician pursues simplified management both at the bedside and in the design of clinical trials can the elusive goal of therapeutic optimization be achieved. The purpose of this paper is to emphasize simplification in order to promote a balanced, optimized approach to management of the neutropenic oncology patient with unexplained fever (Fig. 1).

Standardization of Empiric Therapy

The first step toward simplification of empiric therapy is standardization within an institution or practice. A decade ago at St. Jude Children's Research Hospital, there was lack of standardization of empiric therapy for febrile, neutropenic children. Each physician had a uniform approach, but varied approaches were applied to similar patients. Consequently, there was diminished opportunity to assure quality and discover trends through data analysis. Residents and the nursing staff were perturbed by the diversity; their familiarity with antimicrobial dosages and adverse effects was limited. The pharmacy was burdened by the need to adjust inventories according to which physician was attending the inpatient unit. Bulk purchase of drugs at reduced cost was undermined. Multiple assays for serum antibiotic concentrations had to be maintained. To address these concerns, the Department of Infectious Diseases formulated a set of guidelines for management of the febrile, neutropenic patient. These guidelines, summarized in Fig. 2, were not intended to discourage individualized patient management, but to encourage consistent management when no cause for exception from the standard plan was discovered upon careful evaluation of the patient. Although adherence to these guidelines was voluntary, their acceptance within the institution was virtually universal. In a similar spirit, guidelines for the use of antimicrobials in neutropenic patients with unexplained fever were recently advocated by a panel assembled through the Infectious Diseases Society of America (Hughes et al. 1990). The development of such broad inter-institutional guidelines, however, are necessarily constrained by significant variations in the pattern of infections and antimicrobial susceptibilities among different institutions. Consequently, several alternative initial empiric regimens were suggested for neutropenic cancer patients with unexplained fever, and factors that indicate or contraindicate use were noted. These empiric regimens are summarized in Table 2. A general management plan for febrile neutropenic patients is outlined in Fig. 3.

Modification of Initial Empiric Therapy

Within an institution, the majority of patients can be managed initially with a single empiric regimen. Subsequently, however, many patients will require

Neutropenia and Unexplained Fever

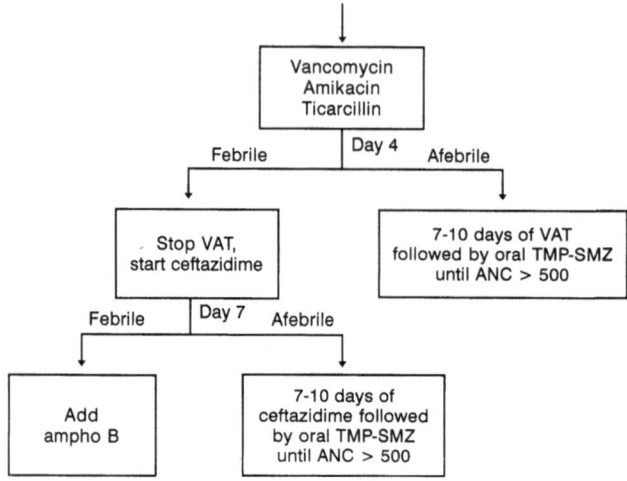

Fig. 2. Standard approach to empiric therapy of neutropenic cancer patients with unexplained fever currently in use at St. Jude Children's Research Hospital. Patients colonized with *Pseudomonas aeruginosa* are continued on amikacin and ticarcillin despite continued fever

Table 2. Suggested initial empiric antimicrobial regimen for neutropenic patients with unexplained fever

Initial regimen(s)	Indication
Monotherapy with ceftazidime or, if renal function is normal, imipenem	ANC > 500; low risk of Gram-positive bacterial and *P. aeruginosa* infection
Aminoglycoside and anti-pseudomonas β-lactam	*P. aeruginosa* infection suspected
Vancomycin plus aminoglycoside and anti-pseudomonal β-lactam or vancomycin plus third-generation cephalosporin[a]	Gram-positive bacterial infection suspected
Ceftazidime or two β-lactams	Renal impairment

[a] This combination was not included in the Infectious Diseases Society of America's guidelines (Hughes et al. 1990), but is listed here because of increasing use with apparently satisfactory outcome.

modification of initial therapy. Therefore, the second necessary step toward streamlining therapy is to reassess initial therapy based on the individual patient's culture results and response to therapy and to modify therapy, but only if indicated. Modifications should be guided by established principles for management of neutropenic cancer patients.

Neutropenia and Unexplained Fever

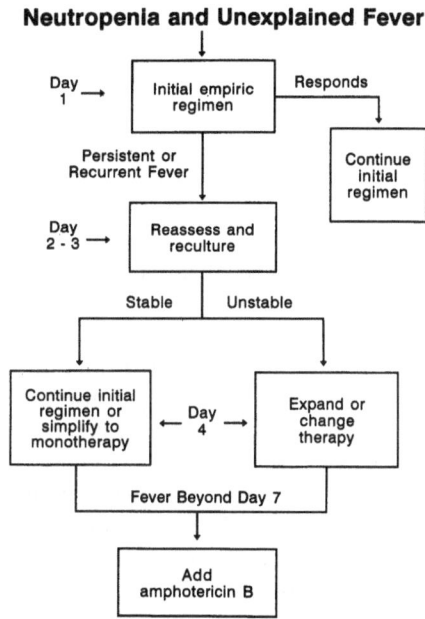

Fig. 3. Generalized approach to the management of neutropenic cancer patients with unexplained fever. Empiric regimen options are listed in Table 2

In the immunocompetent host, antimicrobial therapy is traditionally narrowed in spectrum according to the susceptibility pattern of the culture isolates. In the neutropenic host, however, restricting antimicrobial therapy according to culture isolates can result in second infections with nonsusceptible organisms, especially if therapy is limited to drugs active only against Gram-positive bacteria. For example, Pizzo et al. (1980) reported that among patients with Gram-positive infection, seven of 15 patients (47%) who remained neutropenic for more than 7 days and who were treated with narrow-spectrum antibiotics developed secondary sepsis with a Gram-negative organism. Thus, as a rule, antibiotics with broad activity against Gram-negative bacteria should be included if the neutropenic patient is to receive parenteral antibiotics. However, if cultures are sterile or Gram-negative bacteria are isolated, then consideration can be given to discontinuing antibiotics with activity directed primarily toward Gram-positive bacteria.

Neutropenic patients with sterile initial cultures present a dilemma regardless of whether or not there is an apparent response to empiric therapy (Joshi et al. 1984). If the culture-negative patient defervesces, the physician must consider that a response to the empiric regimen may have occurred. At St. Jude this leads us to continue triple-drug therapy for a minimum of 7 days in patients who defervesce. On the other hand, if the culture-negative patient fails to defervesce within 4 days, we recommend changing to ceftazidime monotherapy (Fig. 2). This change does not appreciably expand cumulative coverage for the likely pathogens, but it does reduce the potential for nephrotoxicity in patients who subsequently require amphotericin B.

Discontinuing empiric therapy before neutropenia resolves is associated with a high risk of infectious sequelae, as was shown in a pivotal study conducted by Pizzo et al. (1979): 16 patients who had become afebrile but remained culture negative were randomized to continue antibiotic therapy and had no infectious sequelae; in contrast, seven of 17 patients (41%) randomized to discontinue antibiotic therapy developed infectious sequelae ($p = 0.007$), including two fatal infections. An approach that appears to be less perilous is the substitution of broad-spectrum oral antibiotics for parenteral drugs. The broad spectrum of ciprofloxacin favors its consideration in neutropenic adults, but concern about the association of quinolones with cartilage dysplasia in growing mammals has curtailed pediatric use. After completion of at least 7 days of parenteral therapy we routinely maintain neutropenic children who defervesced during intravenous therapy with empiric oral trimethoprim-sulfamethoxazole. Trimethoprim-sulfamethoxazole is given at therapeutic doses (10 mg/kg per day of trimethoprim in two divided doses, with a maximal dose of 320 mg daily) until neutropenia resolves (Fig. 2). Parenteral therapy is reinstated if fever recurs, but this is uncommon. In addition, we are currently conducting a randomized trial of continued intravenous therapy versus switching to oral cefixime in consenting patients who have no evidence of bacterial infection other than fever during the first 48 h of parenteral therapy (Fig. 4). Eligible patients lack all of the following risk factors for bacteremia: grade 2 or higher oral mucositis (National Cancer Institute, NCI, common toxicity criteria), grade 2 or higher gastrointestinal mucositis or diarrhea, prolonged neutropenia (>10 days); *Pseudomonas aeruginosa* colonization, or methicillin-resistant staphylococcal colonization. Empiric oral antimicrobial regimens would reduce exposure to contaminated intravenous fluids and would facilitate outpatient management of low-risk patients. Alternatively, outpatient management of low-risk patients can also be achieved through use of programmable intravenous drug delivery systems.

While it may be possible to manage selected immunocompromised patients with oral therapy, other patients will require escalating therapy including amphotericin B, flucytosine, antivirals, growth factor administration, and monoclonal antibody therapy. Carefully formulated institutional guidelines can reduce indiscriminate use of these costly agents. Moreover, a standardized institutional approach has the added advantage of highlighting key therapeutic shortfalls and facilitating the design of discerning clinical trials. For example, we noted several deaths due to systemic mycoses among our cancer patients despite adherence to the guidelines for empiric administration of amphotericin B to neutropenic patients with fever beyond 7 days

Low Risk Febrile Neutropenic Patients

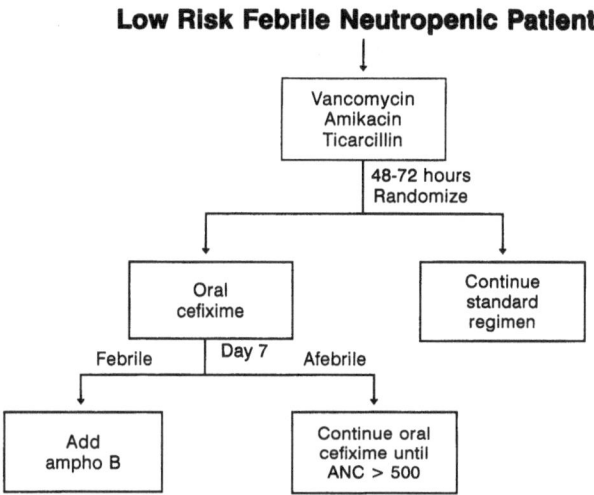

Fig. 4. Outline of a clinical trial currently underway at St. Jude Children's Research Hospital in neutropenic children at relatively low risk for infection. The objective of this study is to assess the strategy of switching to oral antibiotic therapy vs. continuing intravenous antibiotic therapy until neutropenia resolves

of antibiotic therapy (Fig. 2). Consequently, we are conducting a randomized trial in patients at high risk for mycoses, comparing the incidence of fungal infection in patients treated with the standard plan to the incidence in patients treated with amphotericin B every other day (1 mg/kg per day, maximal dose 50 mg daily) initiated on the first day of antibiotic therapy (Fig. 5). We hypothesize that early administration of amphotericin B may not only reduce the incidence of mycoses, but could result in less total exposure to amphotericin B by the avoidance of prolonged courses of therapy. Unique among studies of amphotericin B, this trial is blinded using an infusion of water as a placebo. In a previous study, we observed reactions in only about one third of children receiving open-label amphotericin B without premedication (Gigliotti et al. 1987). In this study investigators are permitted to premedicate patients only if a definitive reaction is documented upon infusion of the study solution. To date only about one fourth of patients have experienced definitive reactions upon infusion, indicating at least half of pediatric patients are not unequivocally reacting to intravenous infusion of 1 mg/kg of amphotericin B given over 4 h.

Periodic Review of Standard Therapy

Once a standard plan is adopted, it requires regular maintenance. The third essential step toward streamlining empiric therapy is the periodic re-

Febrile Neutropenic Patients at
High Risk for Mycoses

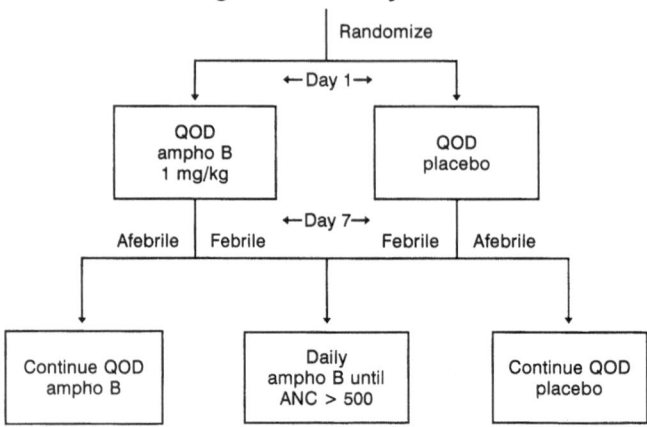

Fig. 5. Outline of a clinical trial currently underway at St. Jude Children's Research Hospital in patients at high risk for mycoses. The objective of this study is to determine if the incidence of fungal infection can be reduced by initiating amphotericin B (*ampho B*) on the first day of empiric antibiotic therapy vs. the standard practice of reserving amphotericin B therapy for patients with fever beyond day 7 of antibiotic therapy

evaluation of the preferred drug regimen for the febrile, neutropenic patient. When indicated, revision of the standard plan should be undertaken. During these periodic reviews it is paramount that simplification of the regimen be afforded equal consideration to that given therapeutic expansion. Are drugs included that are no longer required according to the susceptibilities of recently recovered isolates? Can monotherapy with a third-generation cephalosporin or thienamycin be considered? Can toxicity be reduced by drug substitution without compromising efficacy?

Ideally, fundamental changes to the standard management plan should be assessed by randomized, controlled clinical trials when feasible. At St. Jude, the initial empiric regimen of vancomycin, amikacin, and ticarcillin was selected to provide optimal coverage for the common blood isolates from our patients: coagulase-negative staphylococci, Gram-negative enteric bacilli, and *P. aeruginosa*. While this regimen was highly effective for our pediatric patients, we were concerned about its potential for nephrotoxicity and substantial cost. We hypothesized that vancomycin may not be essential in the initial drug regimen; it could be added to those patients with coagulase-negative staphylococcal infection, which was typically manifest as a bacteremia not associated with hypotension or other life-threatening complications. To test this hypothesis, we randomized consenting patients to receive either the standard regimen or amikacin plus ticarcillin clavulanate in a double-blinded study (Shenep et al. 1988). We were surprised to find that patients receiving the vancomycin-containing regimen fared significantly better, with a higher response rate (85% vs. 62%; $p = 0.010$) and fewer episodes of coagulase-negative staphylococcal and alpha hemolytic streptococcal breakthrough bacteremia (1 vs. 9; $p = 0.006$). One child died from breakthrough streptococcal sepsis despite prompt addition of vancomycin when deterioration was noted on day 3 of ticarcillin clavulanate and amikacin. This experience exemplifies the need for caution and observation when streamlining empiric therapy regimens. Although this attempt to simplify therapy failed, it should nonetheless be recognized that ceftazidime and imipenem monotherapy have been found efficacious and safe in other clinical settings. When applicable, monotherapy has the inherent advantage of eliminating intravenous infusions that could serve as a portal of entry for microorganisms; monotherapy also reduces the workload for nursing and pharmacy personnel (Wade et al. 1986; Pizzo et al. 1986; Shenep et al. 1990).

Critical Evaluation of Each New Agent

The fourth step toward simplifying empiric therapy is the critical evaluation of each new prophylactic and empiric agent. Evaluation should focus on published evidence of efficacy and safety, and applicability of the supporting data to the local institution and individual patient. The addition of empiric drugs without definitive supporting medical literature should be avoided, allowing exceptions only for patients who might otherwise have a dismal prognosis.

A current, striking example of the role of critical evaluation of new agents is the recent introduction of granulocyte colony-stimulating factor (G-CSF) and granulocyte–macrophage CSF (GM-CSF) into management of neutropenic patients before the completion of definitive studies. The high cost of these agents is stressing the health care system, all the more so because the clinician is struggling to define the role for these agents. Only through controlled clinical trials can the relative efficacies of G-CSF versus GM-CSF be determined. Controlled trials will also be necessary to determine if these cytokines decrease mortality from infection, reduce costs through reduction in the incidence of infection, or increase cure rates of cancer by allowing intensification of therapy.

Terminally Ill Patients

For the terminally ill, the goal of maximizing the patient's comfort supersedes the goal of achieving therapeutic optimization. Oral therapy may be quite suitable for the cancer patient receiving terminal care. When the patient's condition warrants it, the physician may appropriately choose not to administer antimicrobials. In this case, laboratory tests such as blood cultures and complete blood counts should be minimized and procedures such as measurement of body temperature and vital signs may be omitted. Streamlined management can greatly enhance the patient's comfort and, for the terminally ill, comfort is paramount.

Conclusion

Ultimately, the clinician's goal is not necessarily simplification, but optimization of empiric therapy (Fig. 1). This objective may require increasingly complex approaches to the severely immunocompromised patient. Nevertheless, therapeutic optimization will only be achieved if opportunities to simplify therapy are pursued with vigilance equal to that afforded the promotion of patented investigational drug use. This increasingly arduous task falls to the clinicians caring for neutropenic cancer patients.

Acknowledgements. This work was supported by National Cancer Institute Center Support (CORE) Grant P30 CA 21765 and the American Lebanese Syrian Associated Charities (ALSAC).

References

Gigliotti F, Shenep JL, Lott L, Thornton D (1987) Induction of prostaglandin synthesis as the mechanism responsible for the chills and fever produced by infusing amphotericin B. J Infect Dis 156:784–789

Hughes WT, Armstrong D, Bodey GP, Feld R, Mandell GL, Meyers JD, Pizzo PA, Schimpff SC, Shenep JL, Wade JC, Young LS, Yow MD (1990) Guidelines for the use of antimicrobial agents in neutropenic patients with unexplained fever. J Infect Dis 161:381–396

Joshi JH, Schimpff SC, Tenney JH, Newman KA, de Jongh CA (1984) Can antibacterial therapy be discontinued in persistently febrile granulocytopenic cancer patients? Am J Med 76:450–457

Pizzo PA, Robichaud KJ, Gill FA, Witebsky FG, Levine AS, Deisseroth AB, Glaubiger DL, Maclowry JD, Magrath IT, Poplack DG, Simon RM (1979) Duration of empiric antibiotic therapy in granulocytopenic patients with cancer. Am J Med 67:194–200

Pizzo PA, Ladisch S, Ribichaud K (1980) Treatment of Gram-positive septicemia in cancer patients. Cancer 45:206–207

Pizzo PA, Hathorn JW, Hiemenz J, Browne M, Commers J, Cotton D, Gress J, Longo D, Marshall D, McKnight J, Rubin M, Skelton J, Thaler M, Wesley R (1986) A randomized trial comparing ceftazidime alone with combination antibiotic therapy in cancer patients with fever and neutropenia. N Engl J Med 315:552–558

Shenep JL, Hughes WT, Roberson PK, Blankenship KR, Baker DK, Meyer WH, Gigliotti F, Sixbey JW, Santana VM, Feldman S, Lott L (1988) Vancomycin, ticarcillin, and amikacin compared with ticarcillin-clavulanate and amikacin in the empirical treatment of febrile, neutropenic children with cancer. N Engl J Med 319:1053–1058

Shenep JL. Combination and single-agent empirical antibacterial therapy for febrile cancer patients with neutropenia and mucositis (1990) Natl Cancer Inst Monogr 9:117–122

Wade JC, Johnson DE, Bustamante CI (1986) Monotherapy for empiric treatment of fever in granulocytopenic cancer patients. Am J Med 80[Suppl 5G]:85–95

Further Reading

Hughes WT, Armstrong D, Bodey GP, Feld R, Mandell GL, Meyers JD, Pizzo PA, Schimpff SC, Shenep JL, Wade JC, Young LS, Yow MD (1990) Guidelines for the use of antimicrobial agents in neutropenic patients with unexplained fever. J Infect Dis 161:381–396

Pizzo PA (1981) Infectious complications in the child with cancer: I. Pathophysiology of the compromised host and the initial evaluation and management of the febrile cancer patient. J Pediatr 98:341–354

Pizzo PA (1981) Infectious complications in the child with cancer: II. Management of specific infectious organisms. J Pediatr 98:513–523

Schimpff SC (1991) Infections in patients with cancer: overview and epidemiology. In: Moossa AR, Schimpff SC, Robson MC (eds) Comprehensive textbook of oncology. Williams and Wilkins, Baltimore, pp 1729–1732

Wade JC (1991) Infections in patients with cancer: treatment. In: Moossa AR, Schimpff SC, Robson MC (eds) Comprehensive textbook of oncology. Williams and Wilkins, Baltimore, pp 1740–1748

Fever and Granulocytopenia: A Viewpoint from an Academic Setting

N.J. Vogelzang[1] and J.P. Flaherty[2]

[1] Section of Hematology/Oncology and Urology, University of Chicago,
5841 S. Maryland Avenue, Chicago, IL 60637-1470, USA
[2] Section of Infectious Disease, University of Chicago, 5841 S. Maryland Avenue,
Chicago, IL 60637-1470, USA

The optimal management of the febrile neutropenic patient continues to be controversial (Pizzo and Meyers 1989). There are numerous factors which must be taken into account when making recommendations for empiric therapy (Talcott et al. 1988; Pizzo et al. 1984). These factors include the age of the patient and the underlying diagnosis, the type of induction regimen used to treat the underlying disease, the presence of concomitant illnesses (i.e., renal/cardiac/hepatic), the expected duration of neutropenia, the nature and duration of prior infectious episodes, the clinical clues which exist to suggest a source for the neutropenic fever, and the expected organisms and their resistance patterns within that particular hospital. Clearly, if prospective clinical trials of antibiotic regimens are available, patients should be entered into such trials (Table 1).

The choices for empiric antibiotic therapy include monotherapy (Pizzo et al. 1986), double beta-lactam therapy, an aminoglycoside plus an antipseudomonal beta-lactam (EORTC International Antimicrobial Therapy Cooperative Group 1987), or "triple" therapy (an aminoglycoside, an antipseudomonal beta-lactam plus an antistaphylococcal agent). Under appropriate clinical conditions the addition of vancomycin (Rubin et al. 1988; Karp et al. 1986), metronidazole, clindamycin, erythromycin or trimethoprim-sulfamethoxazole may be considered: for example, vancomycin when a Gram-positive catheter-related infection is predicted, metronidazole or clindamycin when an intra-abdominal infection is predicted, erythromycin or trimethoprim-sulfamethoxazole when diffuse pneumonitis is present.

The optimal management of such patients takes on an added level of complexity in an academic medical center (Table 2). First, many patients live a considerable distance from the center. Using the example of the University of Chicago Medical Center, a substantial number of acute leukemic, allo- and autotransplant and "solid" tumor patients live in and are referred from the northern suburbs of Chicago (40–50 miles away) or from South Bend, Indiana (100 miles away). As a result, these patients must be carefully

Recent Results in Cancer Research, Vol. 132
© Springer-Verlag Berlin · Heidelberg 1993

Table 1. Factors entering into decisions regarding empiric antibiotics in febrile neutropenic patients

---

- Age and underlying diagnosis
- Type of induction regimen used (i.e., stomatitis inducing?)
- Concomitant illnesses (renal/hepatic/cardiac)
- Expected duration of neutropenia
- Nature and duration of prior infections
- Clinical clues suggesting a source
- Expected organisms within hospital
- Availability of clinical trials

Table 2. Factors contributing to increased complexity of care of febrile neutropenic patients in an academic medical center

---

- Distance from the center
- Local physician resumes care under emergency circumstances
- Third-party payors demand care at a less-expensive local facility
- Fragmentation of care among the outpatient team and inpatient team at academic centers
- Complex patterns of care during inpatient stay (rotating services, different consultant services)

---

instructed in the steps they must take when a fever develops. Of necessity, patients need to be seen urgently by their local physician or local hematologist/oncologist. In the usual setting, these patients are hospitalized locally and empiric antibiotic therapy is instituted by that physician. Thus, the actual treating hematologist/oncologist may be divorced from the immediate supportive care decisions. In some cases (fortunately rare), the local physicians may decide to withhold empiric antibiotic therapy and attribute a reversible infectious disease event to the underlying malignancy. Such fragmentation of care clearly detracts from optimal patient management.

Second, the problem of geographic dispersal of patients means that patients may refuse to return to the medical center for supportive care citing issues such as cost, convenience, and ill-defined concepts of "equivalence" of care. Patients need to be constantly educated regarding the importance of continuity of care plus the added advantage of state-of-the-art supportive care.

Third, third party payors may refuse permission (and have) for patients to receive treatment for neutropenic fever at an "expensive" tertiary center.

Finally, patients treated at academic medical centers may experience anonymity and loss of the sense of control. A common complaint of referral patients relates to the "different stories" which they receive from interns, residents, or fellows as compared to the attending physician. This perception is often well founded, since patients are typically cared for (in the outpatient setting) by a disease (i.e., leukemia)- or modality (phase I drug program)-oriented team. The team is led by an attending physician and usually includes nurses and data managers who are familiar with (and to) the patient. Direct outpatient care is usually provided by fellows, either first- or second-year trainees in hematology/oncology, in association with an attending physician, both of whom are fully aware of the intricacies of a given disease or modality protocol. The fellow or nurse is typically responsible for organizing the emergency admission of such patients. If the patients have been previously admitted, they have some familiarity with the medical student/intern/resident structure of a teaching hospital. If the patients have not previously been admitted, such structures are bewildering to many patients and increase their sense of "loss of control" and anonymity. The possibility of bewilderment increases when the patient meets a different fellow and attending physician who are on the inpatient service for that month. In some cases that inpatient team may not be fully aware of protocol intricacies. Bewilderment may lead to anger and resentment, especially if patients are admitted during a "switch" weekend or by a "short call" service and transferred the next day to another team yet again.

In the setting of fever and neutropenia, most patients are aware of the emergent nature of their illness and tolerate the anonymity and loss of control if they experience complete and consistent care. One of the most critical needs then in the management of such patients in an academic practice oriented to student, intern, resident, and fellow teaching is the algorithm or protocol for diagnosis and treatment.

These algorithms are preferably written and should be part of the intern "hand-outs" at the start of each year (Table 3). Although there are constant pressures from pharmaceutical representatives to try to change those algorithms by adding the "newest and best" antibiotic (usually their product!) to the protocol, such pressures must be resisted. Alternatively, institutional antibiotic susceptibility data should be periodically reviewed and protocol changes made when indicated. Updates on hospital-wide antimicrobial susceptibility patterns for key nosocomial pathogens are provided annually to all University of Chicago medical staff in the form of a pocket-size reference card (Table 4). The heavy use of particular antibiotics in hospitals or oncology units may render them locally obsolete and only through institutional surveillance can this potential threat be recognized. This becomes especially important in neutropenic patients who develop fever while hospitalized or soon after discharge and are at increased risk for infection with resistant hospital-acquired organisms.

It is important from the attending oncologist's point of view that house staff and other members of the patient-care team be taught a consistent and logical approach. It allows for fewer ad hoc decisions and does not lead as frequently to patient questions and concerns. The patient-care team must speak with one voice. Likewise, when a different housestaff service covers at night, each patient with granulocytopenia and a new fever must be fully

Table 3. Recommendations for empiric therapy of the febrile neutropenic patient

These are guidelines and represent one of many possible approaches. Empiric therapy such as this is made necessary by the rapidity at which untreated infection progresses in this patient population. Remember that each patient must be evaluated individually and therapy decisions tailored to each particular situation.

1   Initial empiric therapy
1.1   Ceftazidime 2 g q 8 h or mezlocillin 4 g q 6 h plus tobramycin 2 mg/kg q 12 h
1.2   Penicillin allergy: Aztreonam 2 g q 8 h
           Tobramycin 2 mg/kg q 12 h
           (+/− vancomycin)
1.3   Reserve monotherapy: Ceftazidime 2 g q 8 h or
                 imipenem 500 mg q 6 h for:
1.3.1 Patients expected to have a brief period (<1 week) of neutropenia
1.3.2 Patients who have fever without other signs of sepsis
1.3.3 Patients who have a compelling reason to avoid aminoglycoside therapy
1.4   Add vancomycin 1 g q 12 h to initial regimen when:
1.4.1 There is clinical suspicion of Gram-positive infection (for example, Hickman catheter site infection or fever developing in a patient on quinolone prophylaxis)
1.4.2 The patient is critically ill with overt signs of sepsis
1.4.3 The patient deteriorates after initial response to anti-Gram-negative regimen
1.4.4 The patient has an abnormal cardiovascular site that could be easily seeded by metastatic Gram-positive infection
1.4.5 If an institutional outbreak of Gram-positive infection is taking place

2   Reassess at 48 h
2.1   No bacteremia, duration of neutropenia likely to be brief (<1 week): consider monotherapy (ceftazidime or imipenem)
2.2   Culture negative or Gram-negative isolate susceptible to gentamicin: switch tobramycin to gentamicin
2.3   Gram-positive bacteremia or suspected catheter-related infection: add vancomycin
2.4   Evidence of severe oral mucositis, necrotizing gingivitis or perianal tenderness: add metronidazole 500 mg q 8 h or clindamycin 600–900 mg q 8 h
2.5   Diffuse pneumonitis: institute trial of trimethoprim-sulfa methoxazole 5 mg/kg q 8 h and erythromycin 750 mg q 6 h and add amphotericin B
2.6   Focal pneumonitis: add amphotericin B

3   Reassess at 4–7 days
3.1   Persistent unexplained fever: add amphotericin B 0.5 mg/kg and escalate to 1 mg/kg if patient remains febrile or signs/symptoms suggestive of *Aspergillus* infection develop (e.g., pneumonitis)

4   Discontinue antibiotics
4.1   Afebrile, no known infection
4.2   ANC >500 for 2 consecutive days

Discontinue antibiotics in face of persistent neutropenia in selected circumstances only (i.e., no hint of infection after 7–14 days of antibiotics). Frequent careful monitoring of these patients and a low threshold for reinstituting therapy are essential.

Table 4. Antibiotic susceptibilities of major nosocomial pathogens[a]: University of Chicago Hospitals, July 1990–June 1991

Organism	Total no. of isolates	Isolates susceptible to specified antibiotic													
		AMPI	CZOL	CEFX	CXM	CTRI	CZID	MEZL	TIM	AZ	IMI	SXT	CIP	GENT	TOBR
E. coli	530	54	93	98	95	99	98	60	77	98	100	89	100	95	97
P. aeruginosa	402	0	0	0	0	22	90	71	81	75	92	0	95	84	95
K. pneumoniae	287	0	92	95	94	97	96	78	88	96	100	90	95	92	93
E. cloacae	240	0	4	3	39	59	63	59	55	63	99	91	98	95	94
P. mirabilis	106	42	96	99	98	100	100	96	99	100	100	95	100	95	95
E. aerogenes	97	4	8	4	54	73	74	69	67	79	100	99	100	99	99
S. marcescens	61	0	0	62	7	100	100	97	97	97	97	95	95	97	92
		PEN	METH	CEPH	ERYT	CLIN	VANC	SXT	CIP						
S. aureus	430	7	76	76	65	77	100	89	76						
S. epidermidis	283	4	19	19	22	31	100	46	74						

[a] Includes only isolates recovered initially at least 2 days after admission. Multiple isolates from the same patient at the same site are counted only once.

AMPI, ampicillin; CZOL, cefazolin; CEFX, cefoxitin; CXM, cefuroxime; CTRI, ceftriaxone; CZID, ceftazidime; MEZL, mezlocillin; TIC, ticarcillin; TIM, timentin; AZ, aztreonam; IMI, imipenem; SXT, trimethoprim-sulfamethoxazole; CIP, ciprofloxacin; GENT, gentamicin; TOBR, tobramycin; PEN, penicillin; METH, methicillin; CEPH, cephalothin; ERYT, erythromycin; CLIN, clindamycin; VANC, vancomycin.

evaluated. Such an evaluation must include a history, physical, blood and urine cultures, culture of suspected sites, chest radiograph, and chemistry profile. Successful patient management relies upon meticulous attention to detail. These patients are characteristically difficult to evaluate because the absence of neutrophils mutes the inflammatory process. Local signs and symptoms of infection may be subtle and repeated careful examinations are necessary. Likewise, the microbiologic data should be thoroughly reviewed each day. Using the established algorithms or protocols, prompt initiation of empiric antibiotics is mandatory. "Looks good, feels good" is not an acceptable reason to withhold antibiotics. More than 60% of febrile neutropenic patients are documented to have infection, either by positive cultures or clinical signs, and over 90% of these are bacterial. Empiric antibiotics are necessary because currently available diagnostic tests are not sufficiently rapid or accurate to identify the infecting organism or exclude patients without infection. Untreated, bacterial infection in these patients, Gram-negative bacteremia in particular, is often rapidly fatal. As clearly stated by Pizzo and Meyers (1989), "the empiric regimen must be broad, achieve high bactericidal levels and be as nontoxic and as simple to administer as possible."

Although numerous reviews have attempted to identify "low-risk" and "high-risk" patients, no consistent risk grouping is more effective than the predicted duration of neutropenia; low risk <7 days, high risk >7 days. The currently preferred approach at the University of Chicago is single-agent ceftazidine or imipenem-cilastatin for low-risk patients, young, healthy high-risk patients and those at increased risk of aminoglycoside nephrotoxicity either because of pre-existing renal insufficiency or concomitant use of nephrotoxic medications (e.g., cyclosporine or cisplatin). Ceftazidime or mezlocillin plus tobramycin is used for high-risk patients (Table 3). Owing to bed availability problems, and the low frequency of *Pseudomonas aeruginosa* infections in our institution, occasional low-risk patients are treated as outpatients with "once-a-day" ceftriaxone.

A *consistent* empiric regimen is important for the education of the students, housestaff, and fellows. It allows the attending physician to judge the efficiency and timing of the work-up and to assess the clinical acumen of the housestaff when additions or alterations are made to the basic regimen. The "next-morning" rounds allow early re-evaluation of the chosen regimen. Rarely is infectious disease consultation needed or requested at this stage of management. Rather, the protocol recommendations are discussed and analyzed as part of teaching rounds. Residents who have chosen to modify the protocol are asked to defend their decisions with support from the literature. Departures from the standard protocol, while certainly indicated in individual patients, should be justified by clinical or microbiologic data.

Excessive antibiotic usage and multiple empiric antibiotic changes may be associated with the emergence of resistant organisms and appears to increase the risks of hepatic and renal toxicity without improving outcome

(O'Hanley et al. 1989). The excessive antibiotic usage and multiple antibiotic regimen changes in febrile neutropenic patients can frequently be attributed to housestaff *unease* with persistent unexplained fever. While initial broad-spectrum antibacterial coverage is necessary to prevent death from overwhelming Gram-negative infection and the empiric addition of amphotericin B is indicated in many patients with persistent fever despite broad-spectrum antibacterial therapy, most other empiric antimicrobial additions or substitutions are not warranted in the absence of specific clinical findings or culture results. Housestaff should understand that numerous "blind" changes in a patient's antibiotic regimen complicates the patient's care and may do more harm than good.

The economic costs of empiric therapy are considerable and should be discussed on "next-morning" rounds. Antibiotic cost information has been disseminated as part of an "antibiotic cost/susceptibility card" provided to house staff and medical staff annually for the past 15 years. More recently, drug costs have been incorporated into the house staff manual (Table 5). The ready availability of the data on cost has clearly increased the staff's sensitivity to this issue; nevertheless, escalating drug costs continue to be a serious concern to academic centers which frequently have a large proportion of underinsured patients. Increasing local regulatory pressure from pharmacists and hospital administrators to control such costs is certain.

Fortunately, the early institution of empiric antibiotics has found widespread support within the oncologic and infectious disease specialty areas. Therefore, little controversy is generated in the initial management of such patients. However, many important and vexing problems face the academic oncologist/hematologist and infectious disease specialist in the continuing management of such patients. These include:

1. The timing of empiric antifungal therapy in patients who remain febrile (EORTC Group 1989, 1991; Pizzo 1987).
2. Management of persistent fever and granulocytopenia in patients on both antibiotics and antifungal agents (DiNubile 1988; Hughes et al. 1990).
3. The pressing need for better diagnostic tests for viral and fungal infections (why can't the infectious disease guys come up with simple tests?).

Although the colony-stimulating factors (CSFs) have shortened the duration of neutropenia and hospital stay in patients receiving intensive combination chemotherapy, the problem of cytokine-induced fever may cloud decision-making. (Crawford et al. 1991)

The last major area of need relates to prophylactic antibiotic and antifungal therapy. There are enormous unmet needs for data on prophylactic antibiotic therapy combined with most of the combination chemotherapy regimens in common use. Although randomized trials of the CSFs have been completed for many combination chemotherapy regimens, virtually none has used prophylactic antibiotics in the control arm. Therefore prophylactic antibiotic therapy may be a less costly alternative to the CSFs under some circumstances.

Table 5. Pharmacy cost of selected antibiotics

Antibiotic	Commonly used adult dose[a]	Daily cost to hospital[b] ($)
Intravenous		
Trimethoprim-sulfamethoxazole	10 ml q 8 h	5
Chloramphenicol	750 mg q 8 h	6
Penicillin G	2×10^6 units q 4 h	7
Ampicillin	2 g q 6 h	8
Erythromycin	750 mg q 6 h	8
Gentamicin	100 mg q 8 h	9
Nafcillin	2 g q 6 h	11
Cefazolin	1 g q 8 h	15
Clindamycin	600 mg q 8 h	17
Metronidazole	500 mg q 8 h	19
Tobramycin	100 mg q 8 h	19
Vancomycin	1 g q 12 h	20
Ampicillin-sulbactam[c]	1.5 g q 6 h	22
Amphotericin B	35 mg q 24 h	23
Cefotetan	2 g q 12 h	37
Mezlocillin	4 g q 6 h	38
Cefuroxime	1.5 g q 8 h	41
Timentin[c,d]	3.1 g q 6 h	41
Ganciclovir	5 mg/kg q 12 h	46
Piperacillin[c,d]	4 g q 6 h	48
Ceftriaxone	2 g q 24 h	49
Rifampin[d]	600 mg q 12 h	54
Ceftizoxime[e]	2 g q 8 h	55
Cefoxitin	2 g q 6 h	59
Aztreonam[c,f]	2 g q 8 h	67
Imipenem[d]	500 mg q 6 h	69
Acyclovir	5 mg/kg q 8 h	73
Ceftazidime[g]	2 g q 8 h	77
Pentamidine	300 mg q 24 h	102
Amikacin[d]	500 mg q 8 h	131
Fluconazole[c,d]	400 mg q 24 h	264
Oral		
Doxycycline	100 mg q 12 h	0.14
Trimethoprim-sulfamethoxazole	160 mg/800 mg q 12 h	0.16
Tetracycline	500 mg q 6 h	0.24
Metronidazole	500 mg q 8 h	0.30
Penicillin VK	500 mg q 6 h	0.32
Erythromycin	500 mg q 6 h	0.40
Amoxicillin	500 mg q 8 h	0.52
Dicloxacillin	500 mg q 6 h	0.64
Cephalexin	500 mg q 6 h	1.08
Ketoconazole	400 mg q 24 h	3.10
Acyclovir	200 mg 5 × /d	3.60
Ciprofloxacin	500 mg q 12 h	4.02
Clindamycin	300 mg q 8 h	4.68
Augmentin	500 mg q 8 h	5.16

Table 5. *Continued*

Antibiotic	Commonly used adult dose[a]	Daily cost to hospital[b] ($)
Azidothymidine (AZT)	100 mg 5 × /d	6.10
Cefaclor	500 mg q 6 h	8.80
Fluconazole[c,d]	200 mg q 24 h	9.17
Vancomycin	125 mg q 6 h	12.88

[a] Dosages are for cost comparison and are not intended as recommendations; appropriate dose will depend on many factors.
[b] Costs shown are UCH Pharmacy acquisition costs and include $0.87 per intravenous dose as the cost of preparation time and materials. Patient charges for antibiotics at UCH and retail pharmacies are considerably higher than the costs shown.
[c] Nonformulary.
[d] Usage restricted. Infectious Diseases approval required.
[e] Usage restricted to obstetrics and gynecology.
[f] Usage restricted to Infectious Diseases approval except for neutropenic oncology patients allergic to beta-lactam antibiotics.
[g] Usage restricted to Infectious Diseases approval except for neutropenic oncology patients and patients with cystic fibrosis.

In response to this situation the Cancer and Leukemia Group B respiratory committee will initiate a three-armed trial of chemotherapy in advanced non-small cell lung cancer. The three arms will be prophylactic granulocyte CSF (G-CSF), G-CSF plus ciprofloxacin, and ciprofloxacin alone all administered with a standard intensive chemotherapy regimen of etoposide plus cisplatin (N.J. Vogelzang, personal communication).

Co-operative cancer groups in the United States and Canada must pursue the lead established by the EORTC in developing large-scale prophylactic and therapeutic trials of antibiotics in patients receiving intensive combination chemotherapy. The dissemination of antibiotic protocols into academic medical centers will greatly reduce the complexity of caring for such patients. Active participation in such protocols is urged.

References

Crawford J, Ozer H, Stoller R, Johnson D, Lyman G, Tabbara I, Kris M, Grous J, Picozzi V, Rausch G, Smith R, Gradishar W, Yahanda A, Vincent M, Stewart M, Glaspy J (1991) Reduction by granulocyte colony-stimulating factor of fever and neutropenia induced by chemotherapy in patients with small-cell lung cancer. N Engl J Med 325:164–170

DiNubile JM (1988) Stopping antibiotic therapy in neutropenic patients. Ann Intern Med 108:289–292

EORTC International Antimicrobial Therapy Cooperative Group (1987) Ceftazidime combined with a short or long course of amikacin for empirical therapy of Gram-negative bacteremia in cancer patients with granulocytopenia. N Engl J Med 3771/27:1692–1698

EORTC International Antimicrobial Therapy Cooperative Group (1989) Empiric antifungal therapy in febrile granulocytopenic patients. Am J Med 86:668–672

EORTC International Antimicrobial Therapy Cooperative Group and National Cancer Institute of Canada (1991) Vancomycin added to empirical combination antibiotic therapy for fever in granulocytopenic cancer patients. J Infect Dis 163:951–958

Hughes WT, Armstrong D, Bodey GP, Feld R, Mandell GL, Meyers JD, Pizzo PA, Schimpff SC, Shenep JL, Wade JC, Young LS, Yow MD (1990) Guidelines for the use of antimicrobial agents in neutropenic patients with unexplained fever. J Infect Dis 161:381–396

Karp JE, Dick JD, Angelopulos C, Charache P, Green L, Burke PJ, Saral R (1986) Empiric use of vancomycin during prolonged treatment-induced granulocytopenia. Am J Med 81:237–242

O'Hanley PO, Easaw J, Rugo H, Easaw S (1989) Infectious disease management of adult leukemic patients undergoing chemotherapy: 1982 to 1986 experience at Stanford University Hospital. Am J Med 87:605–613

Pizzo PA (1987) After empiric therapy: what to do until the granulocyte comes back. Rev Infect Dis 9/1:214–219

Pizzo PA, Meyers J (1989) Infections in the cancer patient. In : DeVita V, Hellman S, Rosenberg SA (eds) Cancer: Principles and practice of oncology, sect 5, 3rd edn. Lippincott, Philadelphia, pp 2088–2124

Pizzo PA, Commers J, Cotton D, Gress J, Hathorn J, Hiemenz J et al. (1984) Approaching the controversies in antibacterial management of cancer patients. Am J Med 76:436–449

Pizzo PA, Hathorn JW, Hiemenz J, Browne M, Commers J, Cotton D et al. (1986) A randomized trial comparing ceftazidime alone with combination antibiotic therapy in cancer patients with fever and neutropenia. N Engl J Med 315/9:552–558

Rubin M, Hathorn JW, Marshall D, Gress J, Steinberg SM, Pizzo PA (1988) Gram-positive infections and the use of vancomycin in 550 episodes of fever and neutropenia. Ann Intern Med 108:30–35

Talcott JA, Finberg R, Mayer RJ, Goldman L (1988) The medical course of cancer patients with fever and neutropenia. Arch Intern Med 146:2561–2567

Empiric Antimicrobial Therapy in the Community Hospital Setting for the Cancer Patient with Fever and Neutropenia: The Need for Vigilance and Attention to Detail

J.G. Gallagher

Department of Hematology/Oncology, Geisinger Clinic, Danville, PA 17822, USA

The neutropenic patient who becomes febrile has a 60% probability of being infected. With extremely low neutrophil counts (<100), the likelihood of bacteremia is approximately 20% (Consensus Panel, Immunocompromised Host Society 1990; Klastersky et al. 1988; Hughes et al. 1990; de Pauw et al. 1990; Pizzo 1989; Hathorn 1989; Lazarus et al. 1989). Untreated or inadequately treated, these infections are often rapidly fatal. The timely and effective treatment of these patients with empiric antibiotics requires attention to detail. Initial evaluation with complete history and physical examination may be lacking important elements when done in settings such as the family doctor's office or the emergency department of the community hospital. After admission to the community hospital, the patient may be cared for by a private attending physician who sees the patient briefly once daily. If the patient is on a teaching service in a community hospital, the house staff may have varying levels of confidence and experience in dealing with the rapidly evolving syndromes in immunocompromised hosts. Contrast this with the care given in a major university center. The febrile patient is surrounded by house staff and fellows from the departments of hematology, and oncology and infectious diseases. They are customarily enrolled in the in-house sepsis protocol and reevaluated frequently and cultured extensively.

This attention to detail is important because the early hours of admission for the febrile neutropenic patient are much like the "golden hour" of opportunity for the patient with major trauma. Either early and appropriate attention is paid to important elements of care or there are lapses. If the latter, then outcomes are worse than they could be. Donald Tapley MD in a commencement address (unpublished) has expressed the point I am trying to make: "The importance of paying conscientious and meticulous attention to detail in the management of patients cannot be overemphasized. Without it, intelligence is wasted, factual knowledge is worthless, reasoned judgement is impossible, honesty is irrelevant, and compassion is fraudulent."

Recent Results in Cancer Research, Vol. 132
© Springer-Verlag Berlin · Heidelberg 1993

The major question for treatment in the community hospital or private practice setting is how to ensure this attention to detail. Without it, our patients may go from the early warning sign of fever to established sepsis with hemodynamic compromise and renal, hepatic, or cardiopulmonary failure in less than 24 h. The community hospital oncologist faces this daunting clinical situation with many handicaps to prevent him or her from meeting the standards of care found at a university center. He or she has no fellows in the departments of infectious diseases or oncology, there are few or no house staff to provide night coverage. There are difficulties obtaining bronchoscopies and laboratory services at night, and difficulties getting drug levels. While one could question whether febrile neutropenic patients should be treated in this setting, nevertheless, increasing numbers of patients are presenting for supportive care because of the transfer of primary treatment technology (the initial chemotherapy) to the community centers as National Cancer Institute policy.

Every time I review a new aggressive chemotherapy program with the potential for septic death which is published by major centers such as the National Cancer Institute, Dana Farber Cancer Institute, Memorial Sloan-Kettering Cancer Center, M.D. Anderson Tumor Institute, or Vancouver, I think to myself: "This may go well in Bethesda, New York City, or Boston, but how will it do in Altoona, Bethlehem, or Danville?" While any community hospital hematologist or oncologist can administer a regimen provided in an abstract from the American Society of Hematology (ASH) or American Society for Clinical Oncology (ASCO) meetings, they may not do as well when it comes to dealing with the infectious complications of these regimens. That is the crux of the issue. The supportive care standards have not kept pace with the advances in primary treatment. While aggressive chemotherapy regimens as published often have elaborate grading systems for the toxicities to be expected, they rarely have state-of-the-art protocols for dealing with the toxicities. The standard of care for the expected infectious complications of these chemotherapy protocols is developed in the setting where there is omnipresent house staff coverage and supervision by attending staff physicians with adequate time and interest in clinical research. On the other hand, most community oncologists are not hospital based and must cover several hospitals and an office practice during the course of the day. This makes it impossible for them to reexamine and frequently reassess the patient with impending or established sepsis. Even if competent to manage the febrile neutropenic patients, they are not present for long enough to be effective. New strategies must be devised to improve the amount of attention paid to these patients. House staff physicians or physician extenders such as physicians' assistants and nurse practitioners or oncology nurse specialists may help the interested community oncologist in more frequent monitoring of these patients.

Even where house staff or physician extenders are present, there can be problems in patient management. While house staff may do well with ordering antibiotics for community-acquired pneumonia, for example, they may do very poorly with a compromised host for lack of experience. They do especially poorly with empiric antibiotics for the host who is penicillin allergic or who has concurrent renal or hepatic failure. In a recent review of house staff decision making in the setting of *Pseudomonas aeruginosa* infections, 40% received what was considered inadequate therapy in a quality control study (J.G. Gallagher, unpublished data). Because delayed or inadequate treatment has harmful consequences for compromised hosts, it is necessary to try to reduce the frequency of mistakes in management.

A recent article entitled *Do House Officers Learn from Their Mistakes?* documented that inexperience and lack of supervisory physician input frequently result in mistakes (Wu et al. 1991). In addition, many study chairmen have questioned whether attending staff learn from their mistakes when reviewing the management of the toxicities of chemotherapy by their community affiliates.

If community hospital chemotherapists are going to implement state-of-the-art treatment, they need to have an established protocol for dealing with infectious complications. It seems to me that the only rational solution to the problem of appropriate management of the febrile neutropenic patient in the community hospital is to have either (a) an in-house sepsis protocol; (b) a subsection of the chemotherapy protocol with defined recommendations for infectious complications such as Cancer and Leukemia Group B (CALGB) used to employ in protocols 20 years ago; or (c) cooperative group protocols dealing specifically with febrile neutropenic cancer patients. The International Antimicrobial Therapy Cooperative Group of the European Organization for Research on Treatment of Cancer is a prototype for this approach.

The Geisinger Clinic chose to standardize the approach to febrile neutropenic patients with the EORTC Cooperative Group protocol. With a protocol, the initial evaluation of the patient can be defined, baseline studies demanded prior to release of drugs, rigorous and timely follow-up studies such as drug levels and repeat cultures required, and additional help with patient monitoring made available. In our institution, the house staff and nurses are supplemented for antibiotic protocol patients by two nurse practitioners and the Cancer Center pharmacist who make daily rounds for evaluation of progress and data collection on all enrolled patients. All of the foregoing benefit the patient and help him or her survive the febrile neutropenic episode. Benefits for the private hematologist or oncologist in a community setting include the opportunity to study investigational drugs, new drug combinations, and new strategies for drug delivery. Small institutions which can contribute 10–50 patients per year can participate in these meaningful group trials instead of doing single institution trials with low statistical power and prolonged time to accrue sufficient patients. These minimal criteria for membership are no different from the requirements for most other cooperative oncology groups such as the National Surgical

Adjuvant Breast Project (NSABP), Eastern Cooperative Oncology Group (ECOG), CALGB, or North Central Cancer Treatment Group (NCCTG). We have enrolled 288 patients over a 10-year period. Even for those patients who are ineligible for, or refuse protocol entry, there are benefits when a sepsis protocol is in place. The attending and house staff physicians learn from the protocol more appropriate ways of dealing with the febrile neutropenic patient and do a better job than if there were no such example. They will often employ the control arm of the protocol for off-study patients. Since this is a proven therapy, it is more likely than some ad hoc combinations to be effective.

At the Geisinger Clinic in 1980, a febrile neutropenic patient could have his or her empiric therapy decided by any of eight attending or 12 house staff physicians providing coverage. No two patients were treated alike as there were so many differences of opinion regarding such issues as which aminoglycoside to use, whether or not to use a loading dose of aminoglycoside, how much Gram-positive coccal coverage to provide, whether to worry about anaerobic coverage, whether or not to order drug levels, and when to change therapies. Once protocol therapy was introduced into this chaotic situation and treatment became standardized for most patients, it became clear that there were fewer major drug toxicities such as renal failure, better attention to patient monitoring was being done, more rapid alterations of therapy for failure of initial treatment were made, and there appeared to be fewer fatal infectious episodes overall. The protocol system of management works so well that now the staff become anxious during the intervals between the closing of one protocol and the opening of a new study.

In summary, the febrile neutropenic patient needs vigilant and repetitive assessment for adequate management. The protocol is designed to heighten the "attention to detail" so that vigilance and frequent reassessment are done.

The foregoing material has been an attempt to describe the why – the rationale for belonging to a cooperative group with protocols for empiric therapy and participating vigorously. The following material will define what is actually done at the Geisinger Clinic with febrile neutropenic patients.

The EORTC has just commenced the ninth in a series of major trials dating from 1973. These trials were designed to answer what seem to be the most important questions regarding empiric therapy. As can be seen from the references, the EORTC has compared the efficacy of multiple different drug combinations, examined duration of administration of antibiotics, tried cost-saving single daily drug administration, and examined the addition of empiric amphotericin B to the regimens (Klastersky et al. 1988; Meunier et al. 1991; EORTC International Antimicrobial Therapy Cooperative Group and National Cancer Institute of Canada-Clinical Trials Group 1991; EORTC International Antimicrobial Therapy Cooperative Group 1991). Much of what was learned in the design and analysis of these trials was

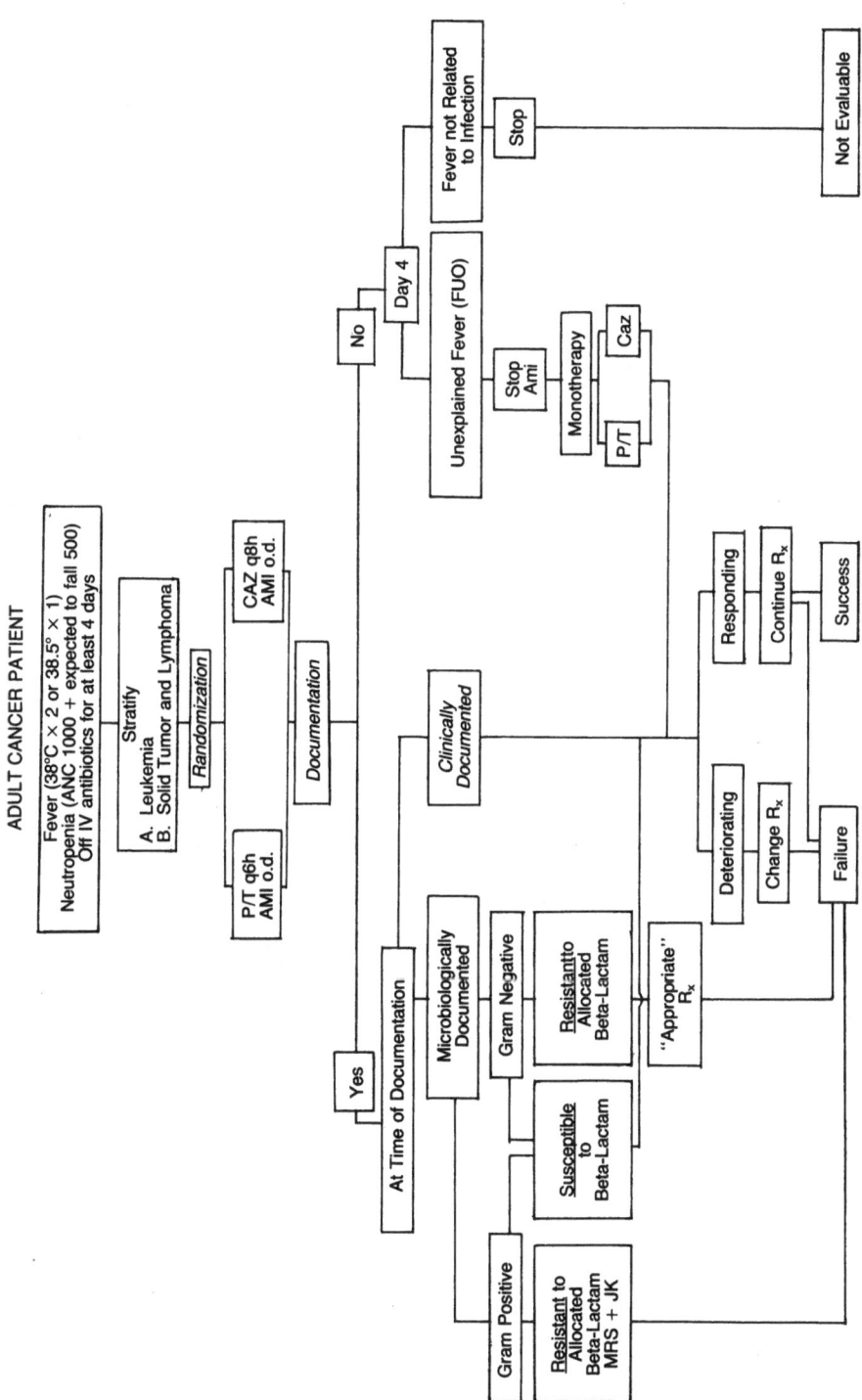

Fig. 1. EORTC Trial IX schema

incorporated into the recommendations of the Immunocompromised Host Society for conducting clinical trials (Consensus Panel, Immunocompromised Host Society 1990). Many of the scientific conclusions from the conduct of these trials have been widely accepted (Klastersky et al. 1988; Hughes et al. 1990). We have collected all of our blood culture isolates in a single reference laboratory and studied them to enhance our knowledge of the microbiology and epidemiology of infection in our cancer patients. The current Trial IX compares tazobactam–piperacillin plus amikacin with ceftazidime plus amikacin (Fig. 1). Since the percentage of Gram-positive bacteremias has more than doubled from 29% in the first trial to 63% in Trial V, it is important to address that issue. Increased activity of third-generation cephalosporins, such as ceftazidime, was obtained at the price of reduced Gram-positive coccal coverage. The investigational piperacillin–tazobactam provides perhaps better broad-spectrum coverage to include the Gram-positive organisms in the initial combination. This may avoid the need for vancomycin or other agents which have nephotoxicity but are controversial as to whether they are of benefit with initial therapy. The algorithm for this Trial IX forces us to pay meticulous attention to the patient. It requires us to be thorough, efficient, and to make timely and rational adjustments in therapy. Instead of learning from personal mistakes in judgement which cost the patient dearly, we apply what was learned from previous clinical trials to today's patients in deciding what to do and what to avoid.

References

Consensus Panel, Immunocompromised Host Society (1990) The design, analysis, and reporting of clinical trials on the empirical antibiotic management of the neutropenic patient. J Infect Dis 161:397–401

de Pauw BE, Feld R, Deresinski S et al. (1990) Multicentre, randomised comparative study of ceftazidime vs piperacillin + tobramycin as empirical therapy for febrile granulocytopenic patients. Proceedings of the 6th international symposium inf immunocomp host (Abstr 116)

EORTC International Antimicrobial Therapy Cooperative Group (1991) Single versus multiple daily doses of amikacin combined with ceftriaxone or ceftazidime for empirical therapy of fever in granulocytopenic cancer patients. Proceedings of the 31st interscience conference on antimicrobial Agents and Chemotherapy, p 292

EORTC International Antimicrobial Therapy Cooperative Group, the National Cancer Institute of Canada – Clinical Trials Group (1991) Vancomycin added to empirical combination antibiotic therapy for fever in granulocytopenic cancer patients. J Infect Dis 163:951–958

Hathorn JW (1989) Empirical antibiotics for febrile neutropenic cancer patients. Eur J Cancer Clin Oncol 25[Suppl 2]:S43–S51

Hughes WT, Armstrong D, Bodey GP, Feld R, Mandell GL, Meyers JD, Pizzo PA, Schimpff SC, Shenep JL, Wade JC, Young LS, Yow MD (1990) Guidelines for the use of antimicrobial agents in neutropenic patients with unexplained fever. J Infect Dis 161:381–396

Klastersky J, Zinner SH, Calandra T et al. (1988) Empiric antimicrobial therapy for febrile granulocytopenic cancer patients: lessons from four EORTC trials. Eur J Cancer Clin Oncol 24[Suppl 1]:S35–S45

Lazarus HM, Creger RJ, Gerson SL (1989) Infectious emergencies in oncology patients. Semin Oncol 16:543–560

Meunier F, Zinner SH, Gaya H, EORTC International Antimicrobial Therapy Cooperative Group (1991) Prospective randomized evaluation of ciprofloxacin versus piperacillin plus amikacin for empiric antibiotic therapy of febrile granulocytopenic cancer patients with lymphomas and solid tumors. Antimicrob Agents Chemother 35:873–878

Pizzo PA (1989) Evaluation of fever in the patient with cancer. Eur J Cancer Clin Oncol 25[Suppl 2]:S9–S16

Wu AW, Folkman S, McPhee SJ, Lo B (1991) Do house officers learn from their mistakes? JAMA 265:2089–2094

Further Reading

Consensus Panel, Immunocompromised Host Society (1990) The design, analysis, and reporting of clinical trials on the empirical antibiotic management of the neutropenic patient. J Infect Dis 161:397–401
A valuable reference to the conduct of clinical trials in this population.

de Pauw BE, Feld R, Deresinski S et al. (1990) Multicentre, randomised comparative study of ceftazidime vs piperacillin + tobramycin as empirical therapy for febrile granulocytopenic patients. Proc 6th Internat Symp Inf Immunocomp Host (abstr 116)
A cooperative group trial of monotherapy versus combination treatment. As with the single institution National Cancer Institute trial by Pizzo, a majority of patients in both arms required modification of therapy for successful outcome. Vigilance and frequent reappraisal of the patient are essential in order to modify therapy in a timely fashion.

Hathorn JW (1989) Empirical antibiotics for febrile neutropenic cancer patients. Eur J Cancer Clin Oncol 25[Suppl]:S43–S51
Discusses monotherapy with imipenem or ceftazidime in a single institution.

Hughes WT, Armstrong D, Bodey GP, Feld R, Mandell GL, Meyers JD, Pizzo PA, Schimpff SC, Shenep JL, Wade JC, Young LS, Yow MD (1990) Guidelines for the use of antimicrobial agents in neutropenic patients with unexplained fever. J Infect Dis 161:381–396
Recommendations regarding initial therapy, changes for persistent fever, duration of antimicrobial therapy, and addition of antifungal therapy. The bibliography and appendices are valuable references.

Klastersky J, Zinner SH, Calandra T et al. (1988) Empiric antimicrobial therapy for febrile granulocytopenic cancer patients: lessons from four EORTC trials. Eur J Cancer Clin Oncol 24 [Suppl 1]:S35–S45
An excellent review of the work of the EORTC International Antimicrobial Therapy Cooperative Group over the last 15 years. This group has consistently large numbers of carefully defined compromised hosts in trials of early empiric broad-spectrum antibiotics. Microbiologically documented infections, especially bacteremias, are emphasized as the best test of efficacy for an empiric regimen in severely or persistently neutropenic patients.

Lazarus HM, Creger RJ, Gerson SL (1989) Infectious emergencies in oncology patients. Semin Oncol 16:543–560

An excellent review of the epidemiology of infections in cancer patients and the initial approach to the febrile neutropenic patient.

Pizzo PA (1989) Evaluation of fever in the patient with cancer. Eur J Cancer Clin Oncol 25[Suppl 2]:S9–S16

A good review of the principles of management of the febrile neutropenic episode.

Observations on the Effects of Hematopoietic Colony-Stimulating Factors on the Clinical Course of Bone Marrow Transplantation

W.P. Peters

Duke University Bone Marrow Transplant Program, Duke University Medical Center, Box 3961, Durham, NC 27710, USA

The use of the hematopoietic colony-stimulating factors (CSF) in clinical oncology and infectious disease has profound implications for the practice of medicine. The ability to influence the hematopoietic system with these factors offers the potential to reduce the morbidity and mortality associated with the use of chemotherapy, particularly intensive chemotherapy, and also to influence the outcome of various nonmalignant disorders of hematopoiesis.

This brief review will make three points: (a) that the cytokines are a family of hierarchically arranged glycoproteins required for the survival, proliferation, and differentiation of hematopoietic progenitors into mature effector cells; (b) that the in vivo use of these compounds involves a complex interaction of the administered cytokine and others that are induced; and (c) that, while the use of bone marrow alone with stimulating by the "late-acting" cytokines is insufficient to result in elimination of the absolute leukopenia after high-dose chemotherapy, CSF-primed peripheral blood progenitor cells are capable of profoundly altering the hematopoietic recovery after autologous bone marrow transplantation.

Hierarchical Arrangement of Cytokines

The hematopoietic CSF overlap in the progenitor cell types affected. For example, both granulocyte-macrophage CSF (GM-CSF) and granulocyte CSF (G-CSF) will affect the proliferation and differentiation to mature neutrophils from late hematopoietic progenitors. Interleukin 3 (IL-3) and GM-CSF overlap extensively in the cell types responsive to their administration but IL-3 will not result in full myeloid mutation alone. In addition, the cytokines are frequently involved in modulating effector function, e.g., GM-CSF has been reported to influence numerous functional capacities of mature neutrophils including oxidative metabolism, the expression of cell surface adhesion molecules, random and directed migration, and phagocytosic activity.

Recent Results in Cancer Research, Vol. 132
© Springer-Verlag Berlin · Heidelberg 1993

This redundancy in action of the cytokines may serve an important role in protecting the hematopoietic organ from failure by allowing substitution when a simple gene mutation inactivates a given factor. Nonetheless, the successful completion of hematopoietic proliferation and differentiation requires that both a potentially responsive hematopoietic progenitor and the appropriate stimulatory cytokine be present simultaneously. The pharmacologic administration of a cytokine may permit the eliciting of a desired physiologic effect, but only if the cell on which the cytokine needs to act is available to respond. In the setting of bone marrow transplantation, the administration of GM-CSF or G-CSF has little apparent effect on hematopoiesis in the first 8–9 days after marrow infusion, apparently because the responsive progenitors are not present. However, this is not to imply that there is no effect from the cytokine, since these drugs may have effects on nonhematopoietic cells. GM-CSF, for example, may be expected to have effects on tissue-resident macrophages, which in general are not completely destroyed by even intensive chemotherapy programs.

Interactions Among Cytokines

The pharmacologic administration of various cytokines will lead to the proliferation and differentiation of hematopoietic progenitors bearing receptors responsive to the administered agent. It can also lead to the secondary secretion of many other cytokines. GM-CSF, for example, is known to be a potent inducer of intracellular tumor necrosis factor (TNF). While such TNF is not immediately released into the circulation, in the presence of a second event, such as a bolus of endotoxin associated with an infection, the TNF may be released into the circulation. Many other cytokines have also been demonstrated to be produced in vitro by exposure to the hematopoietic CSF, and the effects of these agents in vivo will represent the combined effects not only of the agents themselves, but also very likely the effects of the secondary cytokines which they induce. Much investigation needs to be done to elucidate the importance of the induction of these secondary cytokines. It can reasonably be expected that both positive and negative effects will be encountered.

Effects of GM-CSF and G-CSF on Hematopoietic Recovery After Autologous Bone Marrow Transplantation

When bone marrow is harvested and cryopreserved for subsequent use after high-dose chemotherapy, the mature cells are lost in the cryopreservation process. Multiple studies have demonstrated that the number of colony-forming units – granulocyte macrophage (CFU-GM) present in the harvested bone marrow is relatively limited and, thus, cannot be expected

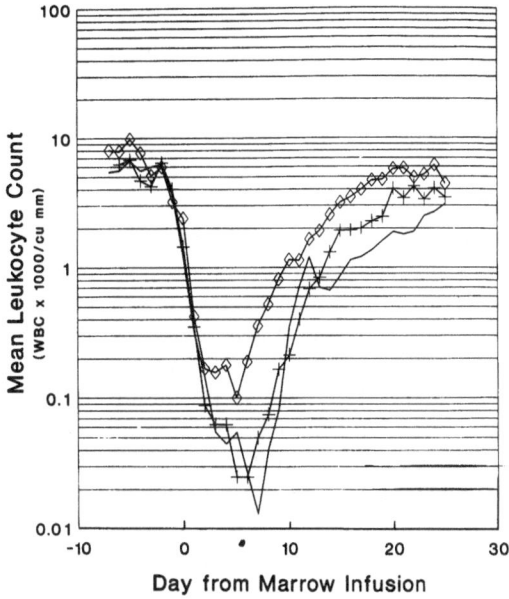

Fig. 1. Hematopoietic recovery following high-dose chemotherapy and autologous bone marrow support. After high-dose cyclophosphamide, cisplatinum, and 1,3-bis(2-chloroethyl)-1-nitrosourea (BCNU), patients were infused with autologous bone marrow and received either no CSF support (*plain line*), GM-CSF (*crosses*), or GM-CSF-primed peripheral blood progenitor cells and recombinant GM-CSF (*diamonds*). Mean leukocyte count nadir is not influenced in these patients by the use of GM-CSF until hematopoietic recovery begins to occur, and then there is an acceleration in the patients receiving GM-CSF. The use of CSF-primed peripheral blood progenitors reduces the severity of the nadir and shifts the hematopoietic constitution curve to the left, resulting accelerated hematopoietic recovery and, in addition, decreased resource utilization

to provide complete and sustained hematopoietic recovery without the added presence of earlier progenitors and stem cells, which are fortunately also found in the bone marrow. The presence of limited numbers of late progenitors in the bone marrow has important implications for the rate of hematopoietic recovery after autologous bone marrow transplantation (ABMT), which has been verified in clinical studies. After high-dose chemotherapy and the administration of autologous bone marrow, there is a period of absolute leukopenia during which peripheral blood is devoid of cells. Beginning, in general, about 8 days after the infusion of bone marrow, the first cells begin to appear in the peripheral blood, and then there is a progressive rise in the level of the peripheral leukocyte count. It has been a general observation that, during the administration of GM-CSF or G-CSF in patients undergoing ABMT, there is no evident impact on hematopoiesis peripherally until about the same time that the first cells would normally appear without cytokine administration. After this time, there is a significant acceleration of the rate of hematopoietic recovery (Fig. 1). Unfortunately, it is during the early period of absolute leukopenia that most of the infections and other complications of bone marrow transplantation begin. Indeed, most studies have been unable to identify a significant reduction in the frequency of confirmed bacterial infections in patients treated with CSF versus untreated patients, although trends in this direction are present in some studies. These findings, which would be predicted from the available data, suggest that alternative methods of supplying the cells which may be responsive to these cytokines might be particularly effective. Indeed, the use of CSF-primed peripheral blood progenitor cells collected after administration of GM-CSF or G-CSF with or without additional chemotherapy has been associated with a profound reduction in the duration of absolute leukopenia and the toxicity associated with transplantation.

The reduction in the period of absolute leukopenia after high-dose chemotherapy using peripheral blood progenitor cells has been associated with a reduction in the toxicity associated with the treatment program. Obvious at the bedside, there are a number of objective parameters that support these observations. The number of days in the bone marrow unit, days in hospital, number of platelet transfusions required, number and duration of antibiotics, and hospital charges were all significantly reduced. The improvement in patient tolerance for the chemotherapy program may be multifactorial. The reduction in duration of the leukopenia and neutropenia directly contributes to a reduction in the number of serious infections as would be predicted from the observations of Bodey in the 1960s. Whether the reduction in toxicity results from the accelerated recovery induced by the progenitor cells alone or whether other factors, such as the schedule of administration of the cytokines, are also important is not addressed by the available data.

The availability of earlier acting cytokines, such as IL-3, IL-1, IL-6, c-kit ligand, or the fusion molecule of IL-3 and GM-CSF called PIXY321, offers additional possibilities for progenitor collection or for the stimulating of marrow either after the high-dose chemotherapy or prior to the harvesting of the marrow or progenitor cell source. For example, IL-3 is capable of enhancing proliferation of an early hematopoietic progenitor in vitro but does not result in the transit of these progenitors to mature effector cells. Thus, it may offer the potential to increase the number of these progenitors in the marrow or peripheral blood before harvesting. When these cells are returned after intensive chemotherapy, they should be immediately responsive to administered (or endogenous) CSF.

In summary, the hematopoietic CSF offer substantial promise as a method of reducing toxicities associated with chemotherapy-induced myelosuppression. The ultimate value for the agents will depend upon their utility in allowing oncologists to improve the outcomes in chemotherapy by either allowing the reduction of toxicity associated with standard chemotherapy programs or allowing an improvement in the therapeutic outcome by dose escalation. While these goals are likely to be achieved in cancer therapeutics augmented by the colony-stimulating agents, such advantages should not be assumed for any particular treatment program.

References

Further Reading

Brandt SJ, Peters WP, Atwater SK, Kurtzberg J, Borowitz MJ, Jones RB, Shpall EJ, Bast RC, Gilbert CJ, Oette DH (1988) Effect of recombinant human granulocyte–macrophage colony-stimulating factor on hematopoietic reconstitution after high-dose chemotherapy and autologous bone marrow transplantation. N Engl J Med 318:869–876

Dinarello CA (1991) Interleukin-1 and interleukin-1 antagonism. Blood 77:1627–1652

Emerson SG, Gale RP (1987) The regulation of hematopoiesis following bone marrow transplantation. Int J Cell Cloning 5:432–449

Peters WP, Atwater S, Kurtzberg J, Borowitz M, Brandt SJ, Coleman RE, Kim CS, Gilbert C, Shpall EJ, Jones RB, Shogan J, Oette D, Stuart A, Coniglio D, Affronti ML, Evans S (1989a) The use of recombinant human granulocyte–macrophage colony-stimulating factor in autologous bone marrow transplantation. Bone marrow transplantation: current controversies. Liss, New York, pp 595–606

Peters WP, Kurtzberg J, Kirkpatrick G, Atwater S, Gilbert C, Borowitz M, Shpall E, Jones R, Ross M, Affronti M, Coniglio D, Mathias B, Oette D (1989b) GM-CSF primed peripheral blood progenitor cells (PBPC) coupled with autologous bone marrow transplantation (ABMT) will eliminate absolute leukopenia following high dose chemotherapy (HDC). Blood 74:178

Petros WP (1992) Pharmacokinetics and administration of colony-stimulating factors. Pharmacotherapy 12:32S–38S

Steinman RM (1988) Cytokines amplify the function of accessory cells. Immunol Lett 17:197–202

Effect of Colony-Stimulating Factors on Granulocyte Function

K. Vollmer and G.L. Mandell

Division of Infectious Diseases, University of Virginia Health Sciences Center, Charlottesville, VA 22908, USA

Phagocytes including polymorphonuclear neutrophils (PMN), monocytes, macrophages, and eosinophils are essential for host defense against certain microbes and probably play an important role in the surveillance and destruction of neoplastic cells. The production, maturation, and function of these cells appear to be regulated in a very complex manner by various cytokines including colony-stimulating factors (CSF) and other immune modulators. We will concentrate on the effect of CSF on the function of PMN.

Three of the CSF which are important in the stimulation of the production and maturation of neutrophils include granulocyte-macrophage CSF (GM-CSF), granulocyte CSF (G-CSF), and interleukin 3 (IL-3). GM-CSF is produced by activated T lymphocytes, macrophages, selected endothelial cells, and fibroblasts. In addition to stimulating the production of neutrophils, GM-CSF also stimulates the production of monocytes and eosinophils. G-CSF is released mostly from mononuclear cells and fibroblasts, and is responsible for stimulating the production and maturation of neutrophils. IL-3 is derived from T lymphocytes and stimulates a wide array of cells including neutrophils, monocytes, eosinophils, and basophils. Mature neutrophils have been found to have specific receptors for only two of these CSF: GM-CSF and G-CSF. Both GM-CSF and G-CSF have been approved for clinical use in certain populations of patients with induced neutropenia, and therefore understanding the effects these factors have on PMN function is important.

CSF were originally defined as hemopoietins based on their ability to stimulate the production and maturation of bone marrow stem cells. However, recent studies have shown that some CSF act as intracellular communication signals that can prime effector cells for enhanced antimicrobial activities. This can be advantageous or deleterious to the patient. In the setting of most localized infections, the PMN is activated by a delicate balance of humoral factors, including CSF. The phagocyte must sense the infectious agent, migrate toward it, and ingest and destroy it without causing widespread

Recent Results in Cancer Research, Vol. 132
© Springer-Verlag Berlin · Heidelberg 1993

tissue destruction. However, in the presence of overwhelming infection, the balanced regulation of the PMN can be upset, and the PMN may become excessively activated causing fever, shock, and the adult respiratory distress syndrome.

Cytokines are cell-derived humoral factors that usually act over short distances and up-regulate or down-regulate effector cells. CSF are a type of cytokine that also have hematopoietic activity. Some cytokines can act directly on the PMN to enhance chemotaxis, phagocytosis, and microbial killing. Others act indirectly through the stimulation of cells such as lymphocytes which release other humoral factors that can then stimulate the activity of PMN.

The PMN's major role in host defense is the phagocytosis and killing of microbes. To effectively perform this function, PMN must be able to sense the presence of a microbe, migrate to the microbe, and ingest and destroy the microbe without causing destruction of surrounding normal tissue. CSF have been found to affect all of these steps.

The ability of the PMN to migrate toward a microbe (chemotaxis) is a complex process requiring that the microbe first signal its presence to the PMN by releasing N-formylated compounds or by stimulating the release of cytokines from cells or generation of active complement factors. Some of these humoral factors are capable of up-regulating PMN surface receptors responsible for adherence such as CD11b/CD18. They allow the PMN to become "sticky" and adhere to the vascular endothelium. The adherence of PMN to the vascular endothelium is a necessary first step in the migration of the PMN out of the vascular space and into the site of infection. GM-CSF has been shown to increase the surface expression of adhesion-promoting surface glycoproteins (Arnaout et al. 1986) The PMN is attracted to the microbe through chemoattractants, and one study has reported that GM-CSF can serve as a chemoattractant (Wang et al. 1987). These factors attract the PMN to the microbe by forming a concentration gradient around the microbe. This chemoattractant gradient is detected by the PMN through a regional difference in the binding of the chemoattractant to specific PMN surface receptors. A second messenger then transmits information from the receptor to the myosin–actin complex in the cell which is in part responsible for the movement of the cell toward the microbe. The adherent PMN then push through the endothelial cell junction and crawl up the chemoattractant gradient toward the microbe.

GM-CSF in physiologic concentrations has been shown by Weisbart et al. (1986) and others to enhance neutrophil chemotaxis under agarose in the presence of the chemoattractant fMLP (f-Met-Leu-Phe). This has been shown to correlate with a rapid increase in the number of high-affinity fMLP receptors present on the surface of the PMN (Weisbart et al. 1986). Increased binding of fMLP to its high-affinity fMLP receptor has been shown to correlate with increased PMN chemotaxis (Sklar et al. 1981). In the absence of a chemoattractant, GM-CSF has been shown to directly inhibit the migration of PMN (Peters et al. 1988). G-CSF and IL-3 do not have significant effects on PMN migration. These findings are based on in vitro studies and their clinical relevance is unknown. Theoretically, it would seem to be advantageous to the host if GM-CSF could prevent the migration of PMN into tissues in the absence of infection and augment tissue migration in the presence of infection.

Once the activated PMN reaches the site of infection, it can phagocytize and kill the microbe. Microbial killing occurs through two major mechanisms: one is the respiratory burst and the other is the deposition of granular contents into the phagosome. The respiratory burst refers to several enzymatic events occurring intracellularly, which leads to the production of metabolic products that are toxic to the microbe. Through the respiratory burst, the PMN is able to convert oxygen into toxic metabolites such as hydrogen peroxide, superoxide anion, hydroxyl radicals, and singlet oxygen which can destroy the microbe. However, if these metabolites are leaked to the outside of the PMN, destruction of normal tissue can occur. Degranulation, or the release of enzymes such as myeloperoxidase from the intracellular primary granules into the phagosome, can also cause destruction of the microbe. These enzymes can add to tissue inflammation if leaked to the outside of the PMN.

CSF have been shown to affect PMN phagocytosis and bactericidal killing. Both GM-CSF and G-CSF have been shown to increase the phagocytosis of bacteria (Fleischmann et al. 1986; Roilides et al. 1991). GM-CSF has been shown to increase the phagocytosis of opsonized yeast as well. GM-CSF and G-CSF have been shown in vitro to directly increase the bactericidal activity of PMN which are adherent to surfaces (Nathan 1989; Roilides et al. 1991). The mechanism for this increase is unknown.

GM-CSF and G-CSF are also able to prime suspended neutrophils for an increased bactericidal activity in response to a second stimulus (Weisbart et al. 1985, 1986). The concept of "priming" of neutrophils for increased activity is important. "Resting" neutrophils have a very low baseline production of superoxide hydrogen peroxide and other toxic metabolites. When these neutrophils ingest particles, their production of superoxide and hydrogen peroxide increases one or two times. However, the neutrophil can be primed for a massive (tenfold) increase in oxygen metabolites with molecules such a tumor necrosis factor (TNF) and interleukin 1 (IL-1). These cytokines do not induce oxidative metabolism by themselves when neutrophils are in suspension but prime the neutrophils for an increased response when they encounter the second stimulus. In contrast, when the neutrophils are already attached to a surface such as fibrin, collagen, or even glass, their incubation with TNF will actually trigger an oxidative burst, thus highlighting differences between resting neutrophils in suspension and neutrophils adherent to surfaces.

GM-CSF and G-CSF can prime suspended neutrophils for an enhanced respiratory burst in response to N-formyl peptides, C5A, and leukotriene B_4

in vitro (Weisbart et al. 1987). It is not known if GM-CSF and G-CSF have similar effects in vivo. Clinically it could be advantageous for a PMN to be in a primed state while circulating in the blood stream en route to a site of infection. Upon reaching the site of infection, various signals such as fMLP or cytokines could then promote microbial killing and thus the containment of the infection. It would seem to be disadvantageous to directly stimulate the respiratory burst of circulating PMN since it could lead to the widespread release of toxic metabolites and destruction of normal tissue.

Thus, in summary, GM-CSF has been shown to enhance the adherence and chemotaxis of PMN in vitro. G-CSF and GM-CSF can activate the bactericidal activity of adherent PMN and prime suspended PMN to undergo oxidative metabolism. GM-CSF and G-CSF have also been shown to increase tumoricidal activity and induce immunoglobulin A (IgA)-mediated neutrophil phagocytosis (Weisbart et al. 1988). GM-CSF can augment antibody-dependant cell-mediated immunity. The mechanism for all of these effects is unknown. GM-CSF has been shown to increase arachidonic acid release, leukotriene B_4 synthesis, as well as change Ca^{2+} fluxes and pH (Denzlinger et al. 1990). These effects may play a role in the mechanism of GM-CSF's effect on the functioning of the PMN. GM-CSF induces the synthesis and release of IL-1, G-CSF, M-CSF, and IL-6 from neutrophils. These molecules could then cause an indirect effect on PMN function (Cicco et al. 1990; Lindemann et al. 1989).

GM-CSF is the most potent of the three growth factors that have effects on the functioning of mature neutrophils. These alterations in PMN function may represent direct effects of the CSF on the PMN or indirect effects through some other humoral factor. The clinical importance of these alterations in PMN function is unknown. It has been noted that in the treatment of neutropenic patients with GM-CSF and G-CSF that adverse side effects such as fever, hypotension, venous thrombosis, pleural effusions, and capillary leak syndrome have occurred. These side effects seem to be more marked with GM-CSF and may be the result of its effect on PMN function. It is unclear at this time whether enhanced PMN function seen with CSF is beneficial to the patient or deleterious. Clinical studies need to be performed to answer this question.

References

Arnaout MA, Wang EA, Clark SG, Sieff CA (1986) Human recombinant granulocyte–macrophage colony-stimulating factor increases cell-to-cell adhesion and surface expression of adhesion-promoting surface glycoproteins on mature granulocytes. J Clin Invest 78:597

Cicco NA, Lindemann A, Content J, Vandenbussche P, Lubbert M, Gauss J, Mertelsmann R, Herrmann F (1990) Inducible production of interleukin-6 by human polymorphonucular neutrolphils: role of granulocyte–macrophage colony-stimulating factor and tumor necrosis factor alpha. Blood 75:2049–2052

Denzlinger C, Kapp A, Grimberg M, Gerhartz HH, Wilmanns W (1990) Enhanced endogenous leukotriene biosynthesis in patients treated with granulocyte–macrophage colony-stimulating factor. Blood 76:1765–1770

Fleischmann J, Golde DW, Weisbart RH, Gasson JC (1986) Granulocyte–macrophage colony-stimulating factor enhances phagocytosis of bacteria by human neutrophils. Blood 68:708–711

Lindemann A, Riedel D, Ostee W, Loems Zeileger-Heitbrock HW, Mertelsmann R, Hermann F (1989) Granulocyte–macrophage colony-stimulating factor induces cytokine secretion by human polymorphonuclear leukocytes. J Clin Invest 83:1308–1312

Nathan CF (1989) Respiratory burst in adherent human neutrophils: triggering by colony-stimulating factors CSF-GM and CSF-G. Blood 73:301–306

Peters WP, Stuart A, Affronti ML, Kim CS, Coleman RE (1988) Neutrophil migration is defective during recombinant human granulocyte–macrophage colony-stimulating factor infusion after autologous bone marrow transplantation in humans. Blood 72:1310–1315

Roilides E, Walsh TS, Pizzo PA, Rubin M (1991) Granulocyte colony-stimulating factor enhances the phagocyte and bactericidal activity of normal and defective human neutrophils. J Infect Dis 163:579–583

Sklar LA, Jesaitis AJ, Painter RG, Chochrane CG (1981) The kinetics of neutrophil activation. J Biol Chem 256:9909

Wang JM, Colella S, Allovema P, Mantovani A (1987) Chemotactic activity of human recombinant granulocyte–macrophage colony-stimulating factor. Immunology 60:439

Weisbart RH, Golde DW, Clark SC, Wong GC, Gasson J (1985) Granulocyte–macrophage colony-stimulating factor is a neutrophil activator. Nature 314:361–363

Weisbart RH, Golde DW, Grassen JC (1986) Biosynthetic human GM-CSF modulates the number and affinity of neutrophil f-Met-Leu-Phe receptors. J Immunol 137:3584–3587

Weisbart RH, Kwan L, Golde DW, Grasson JC (1987) Human CSF-GM primes neutrophils for enhanced oxidative metabolism in response to the major physiologic chemoattractants. Blood 69:18

Weisbart RH, Kacena A, Schuh A, Golde DW (1988) CSF-GM induces human neutrophil IgA-mediated phagocytosis by an IgA Fc receptor activation mechanism. Nature 332:647–648

Further Reading

Golde DW, Baldwin GC, Weisbart RH (1990) Responses of neutrophils to myeloid growth factors. 1990 molecular control of haemopoiesis. Wiley, Chichester. Ciba Found Symp 148:62–75
    GM-CSF activates neutrophils and in their studies, increases chemotaxis.

Nathan CF (1989) Respiratory burst in adherent human neutrophils: triggering by colony-stimulating factors CSF-GM and CSF-G. Blood 73:301–306
    Adherent neutrophils were stimulated by both GM-CSF and G-CSF while nonadherent neutrophils were primed.

Roilides E, Walsh TJ, Pizzo PA, Rubin M (1991) Granulocyte colony-stimulating factor enhances the phagocyte and bactericidal activity of normal and defective human neutrophils. J Infect Dis 163:579–583
    G-CSF enhances the ability of neutrophils to kill staphylococci.

Ruef C, Coleman DL (1990) Granulocyte-macrophage colony-stimulating factor: pleiotropic cytokine with potential clinical usefulness. Rev Infect Dis 12:41–62
    A good review of GM-CSF
Weisbart RH, Gasson JC, Golde DW (1989) Colony-stimulating factors and host defense. Ann Intern Med 110:297–303
    A good overview of GM-CSF.

Invasive Aspergillosis: Host Defenses

R.D. Diamond

Section of Infectious Diseases, The University Hospital and Evans Department of
Clinical Research, Boston University Medical Center, 88 E. Newton Street, Boston,
MA 02118, USA

Though species of *Aspergillus* are among the most common fungi in the
environment, invasive aspergillosis is extremely rare in immunocompetent
individuals. The small conidia of these ubiquitous organisms are inhaled
frequently. However, progressive infections ensue only if conditions permit
these conidia to survive, shed their outermost coatings of hydrophobic
rodlet-like structures, then swell and ultimately germinate, and grow as
potentially pathogenic mycelia. Thus, host defense mechanisms can prevent
invasive aspergillosis by killing or blocking the transition and growth of any
one of these sequential phases in morphogenesis (Levitz and Diamond 1984;
Rinaldi 1983; Waldorf 1986; Schaffner et al. 1982).

In general, successful host responses against invasive aspergillosis appear
to rely predominantly on the fungicidal capacities of "nonimmune" phagocytes, including neutrophils, blood monocytes, and resident tissue macrophages (Schaffner et al. 1982; Waldorf et al. 1984; Levitz and Diamond
1985; Kan and Bennett 1991; Waldorf and Diamond 1985; Levitz et al.
1986; Washburn et al. 1987; Levitz and Farrell 1990). This conclusion is
based on studies performed in vitro and in experimental animal models,
as well as defined associations in patients between increased risks of invasive
aspergillosis and factors that impair phagocyte function. For example,
multivariant analyses of clinical series have revealed significant associations
between invasive aspergillosis complicating granulocytopenia in leukemic
patients or high-dose corticosteroid therapy in transplant recipients (Levitz
and Diamond 1984; Rinaldi 1983; Waldorf 1986). Progressive pulmonary
and extrapulmonary aspergillosis also frequently complicates chronic granulomatous disease, in which oxidant-mediated microbicidal responses of
neutrophils and monocytes are defective due to genetically defined abnormalities (Levitz and Diamond 1984; Rinaldi 1983; Waldorf 1986).

When growing in mycelial phase as a natural saprophyte, species of
Aspergillus release large numbers of airborne, hydrophobic conidia. These
ubiquitous conidia are readily inhaled and small enough in size to favor

Recent Results in Cancer Research, Vol. 132
© Springer-Verlag Berlin · Heidelberg 1993

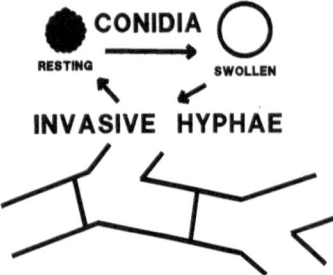

Fig. 1. Life cycle of *Aspergillus* species: small, nongrowing (resting) conidia are released in large numbers by sporulating mycelial phase, filamentous organisms that grow as saprophytes in nature. Upon settling in loci with conditions that favor germination, resting conidia shed their outermost layer of hydrophobic rodlet-shaped structures, swell, and display surface antigens that differ from those of resting conidia. Swollen conidia may then germinate and grow progressively as hyphal filaments that are capable of invading tissues of susceptible hosts. Hyphae within invasive lesions in tissues do not sporulate, though cavitary aspergillomas may provide growth conditions conducive to formation of conidia in vivo, analogous to saprophytic mycelial life cycles in natural habitats

alveolar deposition. If these conidia are deposited at sites where conditions are favorable for growth, they lose their outer surface coats, swell, then germinate to form hyphae which can invade tissues and grow progressively, but only if host defenses fail to function normally (Fig. 1). Differing surface properties of the small, inhaled "resting" conidia, the swollen conidia, and filamentous hyphae evoke distinctive host responses. For example, in the absence of serum opsonins, human neutrophils attach to and ingest resting conidia only minimally (Levitz and Diamond 1985), but human monocytes or murine pulmonary alveolar marcophages readily bind and phagocytose these fungal forms via lectin-like receptors (Kan and Bennett 1991). Activation of complement presumably is crucial to host defenses, both for the genesis of serum-derived chemotactic factors and for opsonization to facilitate neutrophil fungicidal responses (Waldorf et al. 1984; Waldorf and Diamond 1985; Levitz et al. 1986). Compared to swollen conidia and hyphae, resting conidia appear to be relatively inefficient in activating complement and generating C5a-mediated chemotactic activity (Waldorf et al. 1984). While resting conidia activate complement in serum via the alternative pathway, progressive morphogenesis to swollen conidia and hyphae is associated with increasing classical complement pathway activiation (Kozel et al. 1989).

Though opsonization of resting *Aspergillus fumigatus* conidia facilitates phagocytosis by neutrophils, intracellular killing is minimal. In contrast, neutrophils attack and kill opsonized or unopsonized swollen conidia or hyphae (Fig. 2) (Schaffner et al. 1982; Waldorf et al. 1984, Levitz and Diamond 1985; Diamond et al. 1983). Swollen conidia within phagocytic

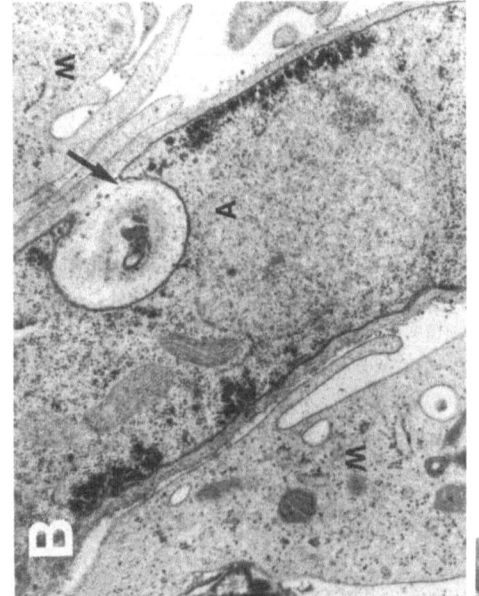

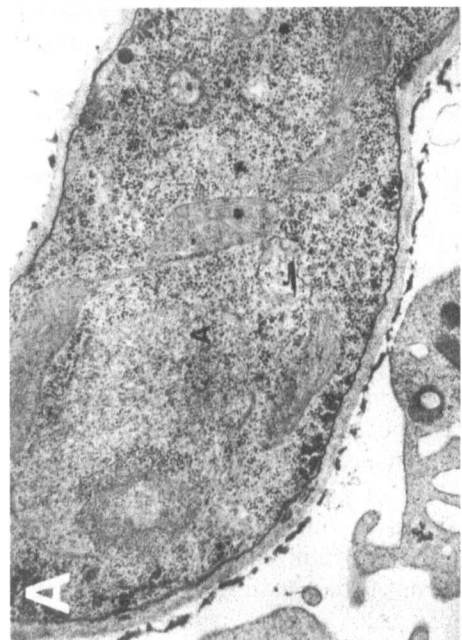

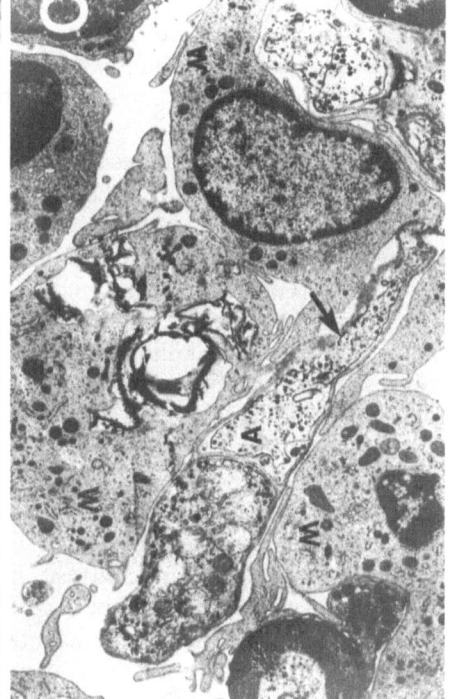

Fig. 2.A–C. Electron micrographs: destruction of large, noningestible *Aspergillus fumigatus* hyphae by cooperative efforts of attacking phagocytic cells. **A** Normal hyphal morphology (*A*) with intact multilayered cell wall, cell membrane, and cytoplasmic organelles prior to attack. **B** Early attack of hypha (*A*) by human peripheral blood monocytes *M*), showing well-defined hyphal cytoplasmic organelles including mitochondria, but areas of cell membrane invagination indicative of beginning damage, C Monocytes *M*) surrounding a destroyed hypha (*A*) after 1 h. Though the hyphal cell wall (including a septum) is clearly demarcated, the cell membrane no longer is closely apposed to the cell wall, mitochondria are disrupted, and neither other organelles nor nuclei are recognizable. (From Diamond et al. 1983)

vacuoles or incompletely ingested hyphae that adhere to neutrophil surfaces both can elicit release of fungicidal products, including oxidants and granule constituents (Levitz et al. 1986; Washburn et al. 1987; Levitz and Farrell 1990). In contrast to normal neutrophils, neutrophils from patients with chronic granulomatous disease cannot generate oxidants and do not kill swollen conidia or hyphae despite unimpaired capacities for surface adherence, ingestion, and degranulation. Similarly, fungicidal activity of normal neutrophils can be ablated by inhibitors of oxidative metabolism or oxidant scavengers (Diamond et al. 1983). Thus, neutrophil fungicidal responses appear to require oxidant generation under normal conditions, though granule constituents such as myeloperoxidase and defensins may have ancillary roles in augmenting the process (Levitz et al. 1986; Washburn et al. 1987; Levitz and Farrell 1990). The inability of mormal neutrophils to kill resting conidia appears to be due to their suboptimal stimulation of neutrophil degranulation and release of oxidants such as superoxide anion, hydrogen peroxide, or hypochlorous acid (Levitz and Diamond 1985; Levitz and Farrell 1990).

Compared to neutrophils, there are distinct differences in responses of mononuclear phagocytes to the various forms of *Aspergillus* (Schaffner et al. 1982; Waldorf et al. 1984; Levitz et al. 1986). Despite their inability to generate oxidants, blood monocytes from patients with chronic granulomatous disease can kill *A. fumigatus* hyphae (Diamond et al. 1983). Human blood monocytes and murine macrophages also have fungicidal activity against resting conidia (Schaffner et al. 1982; Waldorf et al. 1984; Levitz et al. 1986). However, the requirements and time courses for macrophage-mediated killing suggest that swelling of intracellular conidia may be necessary before lethal effects on the organisms can be manifested (Schaffner et al. 1982; Levitz et al. 1986).

The differing capabilities of mononuclear phagocytes and neutrophils provide the potential for cooperative mechanisms in host defenses against aspergillosis. Schaffner et al. (1982) have postulated complementary roles for macrophages and neutrophils in the prevention of invasive aspergillosis. According to that hypothetical model, aspergillosis could progress only under conditions that impaired both macrophage-mediated killing of conidia and neutrophil-mediated killing of hyphae. However, other experimental data suggest complexities in interactions between neutrophils and mononuclear phagocytes. For instance, *A. fumigatus* hyphae can be killed by blood monocytes from either normal subjects or patients with chronic granulomatous disease (Diamond et al. 1983). This monocyte-mediated killing process can be competitively inhibited by the simultaneous addition of neutrophils that lack fungicidal activity either because of genetic defect or by virtue of inhibitory effects. In contrast, mixtures of small numbers of normal neutrophils with larger numbers of neutrophils from patients with chronic granulomatous disease have lethal effects on *A. fumigatus* hyphae, such that the fungicidal activity of these combined cells exceeds hyphal killing by either population of cells separately (Rex et al. 1990).

The hallmark of invasive aspergillosis is pathological evidence of vascular invasion by hyphae, with consequent hemorrhagic necrosis and infarction (Levitz and Diamond 1984; Rinaldi 1983). Thus, though direct data are lacking, it seems likely that vascular endothelium plays a pivotal role in the pathogenesis of invasive aspergillosis. Endothelial cells are endocytic though they appear to lack microbicidal capabilities. In addition, endothelial cells can be triggered to release a wide array of cytokines and other mediators that may modulate both inflammatory responses and thrombotic mechanisms. It will therefore be of critical importance for future studies to begin to define significant interactions of endothelium with *Aspergillus* conidia or hyphae, phagocytic cells, platelets, clotting factors, cytokines, and other potential soluble mediators of inflammation.

The organisms also have the potential to produce a variety of substances that are capable of modifying host responses. For example, *A. fumigatus* hyphae growing in cultures in vitro can release phospholipids that inhibit complement activation (Washburn et al. 1990), in addition to toxins that can inhibit phagocyte function (Eichner et al. 1986), and enzymes with elastase activity that are postulated to enhance invasiveness (Kothary et al. 1984). None of these substances has a firmly established role in the pathogenesis of invasive aspergillosis, but further studies are warranted to determine whether complex interactions between organisms, their products, and host defenses might alter the outcomes of infections in certain circumstances.

Recent studies of patients with chronic granulomatous disease establish that cytokines also can modulate host defenses against aspergillosis. Though data are incomplete and only small numbers of patients have been evaluated, it appears that serious infections in such patients were reduced by administration of $0.05 \, \text{mg/m}^2$ recombinant interferon-gamma three times weekly (International Chronic Granulomatous Disease Study Group 1991). Neutrophils from these interferon-treated patients acquired enhanced abilities to kill *A. fumigatus* hyphae in vitro (Rex et al. 1991).

Clinical experience emphasizes the significant limitations that are inherent in antifungal chemotherapy of opportunistic mycoses in general and invasive aspergillosis in particular. Progressively more detailed characterization of multiple facets of the complex host–parasite interactions in aspergillosis seems likely to increasingly provide new prospects for both prevention and therapy: design of more specific immunosuppressive regimens that reduce risk as well as promising new approaches to augment host responses and enhance the combined efficacy and specificity of antifungal therapy.

References

Diamond RD, Huber E, Haudenschild CC (1983) Mechanisms of destruction of Aspergillus fumigatus hyphae mediated by human monocytes. J Infect Dis 147:474–483

Eichner RD, Al Salami M, Wood PR, Müllbacher A (1986) The effect of gliotoxin upon macrophage function. Int J Immunopharmacol 8:789–797

International Chronic Granulomatous Disease Study Group (1991) A controlled trial of interferon gamma to prevent infection in chronic granulomatous disease. N Engl J Med 324:509–516

Kan LK, Bennett JE (1991) β1,4-Oligosaccharides inhibit the binding of Aspergillus β1,4-oligosaccharides inhibit the binding of Aspergillus fumigatus conidia to human monocytes. J Infect Dis 163:1154–1156

Kothary MH, Chase T Jr, MacMillan JD (1984) Correlation of elastase production by some strains of Aspergillus fumigatus with ability to cause pulmonary invasive aspergillosis in mice. Infect Immun 43:320–325

Kozel TR, Wilson MA, Farrell TP, Levitz SM (1989) Activation of C3 and binding to Aspergillus fumigatus conidia and hyphae. Infect Immun 57:3412–3417

Levitz SM, Diamond RD (1984) Changing patterns of aspergillosis infections. In: Stollerman GH, Harrington WJ, Lamont JT, Leonard JF, Siperstein MD (eds) Advances in internal medicine, vol 30. Yearbook Medical Publishers, Chicago, pp 153–174

Levitz SM, Diamond RD (1985) Mechanisms of resistance of Aspergillus fumigatus conidia to killing by neutrophils in vitro. J Infect Dis 152:33–42

Levitz SM, Farrell TP (1990) Human neutrophil degranulation stimulated by Aspergillus fumigatus. J Leukoc Biol 47:170–175

Levitz SM, Selsted ME, Ganz T, Lehrer RI, Diamond RD (1986) In vitro killing of spores and hyphae of Aspergillus fumigatus and Rhizopus oryzae by rabbit neutrophil cationic peptides and bronchoalveolar macrophages. J Infect Dis 154:483–489

Rex JE, Bennett JE, Gallin JI, Malech HL, Melnick DA (1990) Normal and deficient neutrophils can cooperate to damage Aspergillus fumigatus hyphae. J Infect Dis 162:523–528

Rex JE, Bennett JE, Gallin JI, Malech HL, DeCarlo ES, Melnick DA (1991) In vivo interferon-gamma therapy augments the in vitro ability of chronic granulomatous disease neutrophils to damage Aspergillus hyphae. J Infect Dis 163:849–852, 1991.

Rinaldi MG (1983) Invasive aspergillosis. Rev Infect Dis 5:1066–1077

Schaffner A, Douglas H, Braude A (1982) Selective protection against conidia by mononuclear and against mycelia by polymorphonuclear phagocytes in resistance to aspergillosis: observations on these two lines of defense in vivo and in vitro with human and mouse phagocytes. J Clin Invest 69:616–631

Waldorf AR (1986) Host–parasite relationship in opportunistic mycoses. Crit Rev Microbiol 13:133–172

Waldorf AR, Diamond RD (1985) Neutrophil chemotactic responses induced by fresh and swollen Rhizopus oryzae spores and Aspergillus fumigatus conidia. Infect Immun 48:458–463

Waldorf AR, Levitz SM, Diamond RD (1984) In vivo bronchoalveolar macrophage defense against Rhizopus oryzae and Aspergillus fumigatus. J Infect Dis 150:752–760

Washburn RG, Gallin JI, Bennett JE (1987) Oxidative killing of Aspergillus fumigatus proceeds by parallel myeloperoxidase-dependent and -independent pathways. Infect Immun 55:2088–2092

Washburn RG, DeHart DJ, Agwu DE, Bryant-Varela BJ, Julian NC (1990) Aspergillus fumigatus complement inhibitor: production, characterization, and purification by hydrophobic interaction and thin-layer chromatography. Infect Immun 58:3508–3515

Further Reading

Levitz SM, Diamond RD (1984) Changing patterns of aspergillosis infections. In: Stollerman GH, Harrington WJ, Lamont JT, Leonard JF, Siperstein MD (eds) Advances in internal medicine, vol 30. Yearbook Medical, Chicago, pp 153–174
    General review of clinical aspects of aspergillosis with careful definitions and categorization of infectious and allergic syndromes.
Rinaldi MG (1983) Invasive aspergillosis. Rev Infect Dis 5:1066–1077
    General review of clinical aspects of aspergillosis including excellent summary of mycological aspects.
Waldorf AR (1986) Host–parasite relationship in opportunistic mycoses. Crit Rev Microbiol 13:133–172
    General review of experimental pathogenesis of aspergillosis.

Invasive Aspergillosis: Serologic Diagnosis

V.T. Andriole

Department of Internal Medicine, Yale University School of Medicine,
333 Cedar Street, New Haven, CT 06510, USA

Invasive aspergillosis is a common infection in immunocompromised patients, which, when untreated, is uniformly fatal. Although amphotericin B currently is the drug of choice for invasive aspergillosis, this agent is toxic and is, at times, not successful, particularly in immunosuppressed patients. Early treatment may improve survival (Aisner et al. 1977), but the diagnosis of invasive aspergillosis is difficult to establish because cultures of blood and other body fluids are rarely positive. Serologic techniques have been used in an attempt to establish an antemortem diagnosis of invasive aspergillosis. Initial attempts by our laboratory (Marier et al. 1979) and by others (de Repentigny 1989) were directed at detecting antibody to *Aspergillus*. However, patients at risk for developing invasive aspergillosis often do not develop antibodies to *Aspergillus*, especially early in the course of their infection. Thus, aspergillus antibody has not been helpful as a diagnostic tool for not identifying invasive aspergillosis. Subsequent research in our laboratory, and others, has attempted to diagnose invasive aspergillosis on the basis of circulating aspergillus antigen. The intent has been to develop a reliable method that would establish an early diagnosis which would permit prompt antifungal therapy and an improved clinial outcome.

Aspergillus species are ubiquitous in the environment and are acquired primarily through the respiratory tract, although some cases of disseminated disease have occurred following infection of the skin or gastrointestinal tract. Others have developed as a complication of an invasive procedure, particularly Hickman-type intravenous catheters. *Aspergillus fumigatus* and *flavus* are the most common species that produce infection in humans. Hospital air has often been found to contain aspergillus spores which, when inhaled by immunocompromised patients, may lead to pulmonary infection, sinusitis, and/or disseminated infection. Also, *Aspergillus* spores (conidia) in the operating room air may enter a surgical site for organ transplantation, particularly prosthetic cardiac valves or the eye during cataract surgery. Outbreaks of *Aspergillus* infection have occurred in immunocompromised patients exposed to *Aspergillus* spores during hospital construction. These observations have led to attempts, with some success, to reduce the frequency of *Aspergillus* infection through the use of air filtration.

Although the major cause of invasive pulmonary aspergillosis is thought to be environmental exposure to *Aspergillus* spores, this infection has been thought to occur also as a result of reactivation of endogenous organisms in a few patients during subsequent courses of granulocytopenia (Robertson and Larson 1988).

Since exposure to *Aspergillus* is almost universal, yet this infection is uncommon in nonimmunocompromised patients, normal host defenses appear to be critical in protecting most people from infection. A number of factors, other than environmental exposure, are thought to increase the risk of *Aspergillus* infection. Each of these factors has some detrimental effect on two and possibly three major lines of host defense. Earlier studies have shown that mononuclear phagocytes (macrophages) are a very efficient defense system and kill *Aspergillus* conidia and are thought to constitute the first line of defense. In contrast, polymorphonuclear granulocytes are the main effector cells which provide protection against the mycelial form of *Aspergillus*. Large doses of corticosteroids have been shown to impair killing of conidia by macrophages and to inhibit damage to hyphae by macrophages and mobilization of polymorphonuclear neutrophils (PMNs) around the fungus. Also, impairment of the immune response due to underlying debilitating disease, and/or cytotoxic or immunosuppresive agents may play a role in increasing the risk of *Aspergillus* infection. Recent studies suggest that the most significant of these factors is the duration of granulocytopenia; i.e., the rate of invasive pulmonary aspergillosis increases progressively after the 6th day of granulocytopenia and increases substantially between the 22nd and 36th days of granulocytopenia.

Clinically, infection with *Aspergillus* has been observed in almost every human organ (Denning and Stevens 1990). Invasive aspergillosis is a term used to imply histologic identification of *Aspergillus* hyphae in tissue. Disseminated aspergillosis is used to define active infection in two or more noncontiguous organs. Invasive pulmonary aspergillosis, with or without dissemination, is the most common form of the disease seen in high-risk patients (Saral 1991). Other forms of aspergillosis include cutaneous, paranasal, otomycosis, ocular, osteomyelitis, arthritis, endocarditis, pericarditis, meningitis, brain abscess, epidural abscess, hepatosplenic, adrenal, gastrointestinal, urinary tract, peritonitis, thyroiditis, and lymph node aspergillosis. Diagnosis of invasive aspergillosis is difficult without histologic identification of the organism in tissue. Recent work in our laboratory, however, has demonstrated the utility of a competitive enzyme-linked immunosorbent assay (ELISA) technique which detects small amounts (10 ng/ml) of carbohydrate components of circulating *Aspergillus* antigen in human and rabbit serum (Sabetta et al. 1985). This test is currently being used propsectively to study patients at high risk of developing invasive aspergillosis with the hope that early diagnosis will lead to prompt, aggressive therapy and improve the ultimate outcome of this frequently fatal disease.

Antigen Detection in Invasive Aspergillosis

A number of methods have been developed to detect circulating *Aspergillus* antigen, either free or in the form of immune complexes. Counterimmunoelectrophoresis was used by Lehmann and Reiss (1978) to detect *Aspergillus* polysaccharide antigen in serum. Shaffer et al. (1979a,b) described a radio-immunoassay (RIA) that detected an undefined polysaccharide antigen in the serum of three patients with invasive aspergillosis and in a rabbit model 3 days after infection with *A. fumigatus*. Weiner and Coats-Stephen (1979) also evaluated an RIA to detect circulating *Aspergillus* carbohyrate antigen in experimentally infected rabbits and identified antigen in 78% of animals with invasive aspergillosis. In early clinical studies, Weiner (1980) reported antigenemia detected by RIA in four of seven patients, and in four of six patients in a second study (Weiner et al. 1983). More recently (Talbot et al. 1987), antigen was detected by RIA in 74% of 19 high-risk patients with invasive aspergillosis. They observed that antigenemia was detected prior to clinical suspicion of disease in 30% of patients, and prior to histopathologic or microbiologic evidence of disease in 46% of patients. Their method had a sensitivity of 74%, a specificity of 90%, and a positive and negative predictive value of 82% and 85%, respectively.

Dupont et al. (1987) detected purified *A. fumigatus* galactomannan antigen by RIA and ELISA in the serum of only two of 12 patients, and in the urine of seven of 13 patients with invasive aspergillosis. Furthermore, galactomannan was detected in the serum from only four of 12 lethally infected rabbits, whereas urinary galactomannan was detectable throughout the course of lethal aspergillosis in all 16 rabbits. Both the RIA and ELISA gave comparable results. The difficulty experienced by these investigators in the detection of galactomannan in the serum of lethally infected rabbits was explained by the rapid clearance of *A. fumigatus* galactomannan from the bloodstream via renal excretion and by macrophage mannose receptor-mediated endocytosis by Kupffer cells in the liver (Bennett et al. 1987).

Detection of circulating *Aspergillus* antigen in other experimental animal models of invasive aspergillosis has also been reported by other groups of investigators (Sabetta et al. 1985; de Repentigny et al. 1987; Patterson et al. 1988, 1989b, 1990; Phillips and Radigan 1989; Ste-Marie et al. 1990).

Detection of circulating *Aspergillus* antigen in experimental invasive aspergillosis has been studied extensively in our laboratory (Sabetta et al. 1985; Patterson et al. 1988, 1989b, 1990; Andriole et al. 1992). In our studies, the time course of the appearance of circulating *Aspergillus* antigen following challenge with *A. fumigatus*, as well as the impact of treatment with various antifungal agents on the kinetics of antigenemia and the relationship of antigenemia to the extent of invasive aspergillosis in each animal have been characterized in detail (Sabetta et al. 1985; Patterson et al. 1988, 1989b, 1990; Andriole et al. 1992). Circulating *Aspergillus* antigen is measured by an inhibition ELISA which detects the carbohydrate component of *Aspergillus* antigen in concentrations as low as 10 ng/ml (Sabetta et al. 1985). The antibody used in our method is polyclonal, was prepared in rabbits immunized with *Aspergillus* conidia, and does not cross-react with *Candida* mannan (Sabetta et al. 1985). In no instance are we unable to detect at least 50 ng of *Aspergillus* carbohydrate antigen per milliliter of serum. Thus, our ELISA has been consistently reproducible, with a sensitivity of 63% at 10 ng/ml and 100% at 50 ng/ml. Of note, 500 ng or more of *Aspergillus* carbohydrate antigen per milliliter of serum completely binds all of the available rabbit antibody to *Aspergillus* (Sabetta et al. 1985).

In our rabbit model of invasive aspergillosis, circulating *Aspergillus* antigen first appeared in low concentrations by 48 h after onset of infection, and then in rapidly increasing amounts up to the time of death (Sabetta et al. 1985; Patterson et al. 1988; Andriole et al. 1992). Also, the level of *Aspergillus* antigen in serum correlated with the number of *Aspergillus* organisms per gram of tissue in liver, lung, kidney, and brain. Treatment with the antifungal agents amphotericin B, liposomal amphotericin B, fluconazole, saperconazole, and a combination of amphotericin B plus fluconazole either reduced significantly or eliminated completely the circulating antigen in treated animals as compared with untreated control rabbits. Circulating *Aspergillus* antigen levels in the treated animals correlated directly with the number of *Aspergillus* organisms in tissue and with a reduction in mortality from invasive aspergillosis (Patterson et al. 1988, 1989b, 1990; Andriole et al. 1992). Importantly, the persistence of low levels of *Aspergillus* antigen in the serum of treated animals indicated small numbers of viable *Aspergillus* organisms in tissue. This observation suggested that persistent antigenemia, even at low levels, might be a harbinger of inadequately treated invasive aspergillosis in patients.

A number of investigators (Le Pape and Deunff 1988; Wilson et al. 1987; Johnson et al. 1989; Burnie and Matthews 1989; Rogers et al. 1990), including our own group (Sabetta et al. 1985; Patterson et al. 1989a), have detected circulating *Aspergillus* antigen in patients with proven or highly probable invasive aspergillosis. Some of these patients had localized infection, i.e., invasive pulmonary aspergillosis, whereas others had disseminated infection. This distinction is important with regard to the level of detectable circulating *Aspergillus* antigen, i.e., patients with disseminated disease have higher levels of circulating antigen.

Le Pape and Deunff (1988) found nine of ten patients positive for *Aspergillus* antigen from 28 serum samples using an inhibition ELISA. Wilson et al. (1987) also used an inhibition ELISA to detect *Aspergillus* antigen in three of five bone marrow transplant patients studied retrospectively and one liver transplant patient studied prospectively who died of disseminated aspergillosis proven at autopsy. Circulating antigen was also detected retrospectively in the serum of three other bone marrow transplant patients who died with suspected disseminated aspergillosis. They also observed that tests on single serum samples were often negative, whereas multiple specimens from the same patient increased the frequency of detection. Johnson et al. (1989) detected *Aspergillus* antigenemia, in a retrospective survey, using an inhibition ELISA in three of four bone marrow transplant patients with histopathologically proven invasive aspergillosis and in one patient with suspected infection. No antigen was detected in 17 bone marrow transplant patients without proven or suspected invasive aspergillosis or in 16 healthy control subjects. They also observed that detection of antigen rose with an increasing number of samples tested.

Rogers et al. (1990) evaluated two different inhibition ELISAs to detect serum and urinary *Aspergillus* antigen in 121 neutropenic patients after leukemia therapy or bone marrow transplantation. The anti-*Aspergillus* antibody used was either high-titer human anti-*Aspergillus* serum (polyclonal) or rat IgM monoclonal antibody to *A. fumigatus* galactomannan. Antigen was detected in the serum or urine of 16 of 19 patients early in the course of invasive pulmonary aspergillosis and in 11 of 13 episodes of clinically suspected fungal infection. Significantly more urine samples than sera from patients with invasive pulmonary aspergillosis were positive for antigen. Specifically, with the human anti-*Aspergillus* antibody only 13% of 482 serum samples and 20% of 173 urine samples were positive for antigen; with the rat monoclonal antibody only 18% of 345 serum samples and 44% of 170 urine samples were positive for antigen. Antigen was also detected in one of 90 patients with no evidence of invasive pulmonary aspergillosis. The authors state that antigen detection did not correlate with antifungal therapy or the isolation of *Aspergillus* sp. from sputum or other specimens. However, antigen was detected early in serum or urine in 84% of 19 patients with proven invasive pulmonary aspergillosis, but in only a small percentage of urine and serum samples obtained from these patients throughout the course of their disease. These discordant observations are not easily explained.

In a prospective study in febrile neutropenic patients who failed to respond to broad spectrum antibiotics, Burnie and Matthews (1989) used a latex agglutination method to detect circulating *Aspergillus* antigen. Antigen was detected in the initial serum sample in only five of 20 histopathologically proven cases of invasive aspergillosis, and in seven of 13 with suspected infection, whereas antigen was detected in terminal serum specimens in 12 of the 20 proven cases and in 11 of the suspected cases. Thus an early false-negative result was obtained in 21 of 33 of the proved or suspected cases of invasive aspergillosis. In only 12 cases was there a reasonable level of detectable antigen in the initial serum sample. Currently, a latex agglutination test is commercially available in Europe.

Clinical studies from our laboratory use an inhibition ELISA (Sabetta et al. 1985) which we developed to detect circulating *Aspergillus* carbohydrate antigen in serum. Circulating antigen was detected in 11 of 19 patients with invasive aspergillosis proven histopathologically at autopsy or by biopsy when the method was applied retrospectively to single serum samples from each patient. No circulating antigen was detected in serum from 34 patients with *Candida albicans* sepsis, 28 patients with other non-*Aspergillus* infections, and 18 healthy control hospital personnel. In a follow-up study from our group, Patterson et al. (1989a) determined the positive predictive value of *Aspergillus* antigen testing with our modified inhibition ELISA by reviewing our laboratory records for a 2-year period and identifying all patients with 50 ng or more of antigen detected per milliliter of serum. We identified 30 patients, all of whom were immunosuppressed, with at least one serum sample positive for over 50 ng of *Aspergillus* antigen per milliliter. Histopathologically proven invasive aspergillosis was present in 16 of the 30 patients (57%), and they had maximal antigen values of 70–3500 ng/ml; seven of the 30 had probable invasive aspergillosis defined by a positive culture for *Aspergillus* sp. and a clinical illness compatible with the disease; 20% had an indeterminate diagnosis, defined by no microbiologically proven cause of infection in the presence of persistent fever despite antibiotic therapy; and there was no evidence of invasive aspergillosis in only one of the 30 patients. However, there were no false-positive results in 23 of these 30 patients who had serial serum samples tested and who had 50 ng of antigen or more per milliliter of serum. In addition, when the maximal antigen values detected in patients with proven invasive aspergillosis were analyzed, those with proven *disseminated* aspergillosis had a median antigen value of 600 ng/ml, which was significantly higher than the median antigen value of 93 ng/ml seen in patients with proven invasive *pulmonary* aspergillosis. Also, the course of antigenemia in these patients correlated with outcome. Specifically, 18 of 23 patients with proven or probable invasive aspergillosis had serial serum samples tested for *Aspergillus* antigen. Clearance of antigenemia was seen in five patients and all five survived their infection. In contrast, persistent or rising *Aspergillus* antigen levels were seen in 13 patients and all 13 patients died of invasive aspergillosis. In this study, the positive predictive value of our method for proven or probable invasive aspergillosis was 77% and may be as high as 97% if all patients with a proven, probable, or an indeterminate diagnosis are true positives (Patterson et al. 1989a). Our observations suggest that, with our method, detection of 50 or more ng/ml of aspergillus antigen in the serum of patients is highly predictive of invasive aspergillosis and that a rise or fall in antigenemia correlates with the clinical course of this infection. Furthermore, higher antigen values are seen in disseminated disease.

Significant progress has been made in the serodiagnosis of invasive aspergillosis. The present data does not support serial antibody determinations in patients with invasive aspergillosis as an optimal diagnostic test for the early detection of this infection. In contrast, antigen detection, by the testing of serial samples in serum or urine in high-risk patients by inhibition ELISA or possibly other methods, offers promise as a moderately sensitive but highly specific method of detecting early infection in many high-risk patients. Importantly, the detection of *Aspergillus* antigen in serum and urine is increased by testing frequently obtained samples, dissociating immune complexes in the method employed, and by developing a sensitive assay technique. A major use of antigen detection, at least in our experience, may be in guiding treatment. Although correlation of antigen levels in predicting remission or relapse of infection has not been established, our preliminary observations suggest that falling *Aspergillus* antigen levels in the serum of patients with invasive aspergillosis on proper antifungal therapy correlate with survival from this frequently fatal infection.

References

Aisner J, Schimpff SC, Wiernik PH (1977) Treatment of invasive aspergillosis: relation of early diagnosis and treatment to response. Ann Intern Med 86:539–543

Andriole VT, Miniter P, George D et al. (1992) Animal models: their usefulness for studies of fungal pathogenesis and drug efficacy in aspergillosis. Rev Infect Dis (in press)

Bennett JE, Friedman MM, Dupont B (1987) Receptor-mediated clearance of aspergillus galactomannan. J Infect Dis 155:1005–1010

Burnie JP, Matthews RC (1989) Recent laboratory observations in the diagnosis of systemic fungal infection: Candida and Aspergillus. In: Holmberg K, Meyer R (eds) Diagnosis and therapy of systemic fungal infections. Raven, New York, p 101

Denning DW, Stevens DA (1990) Antifungal and surgical treatment of invasive aspergillosis: review of 2121 published cases. Rev Infect Dis 12:1147–1201

de Repentigny L (1989) Serologic techniques for diagnosis of fungal infection. Eur J Clin Microbiol Infect Dis 8:362–375

de Repentigny L, Boushira M, Ste-Marie L et al. (1987) Detection of galactomannan antigenemia by enzyme immunoassay in experimental invasive aspergillosis. J Clin Microbiol 25:863–867

Dupont B, Huber M, Kim SJ et al. (1987) Galactomannan antigenemia and antigenuria in aspergillosis: studies in patients and experimentally infected rabbits. J Infect Dis 155:1–11

Johnson TM, Kurup VP, Resnick A et al. (1989) Detection of circulating Aspergillus fumigatus antigen in bone marrow transplant patients. J Lab Clin Med 114:700–707

Lehmann PF, Reiss E (1978) Invasive aspergillosis: anti-serum for circulating antigen produced after immunization with serum from infected rabbits. Infect Immun 20:570–572

Le Pape P, Deunff J (1988) Detection of aspergillus glycoprotein antigen in sera of patients with invasive aspergillosis: an enzyme-linked immunosorbent assay inhibition technique. In: Drouhet E, Cole GT, de Repentigny L et al. (eds) Fungal antigens, 1st international symposium. Plenum, New York, p 382

Marier R, Smith W, Jansen M et al. (1979) A solid-phase radioimmunoassay for the measurement of antibody to Aspergillus in invasive aspergillosis. J Infect Dis 140:771–779

Patterson TF, Miniter P, Ryan JL et al. (1988) Effect of immunosuppression and amphotericin B on Aspergillus antigenemia in an experimental model. J Infect Dis 158:415–422

Patterson TF, Miniter P, Andriole VT (1989a) Predictive value of serum Aspergillus antigen detection in the diagnosis of invasive aspergillosis. 89th Annual meeting of the American Society for Microbiology, New Orleans, 14–18 May, 1989, p 458

Patterson TF, Miniter P, Dijkstra J et al. (1989b) Treatment of experimental invasive aspergillosis with novel amphotericin B/cholesterol-sulfate complexes. J Infect Dis 159:717–724

Patterson TF, Miniter P, Andriole VT (1990) Efficacy of fluconazole in experimental invasive aspergillosis. Rev Infect Dis 12:S281–S285

Phillips P, Radigan G (1989) Antigenemia in a rabbit model of invasive aspergillosis. J Infect Dis 159:1147–1150

Robertson MJ, Larson RA (1988) Recurrent fungal pneumonias in patients with acute nonlymphocytic leukemia undergoing multiple courses of intensive chemotherapy. Am J Med 84:233–239

Rogers TR, Haynes KA, Barnes RA (1990) Value of antigen detection in predicting invasive pulmonary aspergillosis. Lancet 336:1210–1213

Sabetta JR, Miniter P, Andriole VT (1985) The diagnosis of invasive aspergillosis by an enzyme-linked immunosorbent assay for circulating antigen. J Infect Dis 152:946–953

Saral R (1991) Candida and aspergillus infections in immunocompromised patients: an overview. Rev Infect Dis 13:487–492

Shaffer PJ, Kobayashi GS, Medoff G (1979a) Demonstration of antigenemia in patients with invasive aspergillosis by solid phase (protein A-rich Staphylococcus aureus) radioimmunoassay. Am J Med 67:627–630

Shaffer PJ, Medoff G, Kobayashi GS (1979b) Demonstration of antigenemia by radioimmunoassay in rabbits experimentally infected with Aspergillus. J Infect Dis 139:313–319

Ste-Marie L, Senechal S, Boushira M et al. (1990) Production and characterization of monoclonal antibodies to cell wall antigens of Aspergillus fumigatus. Infect Immun 58:2105–2114

Talbot GH, Weiner MH, Gerson SL et al. (1987) Serodiagnosis of invasive aspergillosis in patients with hematologic malignancy: validation of the Aspergillus fumigatus antigen radioimmunoassay. J Infect Dis 155:12–27

Weiner MH (1980) Antigenemia detected by radioimmunoassay in systemic aspergillosis. Ann Intern Med 92:793–796

Weiner MH, Coats-Stephen M (1979) Immunodiagnosis of systemic aspergillosis: I. Antigenemia detected by radioimmunoassay in experimental infection. J Lab Clin Med 93:111–119

Weiner MH, Talbot GH, Gerson SL et al. (1983) Antigen detection in the diagnosis of invasive aspergillosis utility in controlled, blinded trials. Ann Intern Med 99:777–782

Wilson EV, Hearn VM, Mackenzie DWR (1987) Evaluation of a test to detect circulating Aspergillus fumigatus antigen in a survey of immunocompromised patients with proven or suspected invasive disease. J Med Vet Mycol 25:365–374

Further Reading

Andriole VT, Miniter P, George D et al. (1992) Animal models: their usefulness for studies of fungal pathogenesis and drug efficacy in aspergillosis. Clin Infect Dis (in press)

Denning DW, Stevens DA (1990) Antifungal and surgical treatment of invasive aspergillosis: review of 2121 published cases. Rev Infect Dis 12:1147–1201 de Repentigny L (1989) Serologic techniques for diagnosis of fungal infection. Eur J Clin Microbiol Infect Dis 8:362–375

Sabetta JR, Miniter P, Andriole VT (1985) The diagnosis of invasive aspergillosis by an enzyme-linked immunosorbent assay for circulating antigen. J Infect Dis 152:946–953

Saral R (1991) Candida and aspergillus infections in immunocompromised patients: an overview. Rev Infect Dis 13:487–492

Aspergillosis in the Immunocompromised: Focus on Treatment

M. Aoun, P. Van der Auwera, J. Gèrain, and J. Klastersky

Service de Médecine Interne et Laboratoire d'Investigation, Clinique Henri Tagnon, Clinique des Maladies Infectieuses et Laboratoire de Microbiologie. Institut Jules Bordet, Centre des Tumeurs de l'Université Libre de Bruxelles, rue Héger-Bordet 1, 1000 Bruxelles, Belgium

Invasive aspergillosis, mainly due to *Aspergillus fumigatus* and *Aspergillus flavus*, is one of the most common fatal infections in the immunocompromised host; 25%–40% of autopsy cases in hematologic malignancies have invasive aspergillosis, with more than 80% of them being unrecognized during life (Young et al. 1970). In the normal host, inhaled *Aspergillus* conidia are first phagocytized by alveolar macrophages. Those which escape phagocytosis sporulate and grow into large branching septated hyphae, which can invade lung tissues, but usually they are destroyed by the tissue neutrophils. Therefore, the patients most susceptible to aspergillosis are those with profound and prolonged granulocytopenia, especially those undergoing induction chemotherapy for acute leukemia, intensive chemotherapy for lymphoma, or bone marrow transplantation (Table 1). Patients with defective neutrophil function, particularly those with chronic granulomatous disease, are also at great risk of aspergillosis, as well as those with impaired macrophage function, such those receiving immunosuppressive therapy for organ transplantation or high-dose corticosteroids for vasculitides or connective tissue diseases. Recently, aspergillosis has been reported increasingly among acquired immunodeficiency syndrome (AIDS) patients; traditional factor risks including neutropenia, hematologic malignancies, and corticosteroid therapy were present in the majority of these patients (Pursell et al. 1992).

The management of invasive aspergillosis remains a challenge because of the frequent delay in diagnosis and the poor response to therapy. Among the factors that influence the outcome, restoration of host defenses is probably the most important: discontinuation of immunosuppressive therapy and acceleration of recovery from neutropenia are determinant but rarely feasible factors. Antifungal therapy acts most likely as a stabilizer rather than effectively eliminating the infection until recovery from neutropenia; patients who do not achieve remission are at great risk of dying from their infection, despite adequate treatment. Arising from a better knowledge and awareness

Recent Results in Cancer Research, Vol. 132
© Springer-Verlag Berlin · Heidelberg 1993

Table 1. Groups at risk of invasive aspergillosis

Neutropenia: PMN < 1000/µl
- Chemotherapy
- Congenital agranulocytosis
- Drug-induced agranulocytosis
- Cyclic neutropenia
- Felty syndrome
- AIDS

Defective neutrophil function
- Chronic granulomatous disease
- Secondary: leprosis, leishmaniasis, cancer, etc.

Defective macrophage function
- Immunosuppressive therapy for organ transplantation
- High-dose corticosteroids

---

of the disease, early initiation of treatment seems to be beneficial (Burch et al. 1987).

The two primary sites of infection are the lungs and the paranasal sinuses. Clinical manifestations include persistent or recurring fever despite broad-spectrum antibacterial therapy, cough, and pleuritic chest pain. Dyspnea and hypoxia appear late (Cohen 1991). Facial swelling and/or tenderness, nasal discharge, and epistaxis indicate acute sinusitis (Talbot et al. 1991). Chest and sinus computed-tomographic scans are superior to standard X-rays and may help early diagnosis and initiation of treatment. Sputum culture is positive in about one third of proven cases. Dissemination of *Aspergillus* to almost all the major organs has been reported in the compromised host, with varying degrees of frequency, and is often an autopsy finding (Young et al. 1970). The hematogenous route has been suggested, although local extension to adjacent tissues, from the lungs to the vertebra, pleura, pericardium, ribs, and chest wall, or from the paranasal sinuses to the orbit and frontal cortex, have all been described.

The treatment of invasive aspergillosis is mainly medical. Adjunctive surgery is indicated in some specific situations (Denning and Stevens 1990).

During the recent years, the armamentarium of antifungal drugs active against *Aspergillus* spp. has grown. In addition to standard amphotericin B, new formulations have been developed including amphotericin B lipid complexes (ABLC) (Clark et al. 1991), amphotericin B colloidal dispersion (ABCD), and amphotericin B entrapped in liposomes. New modalities of local amphotericin B administration are being developed. The amphotericin B nose spray has been well tolerated and decreased *Aspergillus* nasal colonization in neutropenic patients. However, the rate of definite or possible *Aspergillus* infection was not significantly decreased, probably due to *Aspergillus* colonization of the lower respiratory tract. An amphotericin B aerosol might overcome this problem in the future. Encapsulated amphotericin

B in liposomes potentially provides protection against mucosal damage of Fungizone (amphotericin) and the possibility of pulmonary macrophage activation. Lung scintigraphy using a liposomal aerosol labeled with ^{99}mTC demonstrated homogeneous distribution (unpublished results). Among the imidazoles, itraconazole – a new triazole – is the only derivative active against *Aspergillus* spp. Terbinafine, a new synthetic allylamine derivative, is one of the most promising drug against *Aspergillus* spp. based on in vitro activity. Cilofungin, although not active in vitro against *Aspergillus* spp., demonstrated in vivo activity equivalent to amphotericin B in an immuno-competent mouce model of aspergillosis. Concomitantly with the discovery and development of new anti-*Aspergillus* agents, immunotherapy is being applied to the treatment of fungal infections. With the availability of growth factors and cytokines, stimulation of host cells has become a possibility and may become an essential adjunctive therapy of aspergillosis in the future.

Susceptibility Testing and Animal Studies

In vitro susceptibility tests are essential for the monitoring of therapy in serious bacterial infections. Unfortunately, such an application for systemic fungal infections, including invasive aspergillosis, is still not reliable.

Three methods have been applied to *Aspergillus* susceptibility testing: broth dilution, agar dilution, and disk sensitivity tests (Shadomy and Pfaller 1991). Recently, a major effort has been made to standardize these methods by fixing the inoculum size by spectrophotometry; and standardizing the medium composition and its pH, the temperature of incubation, and the time of reading. Antifungal drugs do not give clear-cut MIC endpoints and tend to show partial inhibitory activity over a wide range of concentration. Expected ranges of MIC and minimal fungicidal concentration (MFC) values of amphotericin B against *Aspergillus* spp. including *Aspergillus fumigatus* vary between 0.05 to 8 µg/ml, and 6.25 to more than 100 µg/ml, respectively (Shadomy and Pfaller 1991). MIC values above 2.5 µg/ml suggest possible resistance since achievable serum concentrations for conventional ampho-tericin B do not exceed this value. Using a microdilution method, Anaissie et al. (1991) found comparable MIC values of conventional and liposomal amphotericin B against 13 *Aspergillus* spp. Mean values were 2.5 and 1.25 µg/ml, respectively (Anaissie et al. 1991).

MIC values for 5-fluorocytosine vary between 0.2 and 1.56 µg/ml and MFC values are above 100 µg/ml (Shadomy and Pfaller 1991). 5-Fluorocytosine resistance among *Aspergillus* strains is not an uncommon finding. Itraconazole is highly active in vitro against *Aspergillus* spp. with MIC values ranging between 0.3 and 2.5 µg/ml and MFC values between 0.3 and >10 µg/ml.

Terbinafine is an inhibitor of squalene epoxidase, a key enzyme in ergosterol biosynthesis. Both free terbinafine and liposome-encapsulated terbinafine showed comparable MIC values ranging between 1.2 and 2.5 µg/ml against

20 strains of *Aspergillus fumigatus*. The addition of human serum to the medium significantly increased the MIC values. No fungicidal activity has been detected (unpublished results).

In vitro synergy between amphotericin B and 5-fluorocytosine is well established against *Cryptococcus neoformans* and *Candida* spp. Against *Aspergillus* spp. the situation is less clear. Lauer et al. (1978) found only indifference when this combination was tested against *Aspergillus* spp., while Kitahara et al. (1976) demonstrated synergistic activity against *Aspergillus fumigatus*, but only additive activity against *Aspergillus flavus*. A combination of itraconazole and 5-fluorocytosine, when tested in vitro against *Aspergillus* spp., resulted in variable effects; synergistic inhibitory activity was demonstrated with some isolates, while additive effects or indifferences were found with others. Possible fungicidal antagonistic activity was observed in some isolates of *Aspergillus fumigatus*.

Correlation between MIC values and clinical outcome has been suggested for *Candida* spp. by the reports of Powderly et al. (1988) and Radetsky et al. (1986). To the best of our knowledge, there is no such information for *Aspergillus* spp. Several animal models of aspergillosis have been developed. Few of them are relevant for human disease, except a pneumonia model in which amphotericin B, at doses varying between 1 mg/kg per day and 5 mg/kg per day, demonstrated efficacy in the immunocompromised guinea pig, the neutropenic rabbit, and mice. Invasive aspergillosis in a rabbit model has been successfully treated with amphotericin B–cholesterol sulfate complexes. ABLC was as effective as Fungizone in an immunosuppressed murine model in terms of increased survival time and decreased fungal burden in kidneys and lungs (Clark et al. 1991). The activity of 5-fluorocytosine in animal models of aspergillosis has been minimal (Denning and Stevens 1990). Itraconazole was reported to be effective in a murine model of aspergillosis when the conidia were injected intravenously, while intranasal administration resulted in failure. In another experiment where mice, immunosuppressed with triamcinolone, were challenged intravenously with 10^5 spores of *Aspergillus fumigatus*, itraconazole failed to prolong survival or clear the lungs (Clark et al. 1991). In a neutropenic guinea pig model, following intravenous challenge with *Aspergillus fumigatus*, and in a rabbit model of *Aspergillus* endocarditis, itraconazole at 5 mg/kg per day was superior to amphotericin B.

Management

The term "immunocompromised" encompasses quite a few different situations. They are illustrated by the many variables that influence the outcome of invasive aspergillosis:

1. The nature of underlying diseases: lymphoma and leukemia are associated with poor response; kidney transplant recipients have a better outcome (Green et al. 1991).
2. The status of a given underlying disease: patients in remission have a better prognosis than those who are not.
3. The degree of neutropenia and/or immunosuppression: patients with a decreasing WBC at the time of infection have a poorer outcome than those whose WBC is increasing.
4. The primary site of infection and sites of dissemination: cerebral involvement has the most severe outcome (Green et al. 1991).
5. The time of initiation of the antifungal treatment: early initiation resulted in a better outcome (Burch et al. 1987).

These variables probably account for the discrepancies in mortality rates reported in the literature which vary from 13% to more than 80%. Therefore, all these parameters must be taken into account when evaluating the efficacy of antifungal drugs in the treatment of invasive aspergillosis.

Amphotericin B

The recommended daily dose of amphotericin B in invasive aspergillosis has increased during the recent years, up to 1–1.5 mg/kg per day, based on the fact that pulmonary aspergillosis has still developed in neutropenic patients receiving a dose of 0.5 mg/kg per day. As far as amphotericin B administration is concerned, a test dose of 1 mg diluted in 100 ml 5% dextrose is usually infused over 30 min. If tolerated, the full dose is then given, without escalation, over 6 h. Some patients tolerate the drug well without any premedication. Patients who develop acute toxicity, with fever, chills, nausea, or vomiting should be premedicated with pethidine and antiemetics; hydrocortisone administration is avoided as much as possible. Saline loading seems to be protective against nephrotoxicity; potassium leakage will be replaced as needed. Increase of serum creatinine of more than 3 mg/dl precludes further administration as long as the serum creatinine level is above that value and, if needed after a transitory withdrawal, amphotericin B can be resumed at a lower daily dose. In general, with a total dose lower than 4 g, nephrotoxicity is reversible. The optimal duration of treatment is not well defined; it is calculated in terms of total cumulative dose rather than in days of therapy. A total dose of 2 g has been recommended in neutropenic patients, provided that all signs and symptoms of infection have disappeared.

The interpretation of the chest X-ray might be more problematic. In general, a fibrotic scar may persist for months and is only indicative of a sequella. A nodular lesion with a halo sign on a chest computer-tomographic scan or a cavitary lesion are indicative of an active lesion. In some cases, invasive aspergillosis will result in a persisting aspergilloma, which is refractory to medical treatment and may require surgical removal.

When compared to conventional amphotericin B in healthy volunteers, ABLC caused fewer acute adverse events, except for mild somnolence. Ambisomes, at a daily dose of 3–5 mg/kg, have been well tolerated and nephrotoxicity was unusual, occurring only in conjunction with simultaneous nephrotoxic drugs such as aminoglycosides and cyclosporine (Meunier et al. 1991). No controlled study has yet established the efficacy of these new formulations in comparison to conventional amphotericin B; a few uncontrolled trials have reported success in cases of proven invasive aspergillosis. Of five neutropenic patients who failed to respond to conventional amphotericin B, three responded to further Ambisome therapy (Chopra et al. 1991). Ringden et al. (1991) has administered Ambisomes to 28 immunocompromised patients with proven aspergillosis; 32% of them were cured, although these patients had received various amounts of conventional amphotericin B prior to Ambisome therapy initiated for nephrotoxicity rather than for failure in most of the cases.

Serum amphotericin B levels of the new lipid preparations have been variable. Some preparations (Ambisome, ABLC) resulted in higher concentrations than the conventional preparation, while others (ABCD) resulted in lower levels. In aspergillosis, tissue concentrations might be more important for the outcome; however, we and others have shown that only a small fraction of the tissue-bound amphotericin B is bioactive (Christiansen et al. 1985). Similar findings were observed with ampholiposomes prepared in our institution (Collette et al. 1991).

With Ambisomes, the tissue distribution of amphotericin B shows high concentrations in liver and spleen, whereas low concentrations are found in the kidneys and lungs as compared with the conventional drug; this may explain the relatively modest cure rate of 32% with Ambisome in aspergillosis (Ringden et al. 1991).

Itraconazole

Preliminary clinical experience is encouraging. Oral treatment with 200 or 400 mg itraconazole daily has been successful in treating invasive aspergillosis in organ transplant recipients and patients with hematologic malignancies; 60%–80% response rates have been reported. Higher doses, 600 mg daily, were given to a limited number of patients with serious fungal infections; adrenal insufficiency was noted in one patient; hypokalemia, mild edema, and hypertension in five. This probably constitutes the upper limit of what can be given (Sharkey et al. 1991). Variable absorption between individuals, as well as in the same individual over time, has been reported; poor absorption in neutropenic patients has been documented. Reduced gastric acidity decreases the absorption of itraconazole; it is better absorbed after food intake. The half-life is approximately 17 h and the protein-binding about 98%. An intravenous formulation has recently become available for clinical trials: this may overcome the problem of erratic absorption of the oral drug.

Surgery

In some specific situations, surgery is a major contribution to the management of aspergillosis. In *Aspergillus* endophtalmitis, vitrectomy is helpful for diagnosis and treatment, allowing slow instillation of 5 or 10 µg amphotericin B. This is essential because the penetration of systemically administered amphotericin B into the eye is poor (Roney et al. 1986).

Aspergillus endocarditis is more frequent in the nonimmunocompromised, usually affecting prosthetic valves, but it can also occur in the neutropenic patient with disseminated disease; early valve replacement is indicated. Surgical debridement in *Aspergillus* osteomyelitis and resection of epidural abscess are indicated and resection of a well-encapsulated accessible brain abcess constitutes an adequate approach; mycotic aneurysm is also an indication for surgery. Unfortunately, the majority of cases of cerebral aspergillosis in the immunocompromised patient are part of a disseminated disease, with multiple abcesses in many organs. In addition, these patients are often thrombopenic, and it is not uncommon that cerebral aspergillosis goes undetected until premortem hemorrage occurs.

A localized pulmonary nodule, persisting after an episode of invasive aspergillosis and prior to further chemotherapy-induced neutropenia or before marrow transplantation, can be considered for surgery; aspergilloma, with recurrent hemoptysis, is another indication for surgery.

Enhancement of Host Defenses

In order to palliate the relative lack of efficacy of antifungal drugs in the immunocompromised host with aspergillosis, investigators have tried to enhance host defenses. Historically, granulocyte transfusion was the first to be applied in this setting; many factors have contributed to discredit it: (a) the high number of granulocytes required daily; (b) the functional effectiveness of these cells, depending on the method of harvesting; (c) the risk of cytomegalovirus transmission; (d) the danger of allo-immunization; (e) the lecoagglutinin reactions with pulmonary edema; and (f) the lack of controlled studies. Colony-stimulating factors (CSF; granulocyte CSF, G-CSF; macrophage CSF, M-CSF; and granulocyte–macrophage CSF, GM-CSF) are glycoproteins which are responsible for the proliferation and maturation of progenitor cells into fully differentiated phagocytes. In vitro, enhancement of respiratory burst activity and microbial killing by neutrophils (G-CSF and GM-CSF) and macrophages (M-CSF and GM-CSF) have been reported. In vivo, shortening the period of neutropenia and enhancement of the phagocytic cell functions should theoretically result in a better outcome of patients with invasive fungal infections.

A few cases of *Aspergillus* infections, treated concomitantly with antifungal drugs and growth factors, have been reported. Nemunaitis et al. (1991) treated five patients with $100-2000\,\mu g/m^2$ per day of recombinant human (rh) M-CSF; three had a resolution of infection but one patient failed to respond and another was not evaluable. Of concern was the dose-related thrombocytopenia observed in that study. Another trial using rh GM-CSF reported two cases of treated invasive aspergillosis; one patient improved and the other died from the infection (Anaissie et al. 1989). In summary, definitive conclusions must await the results of controlled ongoing trials.

Interferon-γ can enhance the oxidative metabolism and the bactericidal activity of phagocytes in patients with leishmaniasis, cancer, leprosy, AIDS, and in some, but not all, patients with chronic granulomatous disease (CGD). Invasive aspergillosis accounts for 16% of all infections in CGD patients, with a mortality rate approaching 50%. A controlled trial of interferon-γ vs. placebo in the prevention of infection in CGD clearly showed a benefit in favor of interferon-γ therapy. Aspergillosis occurred in 1.6% of the interferon-γ group in comparison to 6% in the placebo group (International CGD Cooperative Study Group 1991). Recombinant human interferon-γ has also been used successfully in the treatment of a CGD patient with invasive aspergillosis unresponsive to conventional amphotericin B. Larger trials are needed in order to confirm these encouraging preliminary data and to determine whether other groups at risk could benefit from interferon-γ therapy.

Conclusion

It has become clear that in future the management of invasive aspergillosis will be based on a multidisciplinary approach. Antifungal therapy and enhancement of host defenses will have to be conducted simultaneously, with adjunctive surgery when indicated.

References

Anaissie E, Bodey GP, Obrien S, Gutterman J, Vadhan-Raj S (1989) Effect on granulocyte-macrophage colony-stimulating factor (GMCSF) on myelopoiesis and disseminated mycoses in neutropenic patients with hematologic malignancies. Blood 74 [Suppl 1]:15A

Anaissie E, Paetznick V, Proffitt R, Adler-Moore J, Bodey GP (1991) Comparison of the in vitro antifungal activity fo free and liposome-encapsulated amphotericin B. Eur J Clin Microbiol Infect Dis 10:665–668

Burch PA, Karp JE, Merz WG, Kuhlman JE, Fishman EK (1987) Favorable outcome of invasive aspergillosis in patients with acute leukemia. J Clin Oncol 5:1985–1993

Chopra R, Blair S, Strang J, Cervi P, Patterson KG, Goldstone AH (1991) Liposomal amphotericin B (Ambisome) in the treatment of fungal infections in neutropenic patients. J Antimicrob Chemother 28 [Suppl B]:93–104

Christiansen KJ, Bernard EM, Gold JWM, Armstrong D (1985) Distribution and activity of amphotericin B in humans. J Infect Dis 152:1037–1043

Clark JM, Whitney RR, Olsen SJ, George RJ, Swerdel MR, Kunselman L, Bonner DP (1991) Amphotericin B lipid complex therapy of experimental fungal infections in mice. Antimicrob Agents Chemother 35:615–621

Cohen J (1991) Clinical manifestations and management of aspergillosis in the compromised patient. In: Warnock DW, Richardson MD (eds) Fungal infection in the compromised patients. Wiley, New York, pp 118–152

Collette N, van der Auwera P, Meunier F, Lambert C, Sculier JP, Coune A (1991) Tissue distribution and bioactivity of amphotericin B administered in liposomes to cancer patients. J Antimicrob Chemother 27:535–548

Denning DW, Stevens DA (1990) Antifungal and surgical treatment of invasive aspergillosis: review of 2.121 published cases. Rev Infect Dis 12:1147–1201

Green M, Wald ER, Tzakis A, Todo S, Starzl TE (1991) Aspergillosis of the CNS in a pediatric liver transplant recipient: case report and review. Rev Infect Dis 13:653–657

International Chronic Granulomatous Diseases Cooperative Study Group (1991) A controlled trial of interferon gamma to prevent infection in chronic granulomatous disease. N Engl J Med 324:509–516

Kitahara M, Seth VK, Medoff G, Koboyashi GS (1976) Activity of amphotericin B, 5-fluorocytosine, and rifampicin against six clinical isolates of Aspergillus. Antimicrob Agents Chemother 9:915–919

Lauer BA, Reller LB, Schroter GP (1978) Susceptibility of Aspergillus to 5-fluorocytosine and amphotericin B alone and in combination. J Antimicrob Chemother 4:375–380

Meunier F, Prentice HG, Ringden O (1991) Liposomal Amphotericin B (Ambisome): safety data from a phase II/III clinical trial. J Antimicrob Chemother 28 [Suppl B]:83–92

Nemunaitis J, Meyers JD, Buckner CD, Shannon-Dorcy K, Mori M, Shulman H, Bianco JA, Higano CS, Groves E, Storb R, Hansen J, Appelbaum FR, Singer JW (1991) Phase I trial of recombinant human macrophage colony-stimulating factor in patients with invasive fungal infections. Blood 78:907–913

Powderly WG, Kobayashi GS, Herzig GP, Medoff G (1988) Amphotericin B-resistant yeast infection in severely immunocompromised patients. Am J Med 84:826–832

Pursell KJ, Telzak EE, Armstrong D (1992) Aspergillus species colonization and invasive disease in patients with AIDS. Clin Infect Dis 14:141–148

Radetsky M, Wheeler RC, Roe MH, Todd JK (1986) Microtiter broth dilution method for yeast susceptibility testing with validation by clinical outcome. J Clin Microbiol 24:600–606

Ringden O, Meunier F, Tollemar J, Ricci P, Tura S, Kuse E, Viviani MA, Gorin NC, Klastersky J, Fenaux P, Prentice HG, Ksionsky G (1991) Efficacy of amphotericin encapsulated in lipsomes (Ambisome) in the treatment of invasive fungal infections in immunocompromised patients. J Antimicrob Chemother 28 [Suppl B]:73–82

Roney P, Barr CC, Chun CH, Raff MJ (1986) Endogenous Aspergillus endophtalmitis. Rev Infect Dis 8:955–958

Shadomy S, Pfaller MA (1991) Laboratory studies with antifungal agents: susceptibility tests and quantitation in body fluids. In: Balows A, Hausler WJ Jr, Herrmann

KL, Isenberg HD, Shadomy HJ (eds) Manual of clinical microbiology. American Society for Microbiology, Washington

Sharkey PA, Rinaldi MG, Dunn JF, Hardin TC, Fetchick RJ, Graybill JR (1991) High-dose itraconazole in the treatment of severe mycoses. Antimicrob Agents Chemother 35:707–713

Talbot GH, Huang A, Provencher M (1991) Invasive aspergillus rhinosinusitis in patients with acute leukemia. Rev Infect Dis 13:219–232

Young R, Bennett JE, Vogel R, Carbone P, DeVita V (1970) Aspergillosis: the spectrum of disease in 98 patients. Medicine (Baltimore) 49:147–173

Further Reading

Denning DW, Stevens DA (1990) Antifungal and surgical treatment of invasive aspergillosis: review of 2121 published cases. Rev Infect Dis 12:1147–1201
An extensive and detailed analysis of all forms of invasive aspergillosis treatment, including the review of 379 cases in the literature with sufficient treatment information. Unfortunately, exclusion of patients who received less than 14 days of treatment somewhat decreases the accuracy of results.

Talbot GH, Huang A, Povencher M (1991) Invasive Aspergillus rhinosinusitis in patients with acute leukemia. Rev Infect Dis 13:219–232
Excellent review that stresses the importance of *Aspergillus* rhinosinusitis, another major site of *Aspergillus* infection in leukemic patients, and discusses its different modalities of treatment and prevention.

Cohen J (1991) Clinical manifestations and management of aspergillosis in the compromised patient. In: Warnock DW, Richardson MD (eds) Fungal infection in the compromised patients. Wiley, New York, pp 118–152
The clinical presentation of invasive aspergillosis according to the site of infection is well summarized in this article. The different methods of diagnosis are reviewed. Amphotericin B remains the drug of choice. Combination with 5-fluorocytosine is not recommended, according to the author's view.

Collette N, van der Auwera P, Meunier F, Lambert C, Sculier JP, Coune A (1991) Tissue distribution and bioactivity of amphotericin B administered in liposomes to cancer patients. J Antimicrob Chemother 27:535–548
This is the first study that evaluates the tissue distribution of amphotericin B entrapped in liposomes. Tissue distribution and bioavailability of amphotericin B do not seem to be altered by the liposomal formulation.

Invasive Candidiasis During Granulocytopenia

E. Anaissie and H. Pinczowski

The University of Texas M. D. Anderson Cancer Center, Texas Medical Center,
1515 Holcombe Boulevard, Houston, TX 77030, USA

Candidiasis remains the most frequently encountered fungal infection in granulocytopenic patients (Horn et al. 1985; Crislip and Edwards 1989). Its increasing frequency has been documented from several institutions and seems highest among patients with acute leukemia. With the advent of newer forms of anticancer therapy, disseminated candidiasis is now more frequently recognized in patients with chronic lymphocytic leukemia receiving fludarabine phosphate and in patients with various malignancies treated with high doses of cytotoxic chemotherapy with autologous bone marrow transplantation.

For many years, *Candida albicans* and *Candida tropicalis* were responsible for the vast majority of these infections. In recent years, other species such as *Candida parapsilosis*, *Candida lusitaniae*, *Candida krusei*, and others have emerged as important pathogens in cancer patients (Maksymiuk et al. 1984). While these agents are less virulent than *C. albicans* or *C. tropicalis*, they can, in the host at risk, cause life-threatening infection. With the introduction of antifungal prophylaxis with the newer triazoles, it is possible that this trend for infection with non-*C. albicans* species will further accentuate, and that *C. krusei* and *Torulopsis glabrata* will account for an increasing number of cases of disseminated candidiasis.

Several factors predispose patients to disseminated candidiasis. Cellular defects and ulcerations of the skin, oropharynx, and gastrointestinal tract are all known predisposing factors. Any defect in one of these factors may predispose to infections, although it is not unusual that patients suffer from multiple defects simultaneously. Neutropenia is probably the most important factor responsible for the increased frequency of disseminated candidiasis (Bodey 1966). Patients are at greatest risk for disseminated candidiasis when their neutrophil count falls below 100 cells per microliter and when this profound neutropenia persists for more than 1 week. In addition, the trend of neutrophil count is an important determinant of the course of this infection: a rising count during therapy is associated with a more favorable prognosis

Recent Results in Cancer Research, Vol. 132
© Springer-Verlag Berlin · Heidelberg 1993

than a count that continues to decrease or one that remains low. The ulcerations caused by cancer chemotherapeutic agents in the oropharynx and along the entirety of the gastrointestinal tract set the stage for colonization and invasion by *Candida* species. It is well established that broad-spectrum antibacterial agents, particularly those that achieve a high concentration in the gastrointestinal tract and that have good activity against Gram-negative anaerobes, result in a substantial increase in the gastrointestinal concentrations of *Candida* species. This increased concentration, together with ulcerations following cytotoxic chemotherapy, may lead to disseminated candidiasis.

Other factors known to predispose to *Candida* infection in cancer patients include adrenal corticosteroids, abdominal surgery, and concomitant diabetes mellitus. Whether central venous catheterization and the administration of total parenteral nutrition predispose to disseminated candidiasis remains controversial, although most reviews implicate these factors in the pathogenesis of disseminated infection.

Once colonization with *Candida* species occurs, infections may disseminate to various organs. The most frequent source of disseminated infection is the gastrointestinal tract (Rose and Kurup 1977) as the integrity of the oropharyngeal and gastrointestinal epithelium is disrupted by chemotherapeutic agents such as cytosine arabinoside. After colonizing the injured areas, fungi migrate into the bloodstream. Persorption has also been considered as a potential mechanism of disseminated infection (Stone et al. 1973). Persorption of *C. albicans* has been demonstrated in dogs and monkeys, and a surgeon who actually drank the organisms became fungemic and very ill. Intravenous catheters have been implicated as a source of infection. Data to support such hypotheses are, however, lacking.

The spectrum of disseminated candidiasis includes both an acute and a chronic presentation. Acute disseminated candidiasis may be sudden in onset and usually evolves over days with skin lesions, fungemia, and sometimes shock, while the chronic form of the infection – referred to as hepatosplenic candidiasis – extends over several months and is characterized by progressive debilitation. Despite these differences, it is wise to consider these two aspects of disseminated candidiasis as a continuum. While it is believed that the chronic infection usually follows an acute episode, the chronic syndrome may also convert into an acute infection when the patient's immune status suffers further deterioration. Chronic disseminated candidiasis is being recognized with increasing frequency (Anaissie et al. 1991). Typically, the patient has a hematological malignancy and acquires the infection after he/she has received myelosuppressive chemotherapy. The infection is usually diagnosed after the patient has recovered from the myelosuppression but has persistent fever, unresponsive to broad-spectrum antibacterial agents. Deep-seated abscesses of liver, spleen, kidneys, and lungs can be best identified by computerized tomography, and the infection confirmed by biopsy or isolation of the organism from an otherwise sterile site. This infection (a) has been reported with increasing frequency; (b) is responsible for significant delays in the therapy for the underlying malignancy; (c) is highly fatal without therapy; and (d) is difficult to diagnose and treat, and frequently requires long-term combination chemotherapy with amphotericin B plus 5-flucytosine. Only 50% of patients respond to amphotericin B with or without 5-flucytosine, with a significant number of patients succumbing to infection despite antifungal therapy (Thaler et al. 1988). While the previously used terminology of "hepatosplenic candidiasis" suggests that the infection is limited to liver and spleen, the clinicopathological features of this syndrome clearly indicate that the infection involves multiple organs. A more appropriate descriptive term is "chronic disseminated candidiasis." This is not a purely semantic issue, but has important diagnostic and therapeutic implications. Rather than focusing on a "hepatosplenic infection," a disseminated process would imply careful clinical and laboratory evaluation of its extension to various organs, and continuing therapy until infection at all sites, including the extraabdominal ones, has responded. A disseminated process would also imply that agents that distribute widely in body tissues should be given serious consideration for the treatment of this infection.

Acute disseminated candidiasis has a more rapidly progressive clinical picture and usually refers to the presence of infection with *Candida* species at two or more noncontiguous sites. In the proper clinical setting, the presence of multiple deep-seated cutaneous lesions due to *Candida* species is also indicative of disseminated infection even if the blood specimens fail to yield the organism (Bodey and Luna 1974). Furthermore, the isolation of *Candida* species from the bloodstream of a patient with persistent profound neutropenia (<100 PMN/μl for more than 7 days) is usually, although not always, indicative of disseminated infection.

Questions may arise as to whether overlap exists between some of the features of chronic disseminated candidiasis and those observed in acute disseminated candidiasis, and whether chronic disseminated candidiasis represents the same disease process as hepatosplenic candidiasis. Significant overlap is expected between the features of chronic disseminated candidiasis and acute disseminated candidiasis as both syndromes represent a continuum of disseminated infection with *Candida* species, with chronic disseminated candidiasis following acute disseminated candidiasis, perhaps as the use of "early amphotericin B may be changing the pattern of disseminated candidiasis in some patients" (Thaler et al. 1988). Similarly, chronic disseminated candidiasis may convert into acute disseminated candidiasis when the patient's immune status suffers further deterioration. An analogy can be made with the syndrome of graft-versus-host disease (GVHD) as chronic GVHD may be an extension of acute GVHD with a different clinical picture and yet significant overlap. Also, the clinicopathological features of chronic disseminated candidiasis presented in this series are no different from those reported in the literature describing hepatosplenic candidiasis. Both syndromes evolve over several months, respond poorly to amphotericin B, have similar histopathological findings, and have evidence of disseminated infection which may include bloodstream, kidneys, lungs, bile, liver, spleen, peritoneal fluid, cerebrospinal fluid, urine, pleural fluid, soft tissue, and heart, as reported in three recently published manuscripts.

The distinction between acute disseminated candidiasis and candidemia may be difficult. Granulocytopenic patients with bloodstream involvement of *Candida* species are very likely to have disseminated candidiasis. The issue of catheter-related candidemia is somewhat confusing and usually refers to the presence of candidemia in a patient with a central venous catheter. Whether the catheter and the hyperalimentation fluids are the primary source of the infection or whether the catheter has been seeded from a remote source remains unknown. Evidence supporting or negating the role of the catheter in the pathogenesis or persistence of the infection is lacking. Hence, optimal management of bloodstream *Candida* infections in this setting remains to be defined. Two studies from the pediatric literature suggest the need for catheter removal because of the then higher rate of complication and death (Eppes et al. 1989; Dato and Dajani 1990). Both studies, however, included very few patients and were retrospective in nature. Furthermore, data on important predictors of outcome in acute disseminated candidiasis – the degree of immunosuppression, the performance status of the host, and the fungal burden – were not available. On the other hand, it is important to recognize that the gastrointestinal tract is the most likely primary source of the infection in the neutropenic cancer patient, that acute disseminated candidiasis can be reproduced in experimental animals after colonization of the gastrointestinal tract with *Candida* species, and that management of bloodstream *Candida* infections in this setting has been successfully done with the catheter left in place (D. Armstrong, personal communication; E. Anaissie, personal experience). Furthermore, it is our personal experience that in this setting of persistent profound neutropenia, repeated removals of central venous catheters fail to improve overall outcome because most patients with disseminated candidiasis in this setting will die of their infection unless recovery from myelosuppression occurs quickly. It should be kept in mind that routine catheter removal may interfere with the medical management of these seriously ill cancer patients by depriving them of much needed and often difficult to replace venous access. It is our opinion that the management of *Candida* bloodstream infections in neutropenic cancer patients does not usually require removal of the central venous catheter unless clearcut evidence of septic thrombophlebitis is present.

In the surgical patient, the most likely primary source of candidiasis appears to be the gastrointestinal tract. The passage of *Candida* through an intact mucosal barrier into the lymphatic or portal venous circulation has been proposed as a mechanism of candidal bloodstream infection. This process is referred to as "persorption." Its clinical relevance, however, remains unclear. What appears to be a more accepted view is the dissemination of *Candida* species via subtle mucosal damage that occurs in a variety of medical and surgical illnesses. An abnormality in nodal killing of translocated organisms has been recognized in patients with serious burns.

A major obstacle to the successful management of disseminated candidiasis is our inability to establish a diagnosis ante mortem. Isolation of *Candida* species from the bloodstream may not always indicate disseminated multiorgan involvement. Yet disseminated infection may be present despite repeatedly negative blood cultures. It is likely that the availability of the lysis–centrifugation technique has increased our ability to diagnose bloodstream *Candida* infections.

Limited information is available regarding the treatment of disseminated candidiasis. Given the inability to establish this diagnosis, empiric therapy with antifungal agents has become standard practice for the management of neutropenic patients with persistent fever unresponsive to antibacterial antibiotics.

One study evaluated neutropenic patients who had fever of unknown origin for 1 week after receiving an antibacterial regimen (Pizzo et al. 1982). Patients were randomly assigned to continue the same antibacterial regimen, to discontinue all antibacterial therapy, or to receive amphotericin B in addition. Significantly fewer fungal infections were documented in the group of patients receiving amphotericin B. Another prospective study randomized patients who remained febrile after 4 days of antibacterial therapy to continue the same antibacterial regimen or to receive amphotericin B in addition. The subsequent response rates were 53% and 69%, respectively ($p = 0.09$) (EORTC International Antimicrobial Therapy Cooperative Group 1989). Empiric amphotericin B therapy is clearly indicated for some patients but, unfortunately, many patients without fungal infection suffer the toxicities of amphotericin B unnecessarily. In addition, amphotericin B deoxycholate may not be well available to fungi. Despite the presence of high drug concentrations in various tissues of cancer patients examined at autopsy, and despite the good in vitro susceptibility of these fungi to the drug, patients still died of disseminated fungal infections and had extensive mycoses at autopsy examination (Christiansen et al. 1985). In another study of cancer patients succumbing to fungal infections, amphotericin B was detected in very small concentrations in kidneys and lungs, which are usual sites of serious mycoses; fungicidal concentrations of the drug were seldom achieved in tissues, and the drug was poorly biodiffusable and bioavailable (Collette et al. 1989). Since no prospective studies have addressed the role of amphotericin B in acute disseminated candidiasis, one must rely on retrospective analysis of patients treated with this drug. Overall, a 45% response rate has been reported from a cumulative review of the literature. A recent study indicated that no significant differences in survival could be observed between patients with disseminated candidiasis who received amphotericin B and those who did not (Koshian et al. 1989). While this was a retrospective study, it nonetheless indicated the serious limitations of amphotericin B, particularly in severely immunocompromised patients. On the other hand, another retrospective study indicated that early use of amphotericin B decreased the mortality related to fungal infection and reduced the incidence of disseminated mycoses and the frequency of persistent fungemia (Lecciones et al. 1989). The apparent lack of activity in severely ill patients has been further compounded by the emergence, albeit rarely, of resistance to amphotericin B in this patient population (Powderly et al. 1989).

Other agents that could be useful for the treatment of systemic mycoses include 5-flucytosine. However, a high failure rate and secondary emergence of resistance have been reported when 5-flucytosine was used alone in cryptococcosis, and serious concerns exist regarding the myelosuppressive potential of this drug. A review of the literature on the activity of 5-flucytosine in acute disseminated candidiasis and candidemia indicates a good response rate. Based on the pharmacokinetics of 5-flucytosine and on the in vitro susceptibility of *Candida* species to the drug, it is likely that much lower doses of 5-flucytosine will maintain serum and tissue levels significantly above the minimal inhibitory concentration (MIC) of most susceptible strains throughout the course of therapy. For example, a dose of 50 mg/kg per day given at 6-h intervals would result in peak serum and trough levels of around 50 and 10 µg/ml, respectively, assuming a steady state and a normal kidney function in a 70-kg male patient. Since the MIC of 5-flucytosine for most susceptible *Candida* species is usually less than 1 µg/ml, such a dosage schedule will probably constitute appropriate therapy, particularly since the drug is used in combination with other antifungals. This approach may decrease the myelosuppressive potential of this drug and may lead to its wider use.

Yet another family of promising antifungal agents is that of the triazoles, such as itraconazole, fluconazole, SCH 39304, and saperconazole. These agents have clearly demonstrated significant in vivo activity against various mycoses (Saag and Dismukes 1988). In our experience, fluconazole achieved an 88% response rate in a series of 16 cancer patients with chronic disseminated candidiasis who had failed to respond to adequate doses of amphotericin B ($\geq$2 g) or had significant dose-limiting toxicities (Anaissie at al. 1991). This good response was even seen in those patients who had failed to respond to large doses of amphotericin B and in patients who continued to receive cytotoxic chemotherapy for their underlying leukemia. Similar responses were seen in another series of patients with the same syndrome. Fluconazole also produced a 70% response rate in a series of patients with acute disseminated candidiasis and/or candidemia cared for at our institution (unpublished observation).

Given the overall poor response of fungal infections to antifungals, novel approaches are required. These include the use of higher, maximal tolerated doses of antifungal agents, combination antifungal therapy, and the addition of colony-stimulating factors to antifungals. In addition, antifungal prophylaxis should be given consideration. In a prospective randomized double-blind placebo-controlled multicenter study in patients undergoing bone marrow transplantation, prophylaxis with fluconazole (400 mg/day) effectively prevented fungal infections including superficial and disseminated candidiasis. The frequent colonization by *T. glabrata* of patients receiving ketoconazole prophylaxis raises the concern regarding the potential for resistant fungal superinfection, such as *C. krusei* and *T. glabrata*. Antifungal prophylaxis with oral polyenes (amphotericin B or nystatin) has not been shown to be consistently effective and is not well tolerated.

Summary

Candidiasis remains the most frequently encountered fungal infection in patients with profound granulocytopenia and appears to be increasing in frequency. In addition, *Candida* infections are occurring earlier during remission induction chemotherapy and can be caused by a variety of species such as *C. albicans*, *C. tropicalis*, and *C. krusei*. The most frequent source of disseminated infection is the gastrointestinal tract, as the integrity of the epithelium is disrupted by chemotherapeutic agents. The spectrum of disseminated candidiasis comprises both an acute and a chronic presentation (also known in the literature as hepatosplenic candidiasis). The management of disseminated infection consists of early empiric antifungal therapy with a standard agent, amphotericin B. Unfortunately, responses in the setting of profound granulocytopenia appear to be poor. Other agents that appear to be useful in the management of disseminated candidiasis include 5-flucytosine and fluconazole. Based on animal experimentation, it appears that the combination of these three classes of agents might produce superior results compared with amphotericin B alone. Removal of the central venous catheter does not appear warranted in the setting of profound granulocytopenia, and the role of colony stimulating factors needs to be defined. Given the severity and high mortality associated with disseminated candidiasis in patients with hematologic malignancies, antifungal prophylaxis appears warranted.

References

Anaissie E, Bodey GP, Kantarjian H (1991) Fluconazole therapy for chronic disseminated candidiasis in patients with leukemia and prior amphotericin B therapy. Am J Med 91:142–150

Bodey GP (1966) Fungal infections complicating acute leukemia. J Chronic Dis 19:667–687

Bodey GP, Luna M (1974) Skin lesions associated with disseminated candidiasis. JAMA 229:1466–1468

Christiansen KJ, Bernard EM, Gold JWM, Armstrong D (1985) Distribution and activity of amphotericin B in humans. J Infect Dis 152:1037–1043

Collette N, Auwera V, Lopez AP, Heymans C, Meunier F (1989) Tissue concentrations and bioactivity of amphotericin B in cancer patients treated with amphotericin B-deoxycholate. Antimicrob Agents Chemother 33:362–368

Crislip MA, Edwards JE (1989) Candidiasis. Infect Dis Clin North Am 1:103–133

Dato VM, Dajani AS (1990) Candidemia in children with central venous catheters: role of catheter removal and amphotericin B therapy. J Pediatr Infect Dis 9:309–314

EORTC International Antimicrobial Therapy Cooperative Group (1989) Empiric antifungal therapy in febrile granulocytopenic patients. Am J Med 86:668–672

Eppes SC, Troutman JL, Gutman LT (1989) Outcome of treatment of candidemia in children whose central catheters were removed or retained. J Pediatr Infect Dis 8:99–104

Horn R, Wong B, Kiehn TE, Armstrong D (1985) Fungemia in the immunocompromised host: changing frequency, earlier onset, and results of therapy. Rev Infect Dis 7:646–655

Komshian SV, Uwaydah AK, Sobel JD, Crane LR (1989) Fungemia caused by Candida species and Torulopsis *glabrata* in the hospitalized patient: frequency, characteristics, and evaluation of factors influencing outcome. Rev Infect Dis 11:379–390

Lecciones J, Witebsky F, Marshall D, Gress J, Pizzo P, Walsh TJ (1989) Catheter-associated fungemia in cancer patients: characteristics and clinical outcome. In: Program and abstracts of the 29th interscience conference on antimicrobial agents and chemotherapy, American Society for Microbiology 112 (abstr 68)

Maksymiuk AW, Thongrasert S, Hopfer R, Luna M, Fainstein V, Bodey GP (1984) Systemic candidiasis in cancer patients. Am J Med 77:20–27

Pizzo PA, Robichaud KJ, Gill FA, Witebsky FB (1982) Empiric antibiotic and antifungal therapy for cancer patients with prolonged fever and granulocytopenia. Am J Med 72:101–111

Powderly WG, Kobayashi GS, Herzig GP, Medoff G (1988) Amphotericin B resistant yeast infection in severely immunocompromised patients. Am J Med 84:826–832

Rose HD, Kurup VP (1977) Colonization of hospitalized patients with yeast-like organisms. Sabouraudia 15:251

Saag MS, Dismukes WE (1988) Azole antifungal agents: emphasis on new triazoles. Antimicrob Agents Chemother 32:1–8

Stone HH, Geheber CE, Kolb LD et al. (1973) Alimentary tract colonization by Candida albicans. J Surg Res 14:273

Thaler M, Pastakia B, Shawker TH, O'Leary T, Pizzo PA (1988) Hepatic candidiasis in cancer patients: the evolving picture of the syndrome. Ann Intern Med 108:88–100

Further Reading

Armstrong D (1989) Problems in the treatment of opportunistic fungal infections. In: Holmberg K, Meyer RD (eds) Diagnosis and therapy of systemic fungal infections. Raven, New York, pp 149–158

This review analyzes the problems in the diagnosis and treatment of serious mycoses in the immunocompromised host imcluding candidiasis, aspergillosis, mucormycosis, cryptococcosis, the endemic mycoses, and the newly emerging pathogens.

Bodey GP (1986) Infection in cancer patients: a continuing association. Am J Med 81 [Suppl 1A]:11–26

A comprehensive review of infections and host defense defects which complements this chaper.

Bodey GP, Fainstein V (1985) Systemic candidiasis. In: Bodey GP, Fainstein V (eds) Candidiasis. Raven, New York, pp 135–168
    Summary article on the frequency of, predisposing factors for, clinical signs and symptoms and management of systemic candidiasis.
Goodrich JM, Reed EC, Mori M, Fisher LD, Skerrett S, Dandliker PS, Klis B, Counts GW, Meyers JD (1991) Clinical features and analysis of risk factors for invasive candidal infection after marrow transplantation. J Infect Dis 164:731–740
    A review of risk factors for invasive candidiasis among 1506 bone marrow transplant patients at the Fred Hutchinson Cancer Research Center. Tissue involvement was associated with a 90% mortality with or without fungemia. Risk factors for infection were increased age, graft-versus-host disease, and donor mismatch.
Klastersky J, Schimpff SC (eds) (1989) International conference on supportive care in oncology. Eur J Cancer Clin Oncol 25:1343–1391
    Based on a symposium which emphasized issues related to intensive chemotherapy of cancer.
Pizzo PA (1988) Diagnosis and management of infectious disease problems in the child with malignant disease. In: Rubin RH, Young LS (eds) Clinical approach to infection in the compromised host. Plenum, New York, pp 439–464
    This chapter discusses the appropriate approach for the management of febrile and granulocytopenic patients, including diagnosis and antibiotic treatment.
Schimpff SC, Klastersky J, Gaya H (eds) (1986) Therapy of immunocompromised hosts (symposium). Am J Med 80:1–119
    A broad-based series covering basic and clinical concerns in therapy with emphasis on granulocytopenic patients and current controversies such as combination versus monotherapy.
Wade JC, Schimpff SC (1985) Epidemiology and prevention of Candida infection. In: Bodey GP, Fainstein V (eds) Candidiasis. Raven, New York, pp 111–133
    This chapter discusses the various aspects of the pathogenesis, mechanisms of infection, protal of invasion, and prevention of candidal infections.
Walsh TJ, Pizzo PA (1988) Treatment of systemic fungal infections: recent progress and current problems. Eur J Clin Microbiol 7:460–475
    This review summarizes the current problems in diagnosing fungal infections and the emergence of newer fungi as serious pathogens and discusses antifungal chemotherapy with special emphasis on specific therapy of the various mycoses.
Zinner SH, Klastersky J (1985) Infectious considerations in cancer. In: Calabresi P, Schein PS, Rosenberg SA (eds) Medical oncology: basic principles and clinical management of cancer. Macmillan, New York, pp 1327–1357

IV. Infections and Cellular Immune Dysfunction

Infections in Cancer Patients with Suppressed Cellular Immunity

J. Klastersky

Service be Médecine Interne et Laboratoire d'Investigation Clinique H. Tagnon, Institut Jules Bordet, 1 rue Héger-Bordet, 1000 Bruxelles, Belgium

Immunologic Effects of Neoplasic Disease

Patients with advanced neoplasms of any type are likely to have nonspecific defects in both humoral and cellular immunity which may contribute to their increased risk of serious infection. More specific defects in T cell- or B cell-mediated immune function may be inherently present in a variety of untreated neoplastic disorders. Abnormalities in the cellular-mediated immune system have been described as inherent features of some untreated neoplasms.

Patients whose primary immune defect is altered cell-mediated immunity are at increased risk of disseminated infections with intracellular bacteria such as *Mycobacterium tuberculosis*, *Listeria monocytogenes*, *Salmonella* species, and *Brucella* species. These patients are also at special risk of contracting DNA viral infections such as cytomegalovirus, herpes simplex virus, and varicella zoster virus. Patients with T cell defects are also at risk of acquiring yeast infections and, in particular, meningitis and pulmonary infection with *Cryptococcus neoformans*, and disseminated infection with *Candida* species, *Torulopsis glabrata*, *Mucor* and *Aspergillus* species. Specific alterations in T cell function, such as altered ratio of T helper to T suppressor lymphocytes, have been associated with increased risk of pneumonia from *Pneumocystis carinii*. Other organisms, such as *Toxoplasma gondii* and Nocardia asteroides, also may cause disseminated infection in these patients.

The acquired immunodeficiency syndrome (AIDS), described in 1981, has been seen primarily in young homosexually active men, intravenous drug addicts, Haitian refugees, and patients with hemophilia. Cases have also occurred in recipients of blood transfusions and in sexual contacts with high-risk persons. These patients present with Kaposi's sarcoma and/or opportunistic infections caused by *P. carinii*, herpes virus hominis, cytomegalovirus, *Candida albicans*, *C. neoformans*, *M. tuberculosis*, *Mycobacterium avium intracellulare*, *Cryptosporidium* species, *Isospora belli*, *Toxoplasma gondii*, and so forth Cerebral and other lymphomas have been described.

Recent Results in Cancer Research, Vol. 132
© Springer-Verlag Berlin · Heidelberg 1993

The syndrome is associated with anergy to recall and new skin test antigens, lymphopenia, with reduced numbers and depressed function of the T4 subset of T lymphocytes. The syndrome is due to a lymphotrophic retrovirus designated as human T lymphotrophic virus III (HTLV-III), AIDS-associated virus (LAV or HIV). Currently, no treatment is available and the mortality rate is mainly associated with opportunistic infections.

Alteration in B lymphocyte immune function is likely to occur in patients with untreated chronic lymphocytic leukemia, multiple myeloma, and Waldenström's macroglobulinemia. Patients with acute myelocytic leukemia and acute lymphocytic leukemia before treatment and patients with Hodgkin's disease before splenectomy, irradiation, or chemotherapy have intact B cell immunity, although the numbers of normal B cells may be reduced in some individuals with lymphocytic leukemia. Since B cell immunity mediates humoral or antibody-related immunity, immunoglobulin antibody levels may be decreased, and these patients may exhibit decreased responsiveness to antigenic stimulation. Patients with multiple myeloma have increased levels of immunoglobulin which dose not react with bacterial antigens and does not protect against infection. These patients, as well as those with Waldenström's macroglobulinemia, have decreased polyclonal immunoglobulin response to bacterial antigens.

Patients with defects in humoral antibody are most susceptible to infection with encapsulated bacteria such as *Streptococcus pneumoniae*, *Haemophilus influenzae*, *Neisseria meningitidis*, and *Klebsiella pneumoniae*.

Radiation therapy, as well as corticosteroids and several chemotherapeutic agents, may produce cellular immune defects by means of lympholytic or other actions. Splenectomy patients may have deficient complement production and may also have limited ability to opsonize and clear bacterial pathogens. Combination of chemotherapy, splenectomy, and radiation therapy may predispose patients to overwhelming infection with encapsulated bacterial pathogens, such as *S. pneumoniae* and *H. influenzae*. Extensive surgery, often necessary for advanced invasive tumors, may predispose to infection by removing large areas of otherwise protective tissue.

Infections in Patients with Impaired Cellular Immunity

Patients with neoplastic disorders may be immunosuppressed for a few days to several weeks or months, depending on the nature of therapy directed at the primary disease. A variety of opportunistic infections may occur, and there is some overlap with infections occurring in neutropenic patients. More than one organism may cause infection at the same or separate sites in immunosuppressed patients. Pathogens are shown in Table 1 and approaches to therapy are shown in Table 2. What follows is a discussion of specific infection types.

Table 1. Some likely pathogens in patients with cancer and impaired cellular immunity

Bacteria
   Legionella pneumophila
   Mycobacterium tuberculosis
   Atypical mycobacteria
   Listeria monocytogenes
   Salmonella species
Fungi
   Cryptococcus neoformans
   Nocardia asteroides
   Candida species
   Torulopsis glabrata
   Aspergillus species
   Mucor species
Protozoa
   Pneumocystis carinii
   Toxoplasma gondii
   Isopora belli
   Cryptosporidium species
Viruses
   Herpes simplex virus
   Varicella zoster virus
Helminth
   Strongyloides stercoralis

Table 2. Treatment of infections in immunosuppressed patients with cancer

Condition or organism	Suggested agents
Legionella pneumophila	Erythromycin, rifampin
Listeria monocytogenes	Ampicillin ± aminoglycoside, erythromycin
Mycobacterium tuberculosis	Isoniazid, rifampin, cthambutol, streptomycin
Nocardia asteroides	Sulfonamides, trimethoprim sulfamethoxazole
Candida species	Oral: nystatin, ketoconazole
	Systemic: amphotericin B, fluoconazole
Aspergillus species	Amphotericin B
Mucor, Rhizopus	Amphotericin B
Crytpococcus neoformans	Amphotericin B
Varicella zoster virus, Herpes simplex virus	Vidarabine, acyclovir
Cytomegalovirus (CMV)	Ganciclovir ± CMV immune globulin
Pneumocystis carinii	Trimethoprim sulfamethoxazole, pentamidine isethionate
Isospora	
Toxoplasma gondii	Pyrimethamine and sulfonamide
Strongyloides stercoralis	Thiabendazole

Pneumonitis

Pulmonary infiltrates are extremely common in febrile patients with depressed cellular immunity *M. tuberculosis*, atypical *Mycobacteria*, *Nocardia asteroides*, *Legionella pneumophila* and other species, *Candida* species, *Phycomycetes*, *C. neoformans*, *Histoplasma capsulatum*, *Coccidioides immitis*, herpes simplex virus, cytomegalovirus, varicella zoster, *P. carinii*, *T. gondii*, and *Strongyloides stercoralis* may produce pneumonitis in these patients. Few specific diagnostic clinical or radiologic clues exist. Fever and nonproductive cough are usually present with all of these infections. Significant early hypoxia is most suggestive of *P. carinii* infection, but this may also occur with cytomegalovirus, varicella zoster, *Legionella* species, and other bacterial infections. X-ray film findings are rarely diagnostic, but certain patterns are suggestive. Lobar or bronchopneumonic infiltrates are consistent with bacterial pneumonia and infection with *Candida* species, *Aspergillus* species, and the *Phycomycetes*. Interstitial infiltrates are usually observed with viral and protozoan infections. Cavitation occurs with mycobacterial and nocardial infections, but may also be seen with *Aspergillus*, *Cryptococcus*, *Phycomycetes*, and, rarely, with *Legionella* infections. Nodular infiltrates may occur with *Mycobacteria*, *Nocardia*, *Aspergillus*, *Cryptococcus*, varicella zoster, cytomegalovirus, *Strongyloides*, and, rarely, with *P. carinii*.

In most series, bilateral diffuse interstitial infiltrates in the immunosuppressed patient are caused by *P. carinii*, but other entities such as cytomegalovirus infection, herpes virus infection, leukemic infiltration, lymphoma, and drug-induced pneumonitis may exist. Lung biopsy used to be almost always necessary to establish the diagnosis in diffuse interstitial pneumonitis. The open-chest technique probably produces the best diagnostic yield and the lowest frequency of complications. In immunosuppressed patients with diffuse bilateral pneumonitis, an open-chest biopsy is diagnostic in about 80% of the patients; complications associated with open-lung biopsy occur in 7%–19% of patients and include hemorrhage, pneumothorax, pneumonia, wound dehiscence, and hemoptysis. Biopsy of the affected lung can also be obtained via the transbronchial approach through the fiberoptic bronchoscope. Broncho-alveolar lavage (BAL) has been recognized more recently as a very effective means to document the microbiological etiology of pneumonia in cancer patients. Its yield is virtually 100% in patients infected with opportunistic pathogens such as *P. carinii*, cytomegalovirus, or *Mycobacterium avium*; BAL can be performed safely in practically any patient.

Central Nervous System Infection

Central nervous system (CNS) infections represent only about 0.2% of admissions to large cancer centers. These infections are most frequent in patients with lymphomas, neurosurgical tumors, neutropenia, and after splenectomy. CNS infections in cancer patients present as meningitis in approximately two thirds of cases, and as cerebral abscess in approximately 25%. Viral encephalitis and encephalomyelitis account for the other cases and are found chiefly in immunosuppressed patients.

Immunocompromised patients develop meningitis caused by a different spectrum of organisms. *L. monocytogenes* is the most frequent bacterial agent in this setting. These patients may have sepsis and bacteremia but minimal CNS findings, or they may present with low-grade fever, headache and, personality change. Still other patients present with fulminant meningitis with nuchal rigidity, seizures, dyskinesis, and coma. The cerebrospinal fluid shows an increased number of polymorphonuclear or mononuclear infiltrates (rarely up to 10 000/mm^3); protein is usually elevated and glucose depressed. The density of organisms may be low, so that Gram stains are only positive for Gram-positive bacilli in approximately 30% of cases. Culture of cerebrospinal fluid, and often blood, will be positive for *L. monocytogenes*.

Cryptococcus neoformans, a yeast-like fungus, is a common cause of meningitis in immunosuppressed patients, especially in those with Hodgkin's and other lymphomas. This infection may be extremely subtle, with low-grade fever and mild headache, but rarely with nuchal rigidity. Subtle cranial nerve findings may be present and diplopia, pupillary abnormalities, mild extraocular muscle dysfunction, blurred vision, facial paralysis, hearing loss, or disturbed taste sensation may be the only neurologic findings. Mild or minimal personality change, confusion, but rarely coma, may occur. The onset of this infection is gradual, over several weeks or months. Cryptococci may also cause lesions in the lung and on the skin.

Lumbar puncture is usually diagnostic, but as much as 10 ml cerebrospinal fluid may be required to demonstrate the organisms on culture because of their low density in the lumbar spinal fluid. Organisms may be seen on Gram-stained or India ink preparations of centrifuged spinal fluid. If the organism is not cultivated on first attemps, another lumbar puncture, with filtration of the cerebrospinal fluid through a millipore filter and subsequent culture of the filter, can increase the diagnostic yield. A lymphocytic pleocytosis (10–500/µl), depressed cerebrospinal fluid glucose, and elevated cerebrospinal fluid proteins are usually present. Latex agglutination tests or crytpococcal antigen are usually positive in cerebrospinal fluid and occasionally in serum.

Varicella zoster and herpes simplex virus may cause meningitis in the immunocompromised patient with cancer. When varicella zoster virus disseminates from a thoracic or abdominal dermatome, CNS involvement is unusual. With cranial nerve zoster, however, spread to the meninges and brain cortex is not uncommon. The cerebrospinal fluid findings are not specific, although a lymphocytic pleocytosis is usual. Cerebrospinal fluid glucose is normal, and the virus is rarely cultured from spinal fluid, but can often be isolated from brain biopsy specimens. Diagnosis is usually apparent from the associated skin vesicles, smears of which reveal multinucleated giant cells and intranuclear inclusion bodies when slide preparations of lesion scrapings are stained with Wright or Giemsa stains.

Toxoplasma gondii may produce a necrotizing meningitis or meningoencephalitis in the immunosuppressed patient. This may result from reactivation of latent cysts in nervous tissue at the time of immunosuppression. Fever, altered consciousness, headache, and seizures may occur, but some patients may be asymptomatic. Diagnosis rests on serologic documentation of a change in antibody titers.

Other agents, such as *L. pneumophila*, *Bacillus* species, *S. stercoralis*, *Mucor* and *Candida* species, may produce meningitis in immunosuppressed patients, and tuberculous meningitis also may occur. Many of the organisms mentioned above may also produce an encephalitic picture clinically.

Patients with neurosurgical tumors may develop meningitis postoperatively as a result of Gram-negative bacilli, including *Pseudomonas aeruginosa* and *K. pneumoniae*, or from *Staphylococcus aureus*, *Staphylococcus epidermidis*, diphtheroids, *Candida tropicalis*, *Candida albicans*, *Aspergillus* species.

Brain abscess, either single or multiple, may be caused by mixed anaerobic, aerobic, Gram-negative, and Gram-positive flora in the neutropenic patient, or by *N. asteroides*, *C. neoformans*, *Aspergillus* species, and occasionally other organisms. *Nocardia* are Gram-positive branching rods that stain weakly acid-fast with dilute sulfuric acid used as the decolorizing agent. Brain abscess is usually associated with involvement of the pulmonary parenchyma, and isolation of the organism from the sputum of a patient with localizing CNS findings is presumptive evidence of nocardial brain abscess. Other infections may coexist, and the diagnosis is confirmed by brain biospy (with subsequent drainage if abscess is confirmed).

Skin Infections

In immunocompromised patients, varicella zoster is probably responsible for most skin infections. Herpes simplex virus frequently produces vesicular lesions in the perilabial area; the severely immunocompromised patient may present with generalized disseminated lesions.

Zoster presumably occurs as a result of reactivation of the virus believed to be dormant in the nervous system ganglia, although controversies exist with regard to the occurrence of zoster as a primary infection. In one series of patients with cancer, 25% of the cases of zoster occurred in patients with Hodgkin's disease; atypical generalized zoster and disseminated varicella zoster infection occurred in 30% of patients. The major predisposing factors for zoster included anergy, recent irradiation, and immunosuppression with corticosteroids or chemotherapy; most cases of zoster developed within 6–12 months after completion of radiation therapy and infection often involved irradiated or tumor-involved dermatomes.

Clinically, zoster begins with burning dermatomal pain, followed by the appearance of vesicles which progress to crusted pustules. New lesions appear for as long as 7 days, and their crusts may persist for 4 weeks. Dissemination may occur at sites distant from the primary dermatome. Mortality from zoster is low, even with dissemination, although considerable morbidity results from neuralgia, superinfection, and neurologic complications. Visceral dissemination may occur.

Hepatitis and Enteric Infections

Hepatitis is a frequent problem in patients with cancer, especially when multiple blood transfusions are required. Viral hepatitis is usually less evident clinically in immunosuppressed patients than in normal patients. In addition to hepatitis caused by viruses B and A, other viruses, most of which have not yet been clearly identified, can cause a similar disease. Most cases of transfusion-associated hepatitis are due to the recently identified non-A, non-B (virus C) hepatitis virus.

Neutropenic and immunosuppressed patients may also have bacterial and fungal hepatitis, including that caused by *C. tropicalis*. The differential diagnosis requires liver biopsy and adequate microbiologic investigation since the clinical and laboratory presentation is not specific. It may be difficult to differentiate B, C, and A viral hepatitits from that caused by cytomegalovirus or from *T. gondii*. Cytomegalovirus is rarely associated with adenopathy, whereas with toxoplasmosis it is almost the rule. Secondary hepatitis may be a direct consequence of disseminated bacteria, fungal, viral or parasitic infection.

Enteritis in cancer patients can be caused by bacterial and viral pathogens. Patients who develop bacteremia with *Salmonella* species often have an underlying illness such as lymphoma, carcinoma, or hemolytic disease. Only 20% of these patients have associated gastrointestinal complaints, whereas symptomatic salmonellosis is more common in patients with no underlying disease. This suggests that immunosuppressed patients can become bacteremic during salmonella infection, even in the absence of overt alimentary abnormalities. In patients with lymphoma and lymphocytic leukemia, infection with *Salmonella typhimurium* and *Salmonella derby* occurs frequently and 35% had associated bacteremia; most of the bacteremic cases had recently received corticosteroids, radiation therapy, or cytotoxic therapy.

Enteritis secondary to herpes simplex virus or cytomegalovirus most often takes the form of esophagitis or colitis. Both of these infections are frequently polymicrobial. *Strongyloides stercoralis* causes enteritis with severe crampy pain, abdominal distention, fever, shock, and neurologic signs. In severely immunosuppressed patients, this infection is often accompanied by bacteremia with multiple organisms of intestinal origin and concurrent pneumonitis.

Duodenal aspirates will yield the organism, which may also be identified occasionally in the sputum.

Conclusions

The main lesson from the study of infections in immunocompromised patients is the wide variety of microorganisms responsible for a few clinical syndromes. This requires high diagnostic sophistication since therapy is organism specific. Other important considerations are the changing nature and characteristics of the pathogens and the availability of effective prevention for many of them.

References

Corey L, Spear PG (1986) Infections with herpes simplex viruses. N Engl J Med 314:686–691, 749–757

Dismukes WE, Cloud G, Gallis HA et al. (1987) Treatment of cryptococcal meningitis with combination amphotericin B and flucytosine for four as compared with six weeks. N Engl J Med 317:334–341

Foon KA, Yale C, Clodfelter K et al. (1980) Posttransfusion hepatitis in acute myelogenous leukemia: effect on survival. JAMA 244:1806–1807

Hughes WT, Rivera GK, Schell MJ et al. (1987) Successful intermittent chemoprophylaxis for Pneumocystis carinii pneumonitis. N Engl J Med 316:1627–1632

Kovatch AL, Jardine DS, Dowling JN et al. (1984) Legionellosis in children with leukemia in relapse. Pediatrics 73:511–515

Lewis JI, Hart CA, Baxby D (1985) Diarrhoea due to Cryptosporidium in acute lymphoblastic leukaemia. Arch Dis Child 60:60–62

Longworth DL, Weller PF (1986) Hyperinfection syndrome with strongyloidiasis. Curr Clin Top Infect Dis 77:53–56

Luff BJ, Remington J (1985) Toxoplasmosis of the central nervous system. Curr Clin Top Infect Dis 315–358

Meyers JD, Flournoy N (1986) Risk factors for cytomegalovirus infection after human marrow transplantation. J Infect Dis 153:478–488

Robertson MJ, Larson RA (1988) Recurrent fungal pneumonias in patients with acute nonlymphocytic leukemia undergoing multiple courses of intensive chemotherapy. Am J Med 84:233–239

Rubin RH, Greene R (1988) Etiology and management of the compromised patient with fever and pulmonary infiltrates. Clinical approach to infection in the compromised host. Plenum, New York, pp 131–157

Stover DE, Zaman MB, Hadju SI et al. (1984) Bronchoalveo larlavage in the diagnosis of diffuse pulmonary infiltrates in the immunocompromised host. Ann Intern Med 101:1–7

Strauss SE (moderator) (1988) Varicella zoster virus infections: biology, natural history, treatment and prevention. Ann Intern Med 108:221–237

Talbot GH, Provencher M, Cassileth PA (1988) Persistent fever after recovery from granulocytopenia in acute leukemia. Arch Intern Med 148:129–135

Thaler M, Pastakia B, Shawker TH et al. (1988) Hepatic candidiasis in cancer patients: the evolving picture of the syndrome. Ann Intern Med 108:88–100

Herpes Simplex Infections

R. Saral

Bone Marrow Transplantation Program, Division of Hematology-Oncology,
Department of Medicine, Emory University School of Medicine, Atlanta,
GA 30322, USA

Herpes simplex infections may cause significant morbidity following bone marrow transplantation (BMT) (Saral 1988). The pathophysiology of these infections was studied in the pre-antiviral era and provided the basis for the development of studies designed to evaluate the efficacy of promising antiviral agents.

Early studies demonstrated that herpes simplex virus infections in BMT recipients represented reactivation of the virus from the latent state (Saral 1988).

Primary infections with the virus were only rarely observed. The incidence of infections in patients with latent virus was shown to be very high. In our original observations in 107 BMT recipients, in the late 1970s, we determined that seropositive patients had a 70% incidence of reactivation of the virus. Reaction of the virus was associated with diseases in virtually 100% of patients. Subsequent studies done in other centers demonstrated similar findings. Approximately 85% of the infections observed occurred in the oral cavity, 10% in the genital area, and 5% of patients developed infection in both the oral cavity and genital area.

Localized infections were severe with extensive ulcerations that caused significant pain and altered the natural mucosal barriers to infection by bacteria and fungi. In many instances, the lesions were atypical and were felt to represent damage secondary to chemotherapy and irradiation. While these agents may cause mucosal damage, one study in BMT recipients demonstrated a positive correlation between the development of mucositis and the presence of herpes simplex virus in the lesions (Seto et al. 1985). This emphasizes the importance of herpes simplex reactivation in causing or potentiating mucosal lesions in this highly immunocompromised patient population.

Prior to the availability of effective and safe antiviral compounds, BMT recipients had significant delays in healing after herpes simplex virus reactivation occurred. In many instances, this delay was attributable to

Recent Results in Cancer Research, Vol. 132
© Springer-Verlag Berlin · Heidelberg 1993

superinfection of involved areas with bacterial and fungal pathogens. In one clinical trial (Wade et al. 1982), the time of onset to the time of healing in the patient population who did not receive antiviral chemotherapy was noted to be a median of 30 days.

In addition to easily observed mucosal infections with herpes simplex virus, patients were at risk for developing herpes simplex esophagitis, and on rare occasions patients developed herpes simplex pneumonia which was universally fatal in the pre-antiviral era.

One striking feature of these infections was their predictable temporal occurrence following BMT. The median time to development of these infections was 8 days following transplantation or 17 days following the initiation of chemotherapy and/or radiotherapy (Saral 1988).

Another group with predictable reactivation following chemotherapy is the acute leukemia patient. At Johns Hopkins, adult leukemia patients with latent herpes simplex virus, as defined by the presence of antibody, were at high risk for reactivating the virus after receiving intensive chemotherapy (Saral et al. 1983). We determined that 60% of these patients reactivated their virus and developed mucosal lesions. This was in contrast to previous reports in the literature which suggested a much lower rate of reactivation in this patient population (Lam et al. 1981); however, subsequent to our report other investigators noted a similar incidence of herpes simplex virus reactivation in seropositive leukemia patients (Greenberg et al. 1987). As with BMT recipients, the time to reactivation of herpes simplex virus was highly predictable. The median time to developing culture-positive herpes simplex virus infection was 18 days after initiation of chemotherapy.

Since other patient populations have not been studied as extensively as BMT recipients and acute leukemia patients, it is difficult to determine the exact incidence and severity of herpes simplex virus infections in other cancer patients receiving chemotherapy or radiation therapy. Yet, in one clinical trial (Anderson et al. 1984), seropositive lymphoma patients who received intensive chemotherapy had a high incidence of reactivation. Further studies are necessary to define the incidence and severity of herpes simplex virus infections in other patient populations. This predictable occurrence and the high incidence in the patient populations discussed was important in designing clinical trials to evaluate the efficacy of potentially effective antiviral therapy.

The synthesis of the deoxyguanosine analog acyclovir heralded a new era of antiviral chemotherapy (Elion et al. 1977). This compound was an effective inhibitor of herpes simplex virus replication in vitro and, because of its selectivity of action, demonstrated very low toxicity in preclinical in vitro studies and in animal trials. When this compound became available for clinical trials, it was apparent that BMT recipients and acute leukemia patients were potential study populations.

We designed a study to evaluate the efficacy of acyclovir in preventing reactivation of herpes simplex virus following BMT (Saral et al. 1981). All seropositive transplant patients were randomized to receive intravenous acyclovir or placebo starting 3 days prior to transplantation.

Patients were continued on study for 18 days or until a culture-positive herpes simplex infection was documented. Because of the high incidence of herpes simplex virus infection and the potent anti-herpes simplex virus activity of acyclovir, we designed the study so that, if the compound was highly effective, we could demonstrate this using a small sample size. After 20 patients had been enrolled in the study, an interim analysis was performed. Seven of ten placebo recipients developed herpes simplex virus infection during the study period. In contrast, none of the 10 patients who received acyclovir developed infection ($p = 0.003$). This trial was one of the first to demonstrate the efficacy of acyclovir against herpes simplex virus. In a trial of acyclovir prophylaxis in adult leukemia patients, those who were seropositive were randomized to receive intravenous acyclovir or placebo starting on day 4 after initiation of chemotherapy. Twenty-nine of 30 patients enrolled in the study were evaluable. Eleven of 15 patients who received placebo developed culture-positive herpes simplex virus infection compared to none in the 14 patients who received acyclovir ($p = 0.0002$). Of the 11 patients who developed herpes simplex virus infection in the placebo group, ten had an infection that was severe enough to warrant treatment with intravenous acyclovir (Saral et al. 1983). Other groups have shown similar results for patients undergoing BMT or receiving therapy for acute leukemia (Hann et al. 1983; Wade et al. 1984).

An alternative to using acyclovir prophylaxis is the use of acyclovir to treat established infection. In a randomized, placebo-controlled study (Meyers et al. 1982), approximately 100 immunocompromised patients with culture-positive herpes simplex virus infection were randomized to receive acyclovir or placebo. Patients who received acyclovir clearly benefitted from treatment with the compound. Viral shedding ceased a median of 2.8 days after starting acyclovir therapy in contrast to a median of 16.8 days in placebo recipients ($p = 0.0002$). This dramatic antiviral effect translated into a statistically significant reduction in pain and a crusting of lesions and to complete healing. The concept of prophylaxis as the approach to minimizing the impact of herpes simplex virus infection became apparent. While treatment was clearly effective, the time to healing in treated patients was 14 days. In contrast, no culture-positive infections developed in patients who received prophylactic acyclovir. Therefore, we were convinced that prophylaxis would be the preferred method to approach BMT patients at risk for developing herpes simplex virus infection.

Since 1982 we have routinely given intravenous acyclovir as prophylaxis against herpes simplex virus infections in seropositive BMT recipients, and since 1984 we have given acyclovir as prophylaxis against herpes simplex virus infections in seropositive acute leukemia patients. Approximately 1200 patients have been treated in this manner, and fewer than 1% of patients have had herpes simplex virus cultured from lesions while receiving prophylactic treatment. Since cost is an issue, we have modified the dose of intravenous acyclovir used for prophylaxis. The original dose schedule employed in our clinical trial was $250 \, mg/m^2$ every 8 h. Subsequently, we have demonstrated equivalent efficacy with $125 \, mg/m^2$ every 6 h and more recently with $62.5 \, mg/m^2$ every 4 h. Several centers have used oral acyclovir as prophylaxis which reduces costs even further. We prefer to use intravenous acyclovir for hospitalized patients, although oral acyclovir may be considered if compliance on the part of the patient is not an issue. If oral acyclovir is prescribed, I currently recommend a dose of 400 mg given five times daily to immunocompromised patients.

Toxicities directly attributable to acyclovir are uncommon, but careful attention to renal function is important, especially when using the intravenous formulations, and, rarely, idiosyncratic central nervous system dysfunction may be observed. A major concern with the introduction of any effective anti-infective agent is the development or emergence of resistant pathogens. Herpes simplex virus resistant to acyclovir has been isolated from many patients, particularly highly immunocompromised patients receiving the compound as treatment for established lesions. We have hypothesized that prophylaxis might diminish the development of resistance but have no definitive proof to support this concept. Most resistant strains are non-pathogenic. However, we and others have observed acyclovir-resistant herpes simplex virus causing clinically significant lesions in BMT recipients. These observations are similar to those made in acquired immunodeficiency syndrome (AIDS) patients. The initial report documented 12 patients who had received acyclovir treatment in the past and had acyclovir – resistant herpes simplex virus cultured from active lesions while on acyclovir treatment (Ehrlich et al. 1989). The strains isolated were deficient in thymidine kinase activity accounting for their failure to respond to treatment. Therapeutic approaches to patients with lesions caused by acyclovir-resistant virus have included: (a) treatment with higher doses of acyclovir – $500-750 \, mg/m^2$ every 8 h; (b) constant infusion therapy with acyclovir; (c) discontinuation of acyclovir treatment; and (d) treatment with foscarnet. The latter approach has been the most successful treatment in this situation and provides the best current therapeutic alternative, although further studies and the development of new agents will be necessary to define the best treatment options in the future (Chatis et al. 1989).

In summary, herpes simplex virus infections have been well studied in bone marrow transplant patients. Acyclovir prophylaxis provides virtually complete suppression of herpes simplex virus replication and is recommended for seropositive allogeneic and autologous bone marrow transplant recipients. Acyclovir is also effective therapy for patients with culture positive lesions. Clinically significant acyclovir-resistant strains of herpes simplex virus are not common but are treatable with foscarnet. The use of acyclovir prophylaxis versus treatment in other patient populations remains controversial. However, we also routinely use acyclovir prophylaxis in seropositive acute leukemia patients receiving chemotherapy.

References

Anderson H, Scarffe JH, Sutton RNP et al. (1984) Oral acyclovir prophylaxis against herpes simplex virus in non-Hodgkin's lymphoma and acute lymphoblastic patients receiving remission induction chemotherapy: a randomized, double-blind, placebo-controlled trial. Br J Cancer 50:45–49

Chatis PA, Miller CH, Schrager LE et al. (1989) Successful treatment with foscarnet of an acyclovir-resistant mucocutaneous infection with herpes simplex virus in a patient with acquired immunodeficiency syndrome. N Engl J Med 320:297–300

Ehrlich KS, Mills J, Chatis P et al. (1989) Acyclovir-resistant herpes simplex virus infections in patients with the acquired immunodeficiency syndrome. N Engl J Med 320:293–296

Elion GB, Furman PA, Fyfe JA et al. (1977) Selectivity of action of an antiherpetic agent, 9-(2-hydroxyethoxymethyl) guanine. Proc Natl Acad Sci USA 74:5716–5720

Greenberg MS, Friedman H, Cohen SC et al. (1987) A comparative study of herpes simplex infections in renal transplant and leukemia patients. J Infect Dis 156:280–287

Hann IM, Premtice HG, Blacklock AH et al. (1983) Acyclovir prophylaxis against herpes virus infections in severely immunocompromised patients: randomized double blind trail. Br Med J 287:384–388

Lam MT, Pazin GT, Armstrong JA et al. (1981) Herpes simplex in fections in acute myelogenous leukemia and other hematologic malignancies: a prospective study. Cancer 48:2168–2171

Meyers JD, Wade JC, Mitchell CD et al. (1982) Multicenter collaborative trial of intravenous acyclovir for treatment of mucocutaneous herpes simplex virus infection in the immunocompromised host. Am J Med 73:229–235

Saral R (1988) Management of mucocutaneous herpes simplex virus infections in immunocompromised patients. Am J Med 85 [Suppl 2A]:57–60

Saral R, Burns WH, Laskin OL et al. (1981) Acyclovir prophylaxis of herpes-simplex-virus infections. A randomized, double-blind, controlled trial in bone marrow transplant recipients. N Engl J Med 305:63–67

Saral R, Ambinder RF, Burns WH et al. (1983) Acyclovir prophylaxis against herpes simplex virus infection in patients with leukemia. A randomized, double-blind, placebo-controlled study. Ann Intern Med 99:773–776

Seto BG, Kim M, Wolinsky L et al. (1985) Oral mucositis in patients undergoing bone marrow transplantation. Oral Surg Oral Med Oral Pathol 60:493–497

Wade JC, Newton B, McClaren C et al. (1982) Intravenous acyclovir to treat mucocutaneous herpes simplex virus infection after marrow transplantation. Ann Intern Med 96:265–269

Wade JC, Newton B, Flournoy N et al. (1984) Oral acyclovir for prevention of herpes simplex virus reactivation after marrow transplantation. Ann Intern Med 100:823–828

Further Reading

Ehrlich KS, Mills J, Chatis P et al. (1989) Acyclovir-resistant herpes simplex virus infections in patients with the acquired immunodeficiency syndrome. N Engl J Med 320:293–296

> Demonstration of clinically significant acyclovir-resistant herpes simplex virus in humans

Saral R (1988) Management of mucocutaneous herpes simplex virus infections in immunocompromised patients. Am J Med 85 [Suppl 2A]:57–60

> An overview of herpes simplex virus infections and their treatment

Saral R, Burns WH, Laskin OL et al. (1981) Acyclovir prophylaxis of herpes-simplex-virus infections. A randomized, double-blind, controlled trial in bone marrow transplant recipients. N Engl J Med 305:63–67
   The first controlled clinical trial demonstrating efficacy of acyclovir

Treatment and Prophylaxis of Cytomegalovirus Infection After Bone Marrow Transplantation

G.M. Schmidt

Department of Hematology and Bone Marrow Transplantation, City of Hope
National Medical Center, Duarte, CA 91010, USA

Introduction

Cytomegalovirus (CMV) is a ubiquitous human herpes virus (Fig. 1) that
can cause primary infection, reactivated infection, or reinfection in recipients
of blood components. CMV-associated interstitial pneumonia (IP) (Fig. 2)
is the most common infectious cause of death following allogeneic bone
marrow transplantation (BMT) for hematologic malignancies and, thus, is
an important factor in limiting the success of this procedure (Neiman et al.
1977; Meyers et al. 1982a; Krowka et al. 1985; Cardozo et al. 1985).

Incidence of CMV-IP in Allogeneic, Syngeneic, and Autologous BMT

An incidence of CMV-IP of 16.7% was reported in a series (Meyers et al.
1982) examining 525 allogeneic BMT recipients over a 10-year period; the
mortality rate was 85%. None of the 100 recipients of syngeneic transplants
in that series developed CMV-IP. In another series, the incidence of CMV-
IP in recipients of allogeneic transplants for severe aplastic anemia was
found to be 9% (Ljungman et al. 1990). CMV infections in autologous
transplant patients were found to occur at a rate comparable to allogeneic
recipients (Yolken et al. 1982; Reusser et al. 1990). On the other hand,
there are conflicting studies on the incidence of CMV-IP among autologous
recipients; one series reported an incidence of 2% (Yolken et al. 1982),
whereas a more recent study found it to be 11% (Reusser et al. 1990).

Pathogenesis of CMV-IP: Implications for Treatment and Prevention

Host factors appear to be important elements for the development of overt
CMV pulmonary disease. For example, the risk of developing IP is signifi-

Recent Results in Cancer Research, Vol. 132
© Springer-Verlag Berlin · Heidelberg 1993

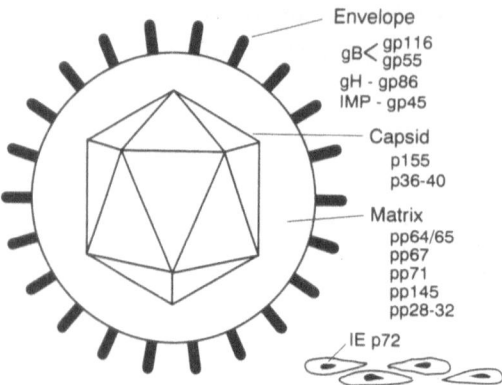

Fig. 1. Immunologically significant proteins of human cytomegalovirus (HCMV) – HCMV virion showing the immediate-early proteins (IE p72) and structural proteins that are thought to be relevant to its immunopathology

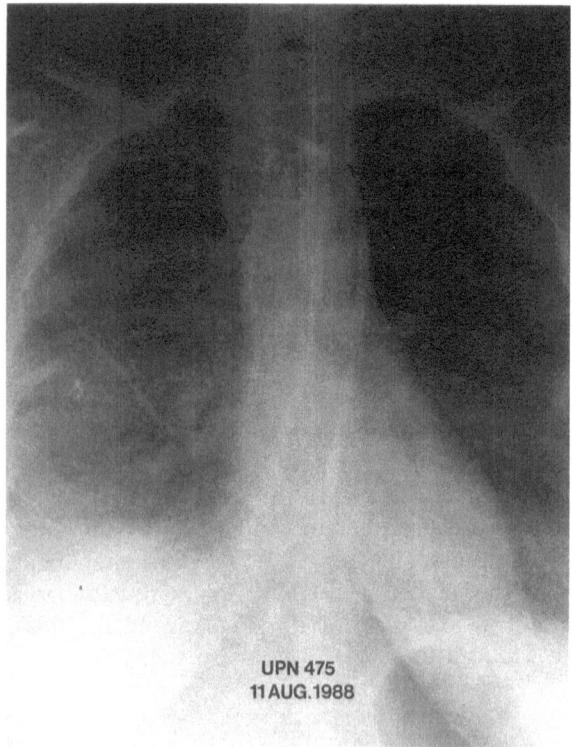

Fig. 2. Interstitial infiltrate in a patient with CMV-IP after bone marrow transplantation

cantly higher in allogeneic recipients with acute graft-versus-host disease (GVHD) and is rare in autologous and syngeneic recipients, as outlined above (Appelbaum et al. 1982; Wingard et al. 1988; Pecego et al. 1986). Exposure to virus, degree of immunosuppression and pulmonary injury have also been found to be important risk factors (Zwaan et al. 1984; Weiner et al. 1986). CMV infection itself, and the risks for infection such as age, seropositivity of donor or recipient, use of blood support from seropositive donors, and use of anti-thymocyte globulin, are all associated with an increased incidence of CMV-IP. Moreover, the association of CMV-IP with total body irradiation and other conditioning agents toxic to lung tissue suggests that nonspecific damage to pulmonary tissues increases the likelihood of CMV-IP. Previous clinical trials for the prevention or the treatment of CMV-IP using antiviral drugs alone or in combination with certain immunotherapeutic agents have not changed the high mortality rate of CMV-IP. However, combined therapy with ganciclovir (GCV) and intravenous immune globulin (IVIG) has been recently shown to improve survival in patients with this disease (Schmidt et al. 1988; Reed et al. 1988). These observations have raised the question of whether CMV-IP can be prevented in the BMT recipient. Asymptomatic pulmonary CMV infection can occur in allogeneic BMT recipients as well as in other severely immunocompromised patients such as solid organ transplant recipients and persons with acquired immuno-deficiency syndrome (AIDS). However, CMV-IP is unique to allogeneic marrow recipients and may therefore not to be attributable to active virus replication alone, but rather to an interaction between host responses and virus. Nevertheless, antiviral therapy, given prior to the postulated immune interaction that leads to disease in the setting of allogeneic BMT may provide an effective prophylactic approach. It is well recognized that reactivation or reinfection of CMV is a very frequent event after BMT which may be associated with subclinical infection in multiple sites. Because of the different epidemiologic mechanisms (primary infection, reactivation, and reinfection), the strategy for the prevention of CMV infection differs markedly. The following is an overview of past and present approaches to the prevention of CMV-IP in allogeneic BMT.

Diagnosis

Detection of CMV in the blood buffy coat, urine, saliva, and bronchoalveolar lavage specimen is accomplished by cytologic, serologic, and culture techniques. In combination with a rise in CMV antibody titer, these essays provide a probable diagnosis of CMV infection (Snydman 1990). The diagnosis of CMV disease is confirmed by the identification of the virus in the bronchoalveolar lavage (BAL) specimen or biopsy material obtained from an organ of concern.

A caveat of serologic testing, however, is that sera from immunocompromised patients often give discordant results by enzyme-linked immunosorbent, radioimmune assay, immunofluorescence, and complement fixation assays (Booth et al. 1989). Therefore there has been an interest in the development of molecular diagnostic techniques. The detection of CMV-specific DNA or RNA sequences by the use of slot-blot hybridization and polymerase chain reaction (PCR) has been recently compared to conventional viral cultures. A high specificity of the PCR assay could be demonstrated by the failure to amplify DNA primers specific for a wide range of other viruses frequently infecting marrow transplant recipients. In contrast to standard viral cultures, the PCR technique allowed detection of the virus very early in the post-transplant period. The incidence of false-positive results was found to be low, and the viral DNA detected appeared to be associated with active viral infection (Einsele et al. 1991). Further studies will have to evaluate the clinical relevance of viral DNA detected early on for the development of CMV disease.

Prevention of Primary Exposure in Seronegative BMT Patients

The use of screened blood products was 96% effective in preventing infection and 99% effective in preventing disease in recipients of allogeneic BMT (Bowden et al. 1987). In the absence of available seronegative blood products, depletion of leukocytes, the site of latent CMV infection, has been recently shown to prevent infection in previously uninfected autologous marrow recipients.

The Role of Immunoglobulin

Intravenous immunoglobulin to prevent primary CMV infection in seronegative BMT patients has been extensively studied with a variety of immunoglobulin preparations, and different doses and schedules. Results have shown a borderline treatment effect for the prevention of infection or pneumonia in four studies (Winston et al. 1985, 1987; O'Donnell et al. 1987; Ringden et al. 1984) but none in three other studies (Meyers et al. 1988; Bowden et al. 1987). Similarly, a study examining the use of immunoglobulin in the setting seropositive BMT recipients showed no effect (Ringden et al. 1987), but a more recent report found that patients who received immunoglobulin had a significant reduction in CMV-IP (Meyers et al. 1988; Sullivan et al. 1990). This was also associated with a reduction in acute GVHD, bacterial infection, and mortality. Although the use of IVIG showed an encouraging reduction in early transplant complications, the long-term benefit, as well as the optimal preparation, dose, and schedule, requires further study (Sullivan et al. 1990).

The Role of Acyclovir in the Prevention of CMV-IP

The role of intravenous acyclovir (ACV) for prophylaxis of CMV infection has been studied in two randomized, double-blind and placebo-controlled clinical trials but showed no effect on the frequency of CMV infection (Ljungman et al. 1986). In a more recent controlled, nonrandomized study, the risk of CMV secretion and disease was found to be significantly reduced in seropositive patients after allogeneic BMT given intravenous ACV at a dose of $500 \, mg/m^2$ three times daily and also improved survival (Meyers et al. 1988). These results have been confirmed in the setting of renal transplant recipients given ACV at a dose of 800 mg orally four times daily and modified for the level of renal funtion. It is clear from these reports that ACV has an antiviral effect against CMV although it is conceivable that immunity to herpes simplex virus has contributed to the protection from CMV. ACV, although associated with a reduced incidence of CMV-IP when used prophylactically, cannot be expected to reduce the incidence to the level associated with more potent antiviral agents such as GCV or foscarnet. ACV prophylaxis in the setting of BMT requires confirmation by a randomized trial.

The Role of GCV in the Prevention of CMV-IP

Three major trials recently investigated the role of GCV prophylaxis in the setting of seropositive allogeneic BMT recipients. At the University of California at Los Angeles the goal was to prevent reactivation or reinfection by administration of GCV before BMT and after engraftment, and in Seattle the emphasis was on those patients with proven CMV infection. At the City of Hope and Stanford we studied whether treatment with GCV could effectively prevent subsequent pulmonary disease in subjects with asymptomatic pulmonary CMV infection randomly assigned to prophylactic GCV or to observation. In addition, we studied the prevalence and clinical relevance of pulmonary CMV detection in subclinical BMT recipients and the natural history of such occult pulmonary CMV infection.

City of Hope-Stanford-Syntex CMV Study Group Results

The use of standard virologic techniques for the detection of CMV infection before the onset of CMV disease has not provided an effective strategy for its prevention (Meyers et al. 1990). It has been suggested that rapid culture methods, such as shell vial cell culture, could determine within 24–48 h whether an individual should receive antiviral treatment (Spector 1990). Our study (Schmidt et al. 1991) addressed the question of whether aggressive diagnostic intervention with early documentation of CMV infection followed

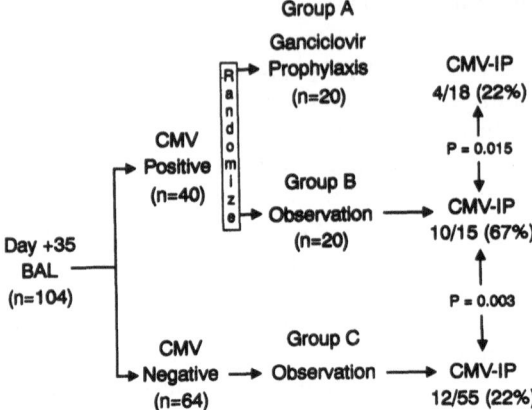

Fig. 3. Study schema, accrual and summary of outcome in the three groups. Sample sizes decrease due to exclusion of inevaluable subjects

by prophylactic treatment of subclinical CMV pulmonary infection could prevent CMV-IP in allogeneic marrow transplant recipients. One-hundred-and-four patients with hematologic malignancies at various stages participated in this study. Forty patients were found to be positive; 20 were randomized to prophylactic ganciclovir and 20 were randomized to observation. An additional 64 patients who were negative for CMV by bronchoalveolar lavage at day +35 were not randomized and observed. The study design and accrual are summarized in Fig. 3.

Effect of GCV Prophylaxis on the Development of CMV Interstitial Pneumonia

Based on the Kaplan-Meier product limit estimates of the probability of developing CMV pneumonia and the logrank test, a large treatment effect was found comparing the two randomized groups ($p = 0.0013$). In addition, the risk of developing CMV pneumonia in the GCV was found to be reduced to the level observed in the nonrandomized group (i.e., patients with a negative BAL on day 35). The risk of treatment failure from CMV interstitial pneumonia or death before day +120 in the GCV group was one third that for the observation group (RR = 0.33, $p = 0.015$). Only four of 18 treated patients (22%) developed CMV interstitial pneumonia or failed to reach the study endpoint, compared to 10 of 15 untreated patients (67%). When all 40 randomized patients were included, a very similar result was seen (25% versus 70%, RR = 0.36, $p = 0.010$). A significantly decreased risk of CMV pneumonia following treatment with GCV was also observed after adjusting for the presence of grade ≥II acute GVHD by logistic

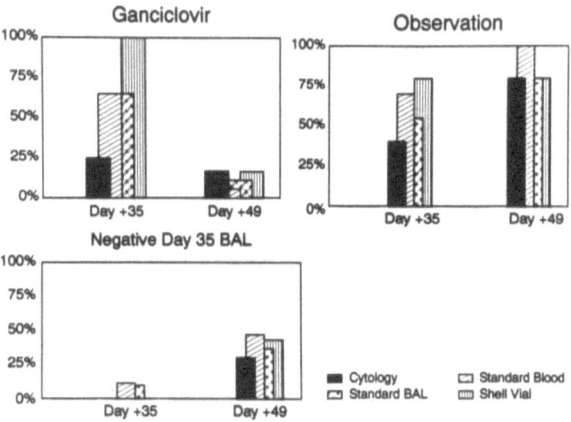

Fig. 4. Virologic results in three study groups

regression ($p < 0.001$). When the analysis of treatment effect was repeated for patients without severe GVHD, the risk of pneumonia in the treatment group was even less compared to patients in the observation group (RR = 0.19). Three out of five patients in the treatment group (60%) with severe GVHD failed while on treatment; among these, one patient did not receive any maintenance GCV, another patient developed CMV pneumonia after only two doses of GCV, and in the third GCV was discontinued after 2 days because of progressive azotemia. Two additional patients in this group died from other causes; thus, no subject who completed the full GCV induction and maintenance therapy developed CMV pneumonia. The details of the virologic test results from day +35 and +49 are summarized in Fig. 4.

Association of CMV Pneumonia with Virologic and Clinical Variables

Seventy-six of the 84 patients in the two non-GCV groups were followed to day +120 or until the development of CMV pneumonia; five patients randomized to observation and nine patients in the group with a negative day 35 BAL were considered inevaluable or died before day +120 without evidence of CMV pneumonia. A risk factor noted to be significantly associated with an increased risk of CMV pneumonia was the presence of CMV in the day +35 BAL specimen based on shell vial culture assay. Nine of 14 positive patients (64%) developed CMV pneumonia, compared with 13 of 56 shell vial culture-negative patients (23%, RR = 2.77, $p = 0.008$). Additional variables found to be significantly associated with the development of CMV pneumonia were a positive conventional CMV culture of the lavage fluid (RR = 5.77, $p < 0.0001$), positive day +35 blood buffy coat culture for CMV (RR = 3.63, $p = 0.0001$), and positive cytology (RR = 2.65, $p =$

0.03). The presence of CMV in the day +35 urine or throat culture was not significantly associated with CMV pneumonia. Also, neither age, preparative regimen (with versus without fractionated total body irradiation), nor presence of active GVHD on day +35 appeared to be significant risk factors for the development of CMV pneumonia.

Characteristics of Patients with Asymptomatic Day +35 CMV Pulmonary Infection

The variables found to be significantly associated with CMV-positive BAL results (i.e., asymptomatic pulmonary CMV infection) in the shell vial culture were: positive blood buffy coat culture for CMV on day +35 (RR = 5.45, p < 0.0001), positive conventional lavage culture (RR = 4.22, p < 0.0001), positive urine culture for CMV (RR = 3.73, p = 0.003), positive throat culture for CMV (RR = 2.90, p < 0.0001), pretransplant CMV titer >1:64 (RR = 2.71, p = 0.002), and age ≤25 (RR = 1.74, p = 0.03). In this study group, radiation was associated only with a marginally increased risk (RR = 1.70, p = 0.15), and diagnosis, disease status, and presence of day +35 grade ≥II acute GVHD were not found to be significantly associated with a positive lavage result.

GCV-Related Side Effects

Only one patient required dose modification during the initial 2 weeks of treatment, whereas most patients required a dose modification as noted above during the maintenance phase. The only toxicity which differed significantly between the treated and untreated groups was the maximal serum creatinine level (p = 0.029). There was a significantly higher proportion of group A patients with a maximal serum creatinine level ≥221 μmol per liter (2.5 mg/dl) between days +35 and +120 (mean observation time: 67.8 days) when compared to group B (mean observation time: 28.4 days). Fourteen patients required a dose modification because of a creatinine ≥133 μmol/l (1.5 mg/dl) and seven patients due to neutropenia of ≤1000 mm³. The median number of patient hospital days after BMT was similar in groups A and B (56.5 and 66.0 days; p = 0.60). However, there was a trend for more patients to have more than two hospitalizations in group B (45%) when compared to group A (15%, p = 0.08). Patients generally tolerated the day +35 BAL without complications. There was no mortality associated with the procedure. The only morbidity consisted of two patients who developed fever and a pulmonary infiltrate in the lavaged lung segments within 24 h following the BAL. In both cases, the abnormalities resolved promptly during administration of broad-spectrum antibiotics.

therapy. Application of shell vial technology to blood cultures, or other rapid methodologies, should be explored in this regard.

With the current clinical progress in the prevention of fatal CMV pneumonia in the allogeneic BMT recipient and the ongoing experimental development in the laboratory, we are now rapidly approaching the goal of eliminating CMV disease in the setting of BMT.

References

Appelbaum FR, Meyers JD, Fefer A et al. (1982) Nonbacterial nonfungal pneumonia following marrow transplantation in 100 identical twins. Transplantation 33: 265–268

Booth JC, Kangro HO, Liu KM, el Mohandes L, Tryhorn YS (1989) Discordant results obtained on testing sera from immunocompromised patients for cytomegalovirus IgG by enzymelinked immunosorbent assay and radioimmunoassay. J Virol Methods 26:77–89

Bowden RA (1989a) Use of leukocyte-poor transfusions to prevent transfusion-associated cytomegalovirus infection after marrow transplantation. Paper presented at the Second International Cytomegalovirus Workshop, 27–30 March 1989, San Diego

Bowden RA (1989b) The role of blood product filtration in the preventio of transfusion associated cytomegalovirus (CMV) infection after marrow transplantation. Paper presented to the American Association of Blood Banks. 21–26 October 1989, New Orleans

Bowden RA, Sayers M, Flournoy N et al. (1986) Cytomegalovirus immune globulin and seronegative blood products to prevent primary cytomegalovirus infection after marrow transplantation. N Engl J Med 314:1006–1010

Bowden RA, Sayers M, Gleaves CA, Banaji M, Newton B, Meyers JD (1987a) Cytomegalovirus/seronegative blood components for the prevention of primary cytomegalovirus infection after marrow transplantation: considerations for blood banks. Transfusion 27:478–481

Bowden RA, Day LM, Amos DE, Meyers JD (1987b) Natural cytotoxic activity against cytomegalovirus-infected target cells following marrow transplantation. Transplantation 44:504–508

Bowden RA, Sayers NM, Gleaves CA, Banaji M, Newton B, Meyers JD (1987c) Cytomegalovirus/seronegative blood components for the prevention of primary cytomegalovirus infection after marrow transplantation: considerations for blood banks. Transfusion 27:478–481

Bowden RA, Dobbs S, Amos D, Meyers JD (1990) Comparison of interleukin 2 and gamma/interferon production by peripheral blood mononuclear cells in response to cytomegalovirus after marrow transplantion. Transplantation 50:38–42

Cardozo BL, Hagenbeek A (1985) Interstitial pneumonitis following bone marrow transplantation: pathogenesis and therapeutic considerations. Eur J Cancer Clin Oncol 21:43–51

Collaborative DHPG Treatment Study Group (1986) Treatment of serious cytomegalovirus infections with 9-(1,3-hydroxy-2-propoxymethyl) guanine in patients with AIDS and other immunodeficiencies. N Engl J Med 314:801–805

Einsele H, Steidle M, Vallbracht A, Saal JG, Ehninger G, Muller CA (1991) Early occurrence of human cytomegalovirus infection after bone marrow transplantation as demonstrated by the polymerase chain reaction technique. Blood 77:1104–1110

Emanuel D, Cunningham I, Jules-Elysee K et al. (1988) Cytomegalovirus pneumonia after bone marrow transplantation successfully treated with the combination of ganciclovir and high dose intravenous immune globulin. Ann Intern Med 109:777–782

Grundy JE, Shanley JD, Griffiths PD (1987) Is cytomegalovirus interstitial pneumonitis in transplant recipients an immunopathological condition? Lancet 2:996–999

Krowka M, Rosenow E, Hoagland HC (1985) Pulmonary complications of bone marrow transplantation. Chest 87:237–246

Leskinen R, Tukainen P, Taskinen P et al. (1984) Bronchoalveolar lavage in the diagnosis of pulmonary complications in bone marrow transplant recipients – preliminary experience. Exp Hematol 12 (Suppl 15):24–25

Ljungman P, Wilczek H, Gahrton G et al. (1986) Long-term acyclovir prophylaxis in bone marrow transplant recipients and lymphocyte proliferation responses to herpes virus antigens in vitro. Bone Marrow Transplant 1:185–192

Ljungman P, Niederwieser D, Pepe MS, Longton G, Storb R, Meyers JD (1990) Cytomegalovirus infection after marrow transplantation for aplastic anemia. Bone Marrow Transpl 6:295–300

Lundgren G, Wilczek H, Lonnqvist B, Lindholm A, Wahren B, Ringden O (1985) Acyclovir prophylaxis in bone marrow transplant recipients. Scand J Infect Dis Suppl 47:137–144

Meyers JD (1989) Prevention of cytomegalovirus infection after marrow transplantation. Rev Infect Dis 11:S1691–S1705

Meyers JD, McGuffin RW, Neiman PE, Singer JW, Thomas ED (1980) Toxicity and efficacy of human leukocyte interferon for treatment of cytomegalovirus pneumonia after marrow transplantation. J Infect Dis 141:555–562

Meyers JD, Flournoy N, Thomas ED (1982a) Nonbacterial pneumonia after allogeneic marrow transplantation: a review of ten years' experience. Rev Infect Dis 4:1119–1132

Meyers JD, Flournoy N, Thomas ED (1982b) Risk factors for cytomegalovirus infection after human bone marrow transplantation. J Infect Dis 153:478–488

Meyers JD, Reed EC, Shepp DH et al. (1988) Acyclovir for prevention of cytomegalovirus infection and disease after allogeneic marrow transplantation. N Engl J Med 318:70–75

Meyers JD, Ljungman P, Fisher LD (1990) Cytomegalovirus excretion as a predictor of cytomegalovirus disease after marrow transplantation: importance of cytomegalovirus viremia. J Infect Dis 162:373–380

Millar AB, Patou G, Miller RF et al. (1990) Cytomegalovirus in the lungs of patients with AIDS. Respiratory pathogen or passenger? Am Rev Respir Dis 141:1474–1477

Neiman PE, Reeves W, Ray G et al. (1977) A prospective analysis of interstitial pneumonia and opportunistic viral infection among recipients of allogeneic bone marrow grafts. J Infect Dis 136:754–767

O'Donnell JJ, Jacobson MA, Mills J (1987) Development of cytomegalovirus (CMV) retinitis in a patient with AIDS during ganciclovir therapy of CMV colitis (letter). N Engl J Med 316:1607–1608

O'Reilly RJ, Reich L, Gold J, Condie RM (1983) A randomized trial of intravenous hyperimmune globulin for the prevention of cytomegalovirus infections following marrow transplantation: preliminary results. Transplant Proc 15:1405–1411

Pecego R, Hill R, Appelbaum FR et al. (1986) Interstitial pneumonitis following autologous bone marrow transplantation. Transplantation 42:515–517

Reed EC, Dandliker PS, Meyers JD (1986) Treatment of cytomegalovirus pneumonia with 9-[2-hydroxy-1-(hydroxymethyl) ethoxymethyl] guanine and high-dose corticosteroids. Ann Intern Med 105:214–215

Reed EC, Bowden RA, Dandliker PS, Gleaves CA, Meyers JD (1987) Efficacy of cytomegalovirus immunoglobulin in marrow transplant recipients with cytomegalovirus pneumonia. J Infect Dis 156:641–645

Reed EC, Bowden RA, Dandliker PS et al. (1988) Treatment of cytomegalovirus pneumonia with ganciclovir and intravenous cytomegalovirus immunoglobulin in patients with bone marrow transplants. Ann Intern Med 109:783

Reusser P, Fisher LD, Buckner CD, Thomas ED, Meyers JD (1990) Cytomegalovirus infection after autologous bone marrow transplantation: occurrence of cytomegalovirus disease and effect on engraftment. Blood 75:1888–1894

Ringden O, Heimdahl A, Lonnqvist B, Malmborg AS, Wilczek H (1974) Decreased incidence of viridans streptococcal septicaemia in allogeneic bone marrow transplant recipients after the introduction of acyclovir (letter). Lancet 1:744

Ringden O, Pihlstedt P, Volin L et al. (1987) Failure to prevent cytomegalovirus infection by cytomegalovirus hyperimmune plasma: a randomized trial by the Nordic Bone Marrow Transplantation Group. Bone Marrow Transplant 2:299–305

Ruutu P, Ruutu T, Volin L, Tukiainen P, Ukkonen P, Hovi T (1990) Cytomegalovirus is frequently isolated in bronchoalveolar lavage fluid of bone marrow transplant recipients without pneumonia. Ann Int Med 112:913–916

Schmidt GM, Kovacs A, Zaia JA et al. (1988) Ganciclovir/immunoglobulin combination therapy for the treatment of human cytomegalovirus associated interstitial pneumonia in bone marrow allograft recipients. Transplantation 46:905–907

Schmidt GM (1988)

Schmidt GM, Horak DA, Niland JC et al. (1991) A randomized, controlled trial of prophylactic ganciclovir for cytomegalovirus pulmonary infection in allogeneic bone marrow transplant recipients. N Engl J Med 324:1005–1011

Schmidt GM (1991)

Shepp DH, Newton B, Meyers JD (1984) Intravenous lymphoblastoid interferon and acyclovir for treatment of cytomegalovirus pneumonia. J Infect Dis 150:776–777

Shepp DH, Dandliker PS, de Miranda P et al. (1985) Activity of 9-[2-hydroxy-1-(hydroxymethyl) ethoxymethyl] guanine in the treatment of cytomegalovirus pneumonia. Ann Intern Med 103:368–373

Snydman DR (1990) Cytomegalovirus immunoglobulins in the prevention and treatment of cytomegalovirus disease. Rev Infect Dis [Suppl 7]:S839–S848

Spector SA (1990) Diagnosis of cytomegalovirus infection. Semin Hematol 27 [Suppl 1]:11–16

Sullivan KM, Kopecky KJ, Jocom J et al. (1990) Immunomodulatory and antimicrobial efficacy of intravenous immunoglobulin in bone marrow transplantation. N Engl J Med 323:705–712

Verdonck LF, de Graan-Hentzen YC, Dekker AW, Mudde GC, de Gast GC (1987) Cytomegalovirus seronegative platelets and leukocyte-poor red blood cells from random donors can prevent primary cytomegalovirus infection after bone marrow transplantation. Bone Marrow Transpl 2:73–78

Volin L, Leskinen R, Taskinen E, Tukianinen P, Ruutu P (1986) Broncoalveolar lavage in the diagnosis of pulmonary complications in bone marrow transplant recipients. Transplant Proc 18:130–131

Wade J, Hintz M, McGuffin R, Springmeiyer SC, Connor JD, Meyers JD (1982) Treatment of cytomegalovirus pneumonia with high dose acyclovir. Am J Med 73:249–256

Weiner RS, Bortin MM, Gale RP et al. (1986) Interstitial pneumonitis after bone marrow transplantation. Ann Intern Med 104:168–175

Wingard JR, Chen DYH, Burns WH et al. (1988) Cytomegalovirus infection after autologous bone marrow transplantation with comparison to infection after allogeneic bone marrow transplantation. Blood 71:1432–1437

Winston DJ, Huang ES, Miller MJ et al. (1985) Molecular epidemiology of cytome-
galovirus infections associated with bone marrow transplantation. Ann Intern
Med 102:16–20
Winston DJ (1987)
Winston DJ, Ho WG, Cheng-Hsien L et al. (1987) Intravenous immune globulin for
the prevention of cytomegalovirus infection and interstitial pneumonia after bone
marrow transplantation. Ann Int Med 106:12–18
Yolken RH, Bishop CA, Townsend TR et al. (1982) Infectious gastroenteritis in
bone-marrow-transplant recipients. N Engl J Med 306:1009–1012
Zaia JA, Forman SJ, Gallagher MT, Vanderwal/Urbina E, Blume KG (1984)
Prolonged human cytomegalovirus viremia following bone marrow transplantation.
Transplantation 37:315–317
Zwaan FE, Lyklema A, Hermans J (1984) Factors associated with the occurrence of
interstitial pneumonitis after bone marrow transplantation. Exp Hematol 12:15–16

Further Reading

Levin MJ, Zaia JA, Spector SA, Bowden RA, Meyers JD, Emanuel D (1990)
Current approaches to the prevention and treatment of cytomegalovirus disease
after bone marrow transplantation (symposium). Semin Hematol 27:1–28
    Proceedings of an educational seminar held December 1, 1989 in conjunction
    with the 31st annual meeting of the American Society of Hematology in
    Atlanta, Georgia.
Rubin RH (1990) Cytomegalovirus infections: epidemiology, diagnosis, and treatment
strategies (symposium). Rev Infect Dis 12:S691–S849
    Based on a symposium held at Cambridge, Massachusetts on November
    10–12, 1988
Zaia JA, Hooper JA (1991) Pathogenesis of cytomegalovirus-associated diseases
(symposium). Transplant Proc 23:1–181
    Based on a symposium which emphasized issues related to cellular and
    immunologic events during cytomegalovirus infection.

Varicella Zoster Infections in Bone Marrow Transplants

S. Feldman

UMC Children's Hospital, University of Mississippi Medical Center,
Jackson, MS 39216, USA

In the 1950s corticosteroids and, shortly thereafter, other antimetabolites were introduced into clinical practice. Within a few years varicella zoster virus (VZV) was recognized as a cause of serious and life-threatening infection in the immunosuppressed host. It is apparent that cytotoxic therapy, administered for a variety of diseases, profoundly affects the host's ability to respond to VZV. The severity and the frequency of VZV infections varies with the intensity and duration of the therapy. Organ transplantation, particularly bone marrow transplantation (BMT), is associated with some of the most intense immunosuppressive regimens and therefore is among the highest-risk categories for life-threatening VZV infection. Patients such as those with cancer, collagen vascular disorders, asthma, nephrotic syndrome, rheumatic heart disease, eczema, etc., treated with single or multiple cytotoxic agents and/or radiotherapy are to varying degrees at risk for serious VZV infections. Even short courses of steroids (≤3 weeks) have been associated with severe and fatal VZV infections.

Clinical syndromes are: primary varicella in the nonimmune host and latent infection in the immune host manifesting either as herpes zoster (HZ) with a dermatome distribution of lesions or varicella-like with diffuse, nonlocalized lesions.

Epidemiology and Pathogenesis

Of adult BMT, surviving 6 months, 30%–50% can be expected to develop VZV infections (Table 1) (Locksley et al. 1985; Schuchter et al. 1989). For pediatric BMT the incidence is 25% (Wacker 1989). The overwhelming majority of VZV infections in adult BMT are HZ (reactivation of the host's latent virus). It is not until adolescence that 85% of children have had their primary VZV infection, thus primary varicella is more common in pediatric BMT. The median time to onset of infection is 5 months with the peak

Recent Results in Cancer Research, Vol. 132
© Springer-Verlag Berlin · Heidelberg 1993

Table 1. Highights of VZV infections in BMT

Infection rate: 30%–50%
Mortality: 5%–10%[a]
  Varicella: ~ 25%
  HZ: ~ 5%
Peak incidence: 2–6 months (median 5 months)
Eighty-five percent of infections occur within 12 months
High risk factors
  GVHD
  Transplant for other than chronic myelogenous leukemia
  Survival for >90 days
  Allogeneic transplant
VZV syndromes
  Primary
    Varicella (negative pretransplant history or serology)
  Latent
    HZ: 75%–85%
    Varicella-like: 15%–25% (positive pretransplant
                            serology or history)
Outcome
  Primary varicella and varicella-like
    Visceral dissemination: 50%
    Fatal visceral dissemination: 50%
Herpes zoster
  Skin dissemination: 25%
    Visceral dissemination: 10%–15%

[a] Preantiviral era (antiviral therapy has dramatically reduced the mortality).

Table 2. Varicella in children who had completed anticancer treatment. (Modified from Feldman and Lott 1987)

Total (n)	30–100 days (n)	4–6 months (n)	7–12 months (n)	1–9 years (n)
74	10	15	20	29

incidence between 2 and 6 months. Over 85% of the infections occur within 12 months of transplantation. Only 5% of the infections are found after 2 years. Morbidity and mortality from infection occurs principally during the 9 months following transplantation. Infection beyond this point is usually self-limiting, with the exception of patients receiving immunosuppressive therapy (e.g., for graft-versus-host disease, GVHD, or relapse of malignancy). Generally the nonlymphopenic and nondebilitated patient who has completed cytotoxic therapy for more than 30–60 days is not at risk for fatal VZV infections (Table 2) (Feldman and Lott 1987).

Primary varicella is limited to the nonimmune BMT (a negative pretransplant history and/or serology). In pediatric transplants nearly 20% of VZV infections will be primary varicella, while in adults primary varicella is responsible for 5%–10% of infections. (By adulthood, 90%–95% of the population has had chickenpox.) For the pretransplant immune host VZV infections will present either as HZ (75%–85%) or a varicella-like syndrome (15%–25%). For immune BMT children, the pattern of reactivation of VZV will be similar to adults. Subclinical infections, evidenced by rises in immunoglobulin G (IgG) or IgM antibodies to VZV have been found in 25% and are not associated with any sequelae.

Unlike herpes simplex virus (HSV) infection, which occurs during the nadir of immunosuppresion, VZV infection tends to occur with the reappearance of immune function. Risk factors for VZV infection are acute and chronic GVHD, transplantation for other than chronic myelogenous leukemia, survival greater than 90 days, and allogeneic transplants. In a series of autologous BMT, the incidence of VZV was reduced to 28% (Schuchter et al. 1989) (versus nearly 50% for allogeneic BMT; Locksley et al. 1985).

Depressed cell-mediated immunity appears to play a key role in the pathogenesis of the infection (Meyers et al. 1980). In vitro lymphocyte responses to VZV are usually absent prior to infection. Following infection, there are cell-mediated and antibody responses to VZV. Neither the presence nor the level of pretransplant antibody protects against infection (Webster et al. 1989). The cell-mediated and antibody responses of the donor are not predictably transferred to the recipient (Kato et al. 1990). The BMT recipient with a negative history and serology for VZV prior to transplant should be considered at risk for primary varicella, irrespective of the status of the donor.

Clinical Features

The overall mortality from VZV infections in BMT is 5%–10% (Locksley et al. 1985). Dissemination of the virus to the lungs, resulting in severe. pneumonitis, is the principal cause of fatal infection.

Varicella, either as the primary infection in the susceptible host or as a diffuse rash in the immune host, will have lesions erupting for 5–7 days. Occasionally new lesions continue to appear for 2–3 weeks. Elevated temperature can be expected during the eruptive phase. It is during the height of new lesion formation and temperature elevation that there is the greatest risk for dissemination of the virus. The rate of visceral dissemination is 50%. VZV hepatitis is usually self-limiting, manifesting as increased liver enzymes and mild elevations in bilirubin, whereas pneumonitis is usually symptomatic, often requiring aggressive respiratory support. Serial chest roentgenograms during the febrile eruptive stage may detect pneumonitis before clinical findings are evident. Although uncommon, acute dissemination

Table 3. Outcome of untreated varicella in children with cancer. (Modified from Feldman and Lott 1987)

Malignancy	Patients (n)	Mortality (n) (%)		VZV pneumonitis (n)	(%)	Mortality for VZV pneumonitis (n)	(%)
Acute leukemia	91	9	10	29	32	9	31
Others	36	0		7	19	0	
Total	127	9	7	36	28	9	25

Table 4. Relationship of absolute lymphocyte count to VZV pneumonitis and mortality in untreated varicella. (Modified from Feldman and Lott 1987)

ALC (/mm^3)	VZV pneumonitis (%)	Fatalities (%)
>500	21	7
	$p = 0.02$	
<500	48	10
<400	49	11
<300	50	15
<200	47	18
<100	71	29

of virus to the CNS may result in fatal encephalitis. Before the availability of antiviral therapy, the mortality from VZV pneumonitis ranged from 25% in children with cancer (Table 3; Feldman and Lott 1987) to over 50% in BMT (Locksley et al. 1985). Thus, for BMT in the preantiviral era, the overall fatality rate from varicella was approximately 25% compared to 7% for varicella in children with cancer. A predisposing factor for VZV pneumonitis appears to be lymphopenia (ALC <500/mm^3) at onset of infection (Feldman and Lott 1987; Feldman et al. 1975) probably reflecting the severe degree of impaired cell-mediated immunity. In children with cancer and ALC ≥500/mm^3 (Feldman and Lott 1987) VZV pneumonitis developed in 21% compared to 50% in those with lower ALC (Table 4) (Feldman and Lott 1987). Furthermore, the mortality increased with the severity of ALC, approaching 30% with ALC <100/mm^3. Secondary bacterial infection develops in 10%–20%. VZV pneumonitis and neutropenia (<1000/mm^3) are high risk factors for this latter complication. Gram-positive organisms are the most common cause of bacterial infection, but, with increasing neutropenia, empiric therapy should include antibiotics for Gram-negative organisms.

Often patients with VZV infection are receiving immunosuppressive therapy at the time of exposure or at onset of the rash. Based on information from children with cancer for the 30 days following chemotherapy, the risk

Table 5. Chemotherapy within the month prior to varicella. (Modified from Feldman and Lott 1987)

Prior to varicella (days)	Pneumonitis (%)
1–7	28
8–26	29
14–26	25

for pneumonitis remains constant (Table 5). Of 74 children with varicella who had completed chemotherapy for 30 days to 9 years, the course of the infection was self-limiting and similar to other otherwise normal healthy children (Table 2; Feldman and Lott 1987). Although interrupting chemotherapy during the incubation period does not appear to reduce the risk for VZV pneumonitis, this should be counterbalanced by the findings of increased risk for dissemination and death with severe lymphopenia due to cytotoxic drugs. This author recommends that chemotherapy should be interrupted during the incubation period of varicella (10–21 days). Exceptions should be made on an individual basis where the risk/benefit ratio favors continuing immunosuppressive therapy. It should be noted that chemotherapy is not administered during the infection and is reinstituted when the child is afebrile and the lesions are scabbed. HZ is the localized manifestation of latent VZV. HZ is responsible for 75%–85% of VZV infections in the immune BMT. New lesions usually erupt for 5–7 days. However, prolonged new lesion formation for 2–3 weeks may occur. Often the infection develops in two or more contagious dermatomes. Bilateral zoster has also been reported and has the same clinical course as unilateral infection. Overall mortality with HZ is only 5% (Locksley er al. 1985; Schuchter et al. 1989). Fatal cases (presumably due to dissemination to the lungs) occur in the first 9 months after BMT. Skin dissemination develops in 25% and is usually self-limiting. Visceral dissemination with HZ develops in only 13%. The primary target of the virus is the lungs. As with varicella, the untreated pneumonitis has significant mortality. Risk for secondary bacterial infection in HZ is high ($\approx$20%) and is related in part to the extent of dermatome involvement and neutropenia. Scarring and postherpetic neuralgia develop in 25% and 20%, respectively. Second episodes of infection have been noted in about 5%. Cranial nerve involvement appears to have a greater risk for morbidity; post-therapeutic neuralgia ($\approx$40%), corneal and facial scarring (33%), hearing loss or tinnitus ($\approx$10%), and VII nerve palsy (15%).

Diagnosis

VZV is usually diagnosed by the clinical presentation: a diffuse, often pruritic, papulovesicular rash for varicella; and a pruritic and/or painful papulovesicular rash, appearing in clusters and conforming to a dermatome distribution, for zoster. During the clear vesicle stage, virus can be readily isolated in tissue culture. However, the typical cytopathic effect of VZV requires 1–2 weeks. Tzanck smear and negative stain electron microscopy of vesicle fluid can be used to identify multinucleated giant cells with intranuclear inclusions and herpes virus particles, respectively. Neither method differentiates HSV from VZV. Recently direct immunofluorescence with monoclonal antibody has become available (Schirm et al. 1989; Gleaves et al. 1988; Sadick et al. 1987). This can be applied directly to a vesicle fluid sample or after 24–48-h incubation to infected tissue culture specimens. The dosage of acyclovir for HSV and VZV is different and, in instances where this factor is critical (e.g., renal disease) and the clinical presentation makes the distinction difficult, the use of immunofluorescent monoclonal antibodies for specific diagnosis should be considered.

Treatment

During the decade of the 1980s, two drugs became available for the treatment of VZV infections – vidarabine (ARA-A) and acyclovir (ACV) (Feldman and Lott 1987; Balfour et al. 1983; Shepp et al. 1986). Antiviral therapy has significantly impacted the outcome of VZV infections (Table 6). Early intervention (preferably within 24–48 h) clearly shortens the cutaneous course of the infection and prevents dissemination (especially pneumonitis). In children with cancer and varicella, no VZV pneumonitis developed after 2 days of ACV treatment (compared to 30% in the ARA-A-treated group) (Feldman and Lott 1987). There is a 10%–20% mortality if treatment is initiated after VZV pneumonitis has developed. Treatment should be administered to those whose infections occur within 9–12 months of BMT. Beyond 1 year post-transplant treatment is optional (and maybe oral) except

Table 6. Antiviral therapy

Acyclovir[a]	
Intravenous	30 mg/kg per day ÷ q8 h
	(≤12 years – 1500 mg/m² per day ÷ q8 h)
Oral (HZ)[b]	800 mg, 4–5×/d
Vidarabine	
Intravenous	10 mg/kg per day, infused over 12 h
Duration	
Treatment within 3 days of onset of rash:	
Minimum 7 days and at least 2 days of no new lesions or fever	
Treatment after 3 days of onset of rash:	
Minimum 5 days and at least 2 days no new lesions or fever	

[a] Drug of choice.
[b] No established oral dose for varicella.

for subjects receiving immunosuppressive therapy for GVHD or reccurrence of malignancy and clinical or laboratory evidence of impaired immune function when antiviral therapy is inducted.

Acyclovir has emerged as the preferred therapy: less toxicity (ARA-A has significant bone marrow toxicity), shortened infusion time (1 h versus 12 h for ARA-A), relative solubility (7 mg/ml versus 0.5 mg/ml for ARA-A), and oral dosing for ACV. The intravenous dose of ACV (Table 6) is 30 mg/kg per day divided q8h (age ≤12 years; 1500 mg/m^2 per day divided q8h. ARA-A dosage is 10 mg/kg per day infused over 12 h. While the duration of treatment has not been firmly established, several regimens have evolved. For VZV infections (varicella or HZ) treated within 24–72 h of onset, ACV (or ARA-A) should be continued for a minimum of 7 days and at least 2 days of no new lesions and fever. For later onset (beyond 72 h) treatment may be reduced to 5 days if at that point there has been no evidence of fever or new lesion formation for at least 2 days. Intravenous ACV is the treatment of choice for varicella. Oral ACV, 800 mg 4–5 times a day has been used successfully for HZ (Huff et al. 1988). Oral therapy should be reserved for subjects with mild zoster and exhibiting recovery of immune functions. At best, the influence of antiviral therapy on postherpetic neuralgia is modest. A word of caution, reccurrence of lesions within a few days or weeks of cessation of antiviral therapy has been reported. All patients should be advised of this possibility so that retreatment can be instituted.

Prophylaxis

For over two decades high-titer VZV antibody preparations have been available for the prevention or modification of primary varicella for the susceptible host with a known exposure. (It should be noted that such preparations are of no benefit for the treatment of varicella or HZ.) A BMT of any age whose pretransplant serology or history is negative, irrespective of the donor's status, and with a known close exposure in the preceding 3–4 days should receive prophylaxis. The risks for infection following a household contact (≥85%), indoor playmate exposure for more than 1 h (≈50%), and hospital contacts are high. The risks from other exposures, while less, are related to the extent of skin involvement (e.g., zoster covered by clothing versus chickenpox in the vesicle stage), physical closeness, duration of contact, indoors versus outdoors, etc. In these latter circumstances, decision for use of prophylaxis must be made on a case by case basis. Varicella-zoster immune globulin (VZIG), the available preparation, is secured through the American Red Cross. The dosage is one vial/10 kg body weight (do not fractionate vials; maximum five vials) (Table 7). VZIG can be expected to prevent or modify infection in the majority of subjects (Zaia et al. 1983). In part, success of prophylaxis is related to the timeliness of VZV

Table 7. VZIG prophylaxis

Dose: 1 vial (1.5 ml)/10 kg, maximum 5 vials administered within 96 h of exposure
High-risk exposures[a]
  Household
  Indoor playmate contact
  Hospital contact: 2–4 bedrooms, adjacent beds in a large ward, prolonged face-to-
    face contact with staff or other patients
Low-risk exposures
  All others: requires case-by-case determination
Outcome
  No clinical infection: 50%
    Subclinical infection: 20%
  Varicella: 50%
    VZV pneumonia: 4%–10%

[a] Contagious period is at least 24 h before rash.

Table 8. Frequency of varicella as related to interval between exposure and prophylaxis with VZIG

Days	Varicella (%)
1–2	25
3–5	42
4–5	75
1–3	25

administration. For the 1-3-day interval between exposure and prophylaxis, varicella developed in 25% versus 75% for those prophylaxed 4–5 days following exposure (Table 8; S. Feldman, unpublished observations). While most breakthrough infections were mild, fatalities have been reported. VZV pneumonitis can be expected to occur in 4%–10% of VZIG recipients (Feldman and Lott 1987; Zaia et al. 1983). There are no clinical or laboratory criteria which will differentiate modified mild varicella from the more progressive and severe infections. This author recommends ACV therapy be initiated for failures of prophylaxis. The course of treatment may be shortened if it appears that the infection has been modified by VZIG. Twenty percent of patients receiving prophylaxis develop subclinical varicella (no lesions). Testing for VZV antibody beyond 2 months will identify this population; however, it is not clear if lasting protection is conferred by subclinical infection. For significant re-exposure beyond 15 days, repeat VZIG prophylaxis is indicated.

ACV has been used to prevent VZV (and HSV) infections in BMT (Perren et al. 1988; Selby et al. 1989). The prophylactic regimen was intravenous

ACV, 5 mg/kg body weight every 8 h, starting on the day before transplantation and continuing for 23 days. This was followed by oral ACV 800 mg q.i.d. GVD for 6 months. For children, the dosage was reduced to 250 mg/m^2 every 8 h followed by 400 mg orally every 6 h. During the 6-month period of ACV prophylaxes, VZV infections were prevented. However, following cessation of ACV, breakthrough infections can be expected to occur.

In summary, VZV is a life-threatening infection for BMT. However, the availability of antiviral therapy has reduced the morbidity and mortality. A live attenuated varicella vaccine is undergoing intensive investigation. The influence of the vaccine on the epidemiology and pathogenesis of VZV infections remains to be determined.

References

Balfour H, Bean B, Laskin O et al. (1983) Acyclovir halts progression of herpes zoster in immunocompromised patients. N Engl J Med 308:1448–1453
Feldman S, Lott L (1987) Varicella in children with cancer: impact of antiviral therapy and prophylaxis. Pediatrics 80:465–472
Feldman S, Hughes WT, Daniel C (1975) Varicella in children with cancer: 77 cases. Pediatrics 56:388–397
Gleaves C, Lee C, Bustamante C et al. (1988) Use of murine monoclonal antibodies for laboratory diagnosis of varicella-zoster virus infection. J Clin Microbiol 26:1623–1625
Huff J, Bean B, Balfour H et al. (1988) Therapy of herpes zoster with oral acyclovir. Am J Med 85 [Suppl 2A]:84–89
Kato S, Yabe H, Yabe M et al. (1990) Studies of transfer of varicella-zoster virus specific T-cell immunity from bone marrow donor to recipient. Blood 73:806–809
Locksley R, Flournoy A, Sullivan K et al. (1985) Infections with varicella-zoster virus after marrow transplantation. J Infect Dis 152:1172–1181
Meyers J, Flournoy N, Thomas E (1980) Cell-mediated immunity to varicella-zoster virus after allogeneic marrow transplant. J Infect Dis 141:479–487
Perren T, Powles R, Easton D et al. (1988) Prevention of herpes zoster in patients by long-term oral acyclovir after allogeneic bone marrow transplantation. Am J Med 85 [Suppl 2A]:99–101
Sadick N, Swenson P, Kaufman R et al. (1987) Comparison of detection of varicella-zoster virus by the Tzanck smear, direct immunofluorescence with amonoclonal antibody, and virus isolation. J Am Acad Dermatol 17:64–69
Schirm J, Meulenberg J, Pastoor G et al. (1989) Rapid detection of varicella-zoster virus in clinical specimens using monoclonal antibodies on shell vials and smears. J Med Virol 28:1–6
Schuchter L, Wingard J, Piantadosi S et al. (1989) Herpes zoster infection after autologous bone marrow transplantation. Blood 74:1424–1427
Selby P, Powles R, Easton D et al. (1989) The prophylactic role of intravenous and long-term oral acyclovir after allogeneic bone marrow transplantation. Br J Cancer 59:434–438
Shepp D, Dandliker P, Meyers J (1986) Treatment of varicella-zoster virus infection in severely immunocompromised patients. N Engl J Med 314:208–212
Wacker P, Hartmann O, Benhamou et al. (1989) Varicella-zoster virus infections after autologous bone marrow transplantation in children. Bone Marrow Transplant 4:191–194

Webster A, Grint P, Brenner M et al. (1989) Titration of IgG antibodies against varicella zoster before bone marrow transplantation is not predictive of future zoster. J Med Virol 27:117–119

Zaia J, Levin M, Preblud S et al. (1983) Evaluation of varicella-zoster immune globulin: protection of immunosuppressed children after household exposure to varicella. J Infect Dis 147:737–743

Further Reading

American Academy of Pediatrics (1991) Report of the Committee on Infectious Diseases, 22nd edn. pp 520–523

Dolin R, Reichman R, Mazur M et al. (1978) Herpes zoster-varicella infections in immunosuppressed patients. Ann Intern Med 89:375–388

Feldman S, Stokes D (1987) Varicella zoster and herpes simplex virus pneumonias. Semin Respir Infect 2:84–94

Feldman S, Hughes WT, Kim HY (1973) Herpes zoster in children with cancer. Am J Dis Child 126:178–184

Holland H, Wingard J, Saral R (1990) Herpesvirus and enteric viral infections in bone marrow transplantation clinical presentations, pathogenesis, and therapeutic strategies. Cancer Invest 8:509–521

Schimpff S, Serpick A, Block J et al. (1972) Varicella-zoster infection in patients with cancer. Ann Intern Med 76:241–254

Straus S, Strove J, Inchauspe G et al. (1988) Varicella-zoster virus infections. Ann Intern Med 108:221–237

Wilson A, Sharp M, Koropchak CM et al. (1992) Subclinical varicella-zoster virus viremia, herpes zoster, and T lymphocyte immunity to varicella-zoster viral antigens after bone marrow transplantation. J Infect Dis 165:119–126

Graft-Versus-Host Disease: Basic Considerations

A.J. Barrett

Department of Haematology, Royal Postgraduate Medical School, University of London, Hammersmith Hospital, Ducane Road, London, W120NN, UK

Introduction

Despite modern matching techniques graft-versus-host disease (GVHD) remains one of the major complications of bone marrow transplantation (BMT). It occurs in up to 80% of patients receiving HLA-matched sibling BMT and is responsible directly or indirectly for about 20% of the mortality seen after BMT. Prevention and treatment of GVHD is only partially successful at present because of both the inefficiency and lack of specificity of treatment. Here the immunopathology of acute and chronic GVHD, and its relationship with infection, is discussed.

Immunopathology of GVHD

Figure 1 illustrates the main stages of GVHD, which are detailed below.

Initiation

A key factor in the initiation of GVHD is the recognition by donor lymphocytes of HLA class I or II antigen differences in the host. This may be due to differences in the HLA types themselves (major antigen mismatch), or minor antigen differences presented by the host through fully matched HLA A, B or DR molecules. Minor histocompatibility antigen differences in the recipient recognised by the donor T lymphocytes are responsible for GVHD occurring between HLA-matched siblings. It is well established that the initiation of GVHD requires the activation of mature (post-thymic) donor T lymphocytes. The most compelling evidence for the central role of T cells in the initiation of GVHD comes from the demonstration, first in animals and then in humans, that T lymphocyte depletion of donor marrow can abrogate

Recent Results in Cancer Research, Vol. 132
© Springer-Verlag Berlin · Heidelberg 1993

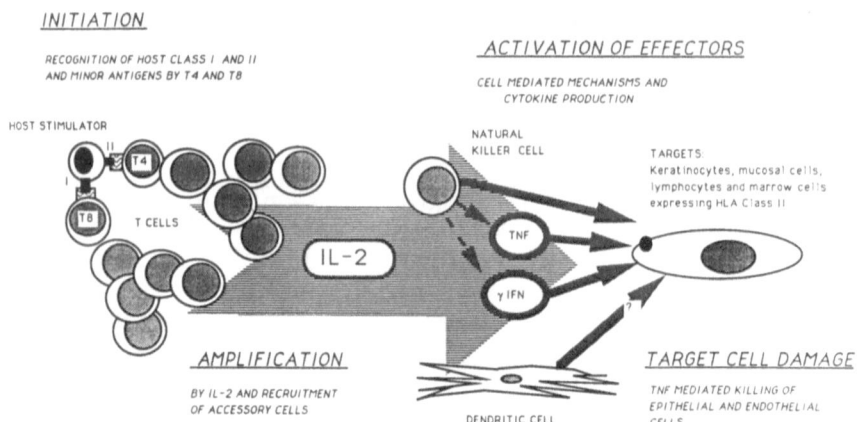

Fig. 1. Immunopathology of GVHD

or reduce the frequency and severity of GVHD. Both helper and suppressor subsets can initiate GVHD. A syndrome histologically indistinguishable from mild skin GVHD may also occur after BMT between identical twins or after autologous BMT. This reaction clearly cannot be due to histocompatibility differences and is thought to be autoimmune. Cyclosporine can induce autologous GVHD in humans by inducing imbalance in the recovery of helper and suppressor T cell subsets after BMT. It appears therefore that immune imbalance is a contributing factor to GVHD (see review by Vogelsang and Wagner 1990).

Amplification

The expression of GVHD depends upon the clonal expansion of T cells recognising host tissues. The lymphokine interleukin 2 (IL-2) produced by T helper lymphocytes is the main factor responsible for amplifying the GVHD reaction. GVHD is induced after allogeneic transplantation in mice by administration of IL-2 but is prevented if the marrow is first depleted of T cells. Recent experiments show that, if the administration of IL-2 is restricted to the first 5 days after BMT, a form of tolerance with no GVHD is induced.

Effector Cells

Both T8 and T4 lymphocyte subsets are found infiltrating GVHD lesions. A constant and early feature of skin GVHD is the detection of enhanced DR antigen expression on the surface of Langerhans cells and neighbouring keratinocytes. It is possible that natural killer (NK) cells are also implicated in the final effector path of the GVHD reaction: antibodies against cells with NK phenotype in mice can partially block GVHD, and in humans the emergence of acute GVHD is accompanied by the rapid appearance of NK cells. In addition to effector cells that cause GVHD, there are also poorly understood regulatory processes that favour the establishment of the tolerant state that characterises a successfully reconstituted immune system. Tolerance may be induced by both recipient- and host-derived suppressor cells.

Target Cells

Although GVHD is a generalised disorder affecting multiple systems, scrutiny of the histological features of the process reveals a pattern of cell damage restricted to proliferating cells of the epithelium and the gastrointestinal tract (with extension into the biliary tree and exocrine glands), and pro-liferating cells of the bone marrow and lymphoid system. Curiously the urothelium is not the site of GVHD reactions. The hallmark of GVHD damage is the appearance of single cell necrosis in the basal layers of the epidermis, the intestinal mucosa or the bile canaliculae. A notable feature is the disparity between the severe disruption of the basal layer of the skin or the submucosa of the gastrointestinal tract, and the paucity of the lymphocyte infiltrate. The bone marrow is also susceptible – severe GVHD being often accompanied by pancytopenia, in part due to marrow suppression.

Cytokines

Tumour necrosis factor (TNF) is a central effector in the cell damage caused by GVHD. In humans skin explant cultures provide a useful model for testing different cytokines in GVHD. Skin biopsies are cultured intact in the presence of lymphocytes previously exposed to recipient lymphocytes. After 6 days of culture the skin is sectioned, stained and examined histologically. Dickenson et al. (1991) showed that the supernatant from mixed lymphocyte reactions contains factors that induce features in the basal layer identical to those seen in GVHD. The changes can be reduced by blocking antibodies to TNF and gamma interferon but not completely abrogated, indicating that other as yet undefined cytotoxic factors are involved.

Chronic GVHD

Chronic GVHD (C-GVHD) usually occurs beyond 100 days from BMT but the acute and chronic forms overlap. Most patients with C-GVHD have a mild to moderate disorder with limited tissue distribution. Occasionally it runs a severe unremitting course with death from lung or liver failure, or infection. The major pathological feature which characterises C-GVHD is an increase in collagen deposition with the development of sclerosis in the dermis and mucosa. C-GVHD is characterised by an immune-deficient state leading to an increased risk of all types of late infection after BMT. There are both cellular and humoral defects leading to immune deficiency: IL-2 and thymic hormone production is decreased. Autoreactive (donor anti-donor) and alloreactive T cells occur leading to autoimmune cytopenia, marrow suppression and decreased T4 subsets. This in turn leads to impaired B cell function with hypogammaglobulinaemia and especially low IgA production (Atkinson 1990). Clinical features and infections associated with chronic GVHD are discussed below.

Clinical Features of GVHD

The manifestations of GVHD vary widely from a mild self-limiting skin rash to extensive and fatal damage to the skin, gastrointestinal tract and liver. Both clinical and histological grading systems have been used to characterise GVHD severity. The clinical I-IV grading is useful as a broad categorisation of severity but it does not convey an accurate description of the pattern of GVHD attack in the individual. GVHD also varies in its site of attack with time: different organ systems become involved at different times. Severity depends upon both the extent of organ involvement as well as the degree of damage sustained.

The Skin

Graft-versus-host disease usually presents as a rash 1–3 weeks after BMT. The rash starts as a maculopapular eruption but may become confluent. Severe GVHD causes blistering and extensive exfoliation. The distribution is variable but typically affects the palms and soles, the face and the trunk. Extensor surfaces of the limbs are particularly affected. The extent of the skin surface affected, as well as the degree of damage sustained, contributes to the overall severity. GVHD may be very localised or affect over 90% of the body surface.

The Gastrointestinal Tract

The first features of GVHD affecting the gastrointestinal (GI) tract are abdominal cramps and diarrhoea often with anorexia, nausea and vomiting. It usually presents later than the skin eruption which may already be resolving at the onset of GI symptoms. The severity varies from a mild transient attack to a life-threatening mucosal shedding with extensive blood and protein loss. Again, the extent of the attack is variable: sometimes the large bowel only is affected, at other times the upper GI tract is the focus of the reaction.

The Liver

Hepatic GVHD is characterised by a progressive rise in alkaline phosphatase and bilirubin. The onset is usually beyond 50 days from BMT. It may resolve or persist as chronic hepatic GVHD distinguished histologically from the acute form only by the presence of fibrosis in addition to the bile duct damage. Hepatic GVHD varies in severity from a mild biochemical perturbation to a lethal hepatic failure from intrahepatic biliary obstruction.

Chronic GVHD

Chronic GVHD presents as several clinical syndromes. It may affect the skin either focally or generally with scleroderma, depigmentation or hyper-pigmentation, lichenplanus-like eruptions or chronic exfoliative dermatitis. Involvement of the GI tract gives rise to chronic diarrhoea, malabsorbtion and weight loss. Salivary and lachrymal glands can be affected causing a sicca syndrome. Chronic liver GVHD leads to persisting liver function abnormalities characterising a mixed hepatocellular–obstructive pattern with a tendency to progress to cirrhosis. Recently the occurrence of chronic GVHD of the lungs has been recognised. This takes the form of a restrictive–obstructive lung damage associated with recurrent infection, and a risk of pneumothorax from bullae formation.

Time Course of GVHD and Infections

Figure 2 illustrates the typical pattern of GVHD evolution and the infectious complications that follow BMT. The pattern of infections seen is intimately bound up with the nature and severity of the GVHD process (see below) and the time elapsed from BMT. Infections can be grouped into those occurring in the neutropenic period after BMT, those occurring in the first 3 months and those occurring later.

Infections in the immediate period after BMT are nowadays usually related to *Staphylococcus epidermidis* invasion from the skin through in-dwelling intravenous catheters. The use of prophylactic antibiotics and the standard practise of treating fevers as presumed bacterial infections with intravenous antibiotics has largely prevented the occurrence of serious Gram-positive and Gram-negative infection.

The subsequent 2–3 months after BMT, when neutrophil counts have largely recovered, is paradoxically the period of greatest danger from life-

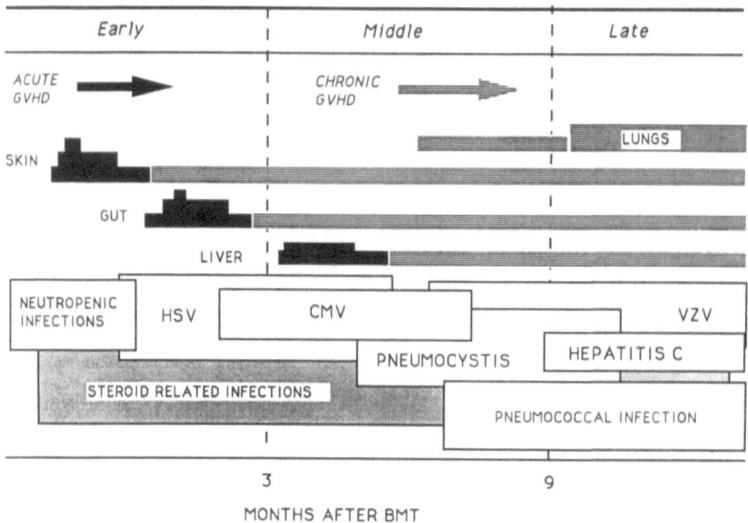

Fig. 2. Time course of GVHD and infection after BMT

threatening infection from all classes of infective agents. At this stage, despite normal counts, neutrophil function is defective, T lymphocyte immunity is low, antibody production has only partially recovered, and finally GVHD or its associated immunosuppressive treatment increases the risk from infection. Viral infections related to reactivation of DNA viruses associated with the depressed cell-mediated immunity are a particular problem. Herpes simplex virus reactivation occurs in the first few weeks after BMT, and cytomegalovirus (CMV) infection usually occurs at 6–12 weeks. Polyoma viruses are often detectable in the urine in the first few months after BMT and occasionally are associated with severe but self-limiting haemorrhagic cystitis. Adenoviruses are responsible for a gastroenteritis-like disorder often difficult to distinguish from the features of GVHD. Fungal infection with *Candida albicans* and *Aspergillus* is seen usually in association with poor neutrophil recovery and continued use of steroids for GVHD treatment. Lastly, *Pneumocystis pneumonia* can occur up to 4 months after BMT.

Infective Processes and GVHD

Infection is a Trigger for GVHD

After BMT, infection by bacteria and viruses can act as a trigger for GVHD (van Bekkum et al. 1974; Lum 1987). Rigorous GI tract decontamination was shown to reduce the risk of GVHD in one study (Storb et al. 1983), and a European survey showed a close statistical association of infecton with the herpes virus group and GVHD (Bostrom et al. 1990). The precise way in which GVHD and infection are linked are not known. Microorganisms may affect the GVHD process at several points in the pathway outlined above.

Initiation. Bacterial and viral antigens acting as minor histocompatibility antigens presented through class I and II MHC molecules of the recipient T cells can precipitate GVHD.

Amplification. Infective processes involving clonal expansion of T cells may increase IL-2 production and exaggerate the GVHD reaction.

Cytokine Production. Infection with bacteria and viruses initiates production of a wide range of cytokines, in particular TNF in Gram-negative bacterial infection and interferons in viral infections. These cytokines both enhance the cytotoxicity of cell-mediated GVHD processes and may increase target cell susceptibility by increasing the expression of HLA molecules on the cell surface of keratinocytes, gut mucosal cells and bile canaliculi.

Infected Target Cells. Reactivation of CMV appears to precipitate acute GVHD (Lonnqvist et al. 1984). This may be related to the enhancing effect of local cytokine release including gamma interferon, the presentation of bacterial or viral peptides by MHC class I or II molecules to donor T cells, or the additive damage to proliferating cells by the infective process. Bacterial colonisation of the GI tract favours the development of GVHD in the same way.

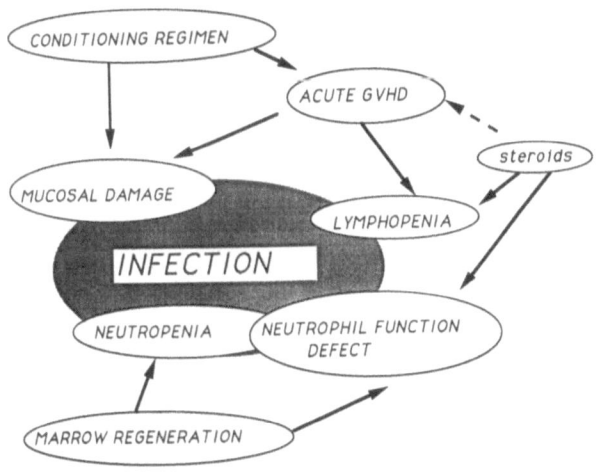

Fig. 3. Acute GVHD and infection early post BMT

Acute GVHD Provokes Infections

At the time when patients develop acute GVHD, a number of factors predispose to infection (Fig. 3): low neutrophil count, defective neutrophil function, inflammation of the GI mucosa, and damage to the skin permitting invasion by skin and gut flora through defective surface barriers. The risk of infection is compounded by the immune dysregulation associated with excessive suppressor lymphocyte activity characteristic of the acute phase of GVHD. The immunosuppressive agents used to prevent GVHD such as methotrexate and steroids used in its treatment further enhance the risk of infection. The more severe and prolonged the GVHD, the more likely is the patient to develop infection as a result of the disease or its treatment. Because of this, infection is frequently an associated cause of death in patients with steroid-resistant acute GVHD (Table 1).

Table 1. Infections facilitated by GVHD

Infection	Precipitating factor
Acute GVHD	
Bacterial and fungal infection	Damaged gut mucosal barriers
	Steroid treatment
	Neutropenia
Reactivation of DNA viruses (HSV, VZV, BK, JC)	Defective cell-mediated immunity
Chronic GVHD	
Disseminated bacterial infection (especially pneumococcus)	Hypogammaglobulinaemia, hyposplenism, neutropenia, defective neutrophil chemotaxis
Fungal infection (*Candida, Aspergillus*)	Steroid treatment; mucosal dysfunction (sicca)
Pneumocystis pneumonia	Low IgA, poor cell-mediated immunity
CMV pneumonitis	Pulmonary damage induced by GVHD and preparative regimen
VZV and HSV reactivation	Defective cell-mediated immunity
Conjunctivitis, sinusitis, stomatitis	Defective mucosal function (sicca)
Staphylococcal skin infections	Exfoliative, GVHD
Bronchopneumonia/pneumonia	Restrictive–obstructive airways disease Low IgA
Viral hepatitis (reactivation)	Defective cell-mediated immunity. Pre-existing liver damage from C-GVHD

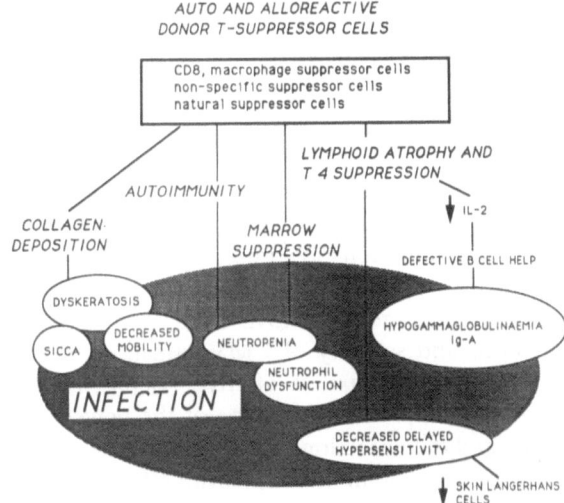

Fig. 4. Immune deficiency in C-GVHD

C-GVHD Provokes Infections

Chronic GVHD induces an immunodeficient state characterised by lymphoid atrophy, splenic hypofunction and autoimmunity. Immunoglobulin levels vary. Serum IgA is typically low. Some patients are neutropenic as a result of a suppressive effect of C-GVHD on the bone marrow or due to an autoimmune neutropenia. The interaction of cell-mediated and humoral immune defects and chronic GVHD tissue damage contributing to the infectious complications of chronic GVHD are shown in Fig. 4.

These multiple abnormalities of immune function predispose particularly to CMV pneumonitis. C-GVHD favours the reemergence of varicella zoster and herpes simplex virus. Low IgA levels and defective cell-mediated immunity predispose to *Pneumocystis* infection but in practise *P. pneumonia* is rare because it is effectively prevented with cotrimoxazole. A long-standing risk for all patients following BMT, but particularly those who develop C-GVHD, is infection from Gram-positive organisms, especially bloodborne pneumococcal infection associated with splenic hypofunction.

Infection Prophylaxis

Because of the major role of infection both in complicating established GVHD and triggering GVHD following BMT, it is important to reduce the risk by preventitive treatment. Treatment to prevent infection are the main stay of day-to-day management of BMT patients. However, firm evidence that all the prophylactic and protective isolation procedures used are effective or useful is hard to come by. Although many expensive and time-consuming protective isolation procedures are commonly used in BMT units, they have not been subjected to rigorous evaluation, and only one trial shows a statistically significant benefit for protective isolation (Storb et al. 1983). Antibacterial prophylaxis has probably contributed more to the reduction of life-threatening neutropenic infection than has protective isolation. Continuous low-dose cotrimoxazole prevents pneumocystis. Infections from herpes simplex virus are preventable by the use of acyclovir, and both acyclovir and ganciclovir have been shown in recent trials to reduce the incidence and severity of CMV infection. It is harder to be sure whether antifungal prophylaxis is effctive. While most clinicians would agree that either oral amphotericin or one of the newer imidazole antifungals prevents most candidal infection, these approaches do little to prevent the more dangerous sinopulmonary infections from *Aspergillus*. Possible approaches are the use of laminar airflow rooms for patients on long-term steroids who are most at risk, and the use of prophylactic intravenous low-dose (20 mg) amphotericin. Infections occurring late after BMT are often seen in patients with C-GVHD with persisting splenic hypofunction. Because of the continuing risk from overwhelming sepsis by encapsulated organisms, many BMT teams have elected to administer penicillin prophylactically for up to 5 years after BMT.

References

Further Reading

Atkinson KA (1990) Chronic Graft-versus-host disease – review. Bone Marrow Transplant 5:69–82
> This is an excellent review of the clinical and pathological features and treatment of chronic GVHD.

Bostrom L, Ringden O, Gratama JW et al. for the Leukaemia Working Party of the European Group for Bone Marrow Tranplantation (1990) A role of herpes virus serology for the development of acute graft-versus-host disease. Bone Marrow Transplant 5:321–326
> A multicenter analysis confirming a strong association of prior herpes virus exposure in patient and donor on subsequent development of GVHD.

Dickenson AM, Sviland L, Dunn J, Carey P, Proctor SJ (1991) Demonstration of direct involvement of cytokines in graft-versus-host reactions using an in vitro human skin explant model. Bone Marrow Transplant 7:209–216
> One of a series of studies using human skin explants to demonstrate histological changes of GVHD in vitro.

Lonnqvist B, Ringden O, Wahren B et al. (1984) Cytomegalovirus infection associated with and preceding chronic graft versus host disease. Transplantation 38:465–468
> A multicentrer statistical review confirming the close association of GVHD with CMV infection.

Lum L (1987) The kinetics of immune reconstitution after human marrow transplantation. Blood 69:369–380

A good review of the pattern of immune recovery after BMT and the impact of GVHD upon it.

Meyers JD, Red EC, Shepp DH et al. (1988) Acyclovir for prevention of cytomegalovirus infection and disease after allogeneic marrow transplantation. N Engl J Med 318:70–75

Schmidt GM, Horak DA, Niland JC et al. (1991) A randomised controlled trial of prophylactic ganciclovir for cytomegalovirus pulmonary infection in recipients of allogeneic bone marrow transplants. N Engl J Med 324:1005–1011

Storb R, Prentice R, Buckner CK et al. (1983) Graft-versus-host disease and survival in patients with aplastic anaemia treated by bone marrow grafts from HLA-identical siblings: beneficial effects of a protective environment. N Engl J Med 308:302–307

This is one of the few studies to show that in clinical practice rigorous bacterial decontamination can affect GVHD incidence and severity.

van Bekkum DW, Roodenburg J, Heidt PJ, van der Waaij D (1974) Mitigation of secondary disease of allogeneic mouse radiation chimeras by modification of the intestinal microflora. J Natl Cancer Inst 52:401–414

The original observation that bacterial microflora predispose to GVHD.

Vogelsang GB, Wagner JE (1990) Graft-versus-host disease. Clin Hemato North Am 4:625–642

A recent review which extensively covers prevention and treatment approaches.

Graft-Versus-Host Disease: Implications

P.J. Tutschka

Bone Marrow Transplantation Program, Hematology/Oncology Division,
Department of Medicine, Room L-3092, University Health Center,
263 Farmington Avenue, Farmington, CT 06030, USA

The intent of the preparative regimen for bone marrow transplantation (BMT) is the destruction of the host tumor cell and the complete ablation of the host lymphohematopoietic system (Thomas 1983). Most aggressive conditioning regimens are applied, usually combining chemo- and radiotherapy, the latter in the form of total body irradiation. This preparative therapy will not only induce complete aplasia, lasting for 3–4 weeks, with severe leukopenia and granulocytopenia, but will also weaken physical defense barriers such as the skin, the oral, esophageal, and gastrointestinal mucosa or the bronchial mucosa (Bearman et al. 1988). The combination of alterations in the integrity of physical defense barriers together with granulocytopenia will permit bacterial infections that quite often express themselves as bacteremia and sepsis. The majority of the organisms ultimately implicated in these infections are derived from the patient's own microflora, two major reservoirs being the gastrointestinal tract with primarily aerobic Gram-negative bacteria and the integument with primarily Gram-positive organisms (Young 1984; Meyers and Atkinson 1983; Winston et al. 1984). Studies published a decade ago demonstrated a greater than 30% incidence and 20% mortality from bacterial sepsis in the 1st month following BMT with Gram-negative organisms derived from the gastrointestinal tract being responsible for the majority of the systemic infections. Over the past 10 years not only has the incidence of bacterial infections been reduced, now demonstrating not more than 15% bacteremia during the first 30 days after transplant, but also a shift from Gram-negative organisms of gastrointestinal provenience to Gram-positive infections derived from the skin has occurred. This is attributable in part to prophylactic measures, such as the application of nonabsorbable antibiotics to reduce the bacterial content of the gastrointestinal tract, and in part due to the increased use of indwelling central catheters placed before marrow transplantation (Meyers 1986).

Fungal infections are much less common during this phase after transplantation and account for no more than 10%–15% of systemic infectious complications. *Candida* species account for the majority of these fungal infections with *Candida albicans* being primarily responsible, followed by *Candida tropicalis* and *Torulopsis glabrata*. Rarely this early after transplantation are infections with *Aspergillus* species seen, a major and sometimes insurmountable barrier for the transplant patient. Apart from the above-described impairment of mucosal barriers through the chemotherapy and post-transplant immunosuppression, e.g., with methotrexate and its associated mucositis, the major predisposing factors for fungal disease are prolonged neutropenia and prolonged use of antibacterial antibiotics.

Viral infections during this phase are frequent but rarely do they contribute to patient mortality. Herpes simplex dermatitis is seen commonly in patients who, preceding transplant, were seropositive for herpes simplex virus (HSV). Although HSV-induced esophagitis can be seen, life-threatening tracheobronchitis and even pneumonia are now rarely observed since acyclovir prophylaxis is commonly instituted in patients who are seropositive to herpes simplex prior to transplantation. Of interest is the high excretion rate of Epstein-Barr virus shortly after transplantation as well as BK papova virus, which might at least in part contribute to early hepatic dysfunction and hemorrhagic cystitis seen not infrequently during the first 3–4 weeks after marrow grafting.

The therapy of systemic infections during the aplastic phase of BMT follows the established guidelines of infectious management in the granulocytopenic patient, the mainstay being the prompt and empiric institution of systemic antibiotics (Pizzo 1985; Rubin 1988). Major efforts in the past years have centered on better prevention of such early infectious complications. Apart from the development of less toxic regimens that hopefully have less impact on the physiological barrier functions and result in shorter bone marrow aplasias, protocols have been instituted aimed at reducing the patient's own microflora. Moreover, frequently, patients are placed into a virtually germ-free environment, providing sterile filtered air, virtually sterile food, and strict protective isolation procedures. Although studies have shown that patients who are placed in such an environment will develop bacterial infections from organisms that have escaped the decontamination process, to date it is not clear if the use of such stringent gnotobiotic principles is justified in BMT. Controlled prospective studies have shown protective environments to be effective only for patients who received transplants for severe aplastic anemia. As a whole, however, these various measures seem to be effective. In our own patient population, the incidence of bacteremia and sepsis has been less than 10%. In fact, in 110 consecutively transplanted patients, sepsis occurred in only three patients (Tutschka 1987, 1988).

There are other febrile illnesses in the early post-transplant phase that might not be infectious in origin. We have recently described a febrile syndrome that seems to be associated with the engraftment process itself (Tutschka et al. 1989). At a median of 9 days after marrow transplantation, 2 days preceding white cell recovery, the patient develops a faint nonpruritic, macular rash over the trunk associated with fever that rapidly evolves into a high-spiking, hectic pattern. Cultures are usually entirely negative and the fever remains unresponsive to multiple antibiotics. The clinical picture is that of sepsis with hypotension, intravascular contraction, renal compromise, and often confusion or even hallucinations. Moreover, a "capillary leak" syndrome is encountered with interstitial edema, weight gain, lung congestion, and even pulmonary compromise that might require mechanical ventilation. The institution of antifungal antibiotics is rarely, if ever, effective, usually leading to severe renal impairment, the necessity to discontinue or at least reduce graft-versus-host disease (GVHD) prophylaxis with cyclosporine, often resulting in a prompt development of acute GVHD with subsequent demise of the patient. An immune-mediated etiology of this syndrome was suspected, the likely etiology being the release of cytokines at high levels early after transplantation. Indeed, we have been able to correlate the excessive release of gamma interferon with this fever pattern and have been able to arrest this syndrome by the institution of a short yet aggressive course of adrenal steroids (Fig. 1) (C.A. Keever, unpublished observations). This syndrome, so far still poorly understood, has been increasingly recognized and has been termed "hyperacute GVHD" by other transplant groups.

The release of cytokines such as gamma interferon or tumor necrosis factor alpha, either as a result of the engraftment process per se or as an indirect result of bacterial or viral infections, might be a major trigger for acute GVHD (Haller et al. 1990). These potent immune modulators will lead to the expression of class I and class II antigens not only on cells of the immune system such as antigen-presenting cells, but on somatic cells as well, rendering them targets for effector cells of GVHD. The effector cells appear to be mature, immunocompetent T cells of donor origin, predominantly of CD 8 phenotype, which have been transferred with the donor bone marrow inoculum.

There is evidence that infections can trigger GVHD. Germ-free rodents which are transplanted in a germ-free environment will not develop GVHD even if they received a mismatched transplant. Conversely, intentional contamination of these chimeric animals will cause GVHD (Pollard et al. 1976). Patients in germ-free environments have a reduced incidence of serious GVHD (Storb et al. 1983). Furthermore, cutaneous GVHD will develop in areas which have tissue damage, especially if this damage is caused by a virus. Finally, viral infections are known to trigger GVHD in rats (Rossie et al. 1988). The incidence of acute GVHD in MHC-matched allogeneic BMT usually exceeds 50%. Over the past years a steady decline has been observed, possibly as a result of not only improved GVHD prophylaxis, but also improved infectious prophylaxis. The use of intravenous immunoglobulins, which cause a reduction in bacterial infections after transplant, is associated with a decrease in the incidence of GVHD, suggestive evidence of the importance of infections in triggering GVHD (Bostrom et al. 1990; Wasserman et al. 1988; Sullivan et al. 1990).

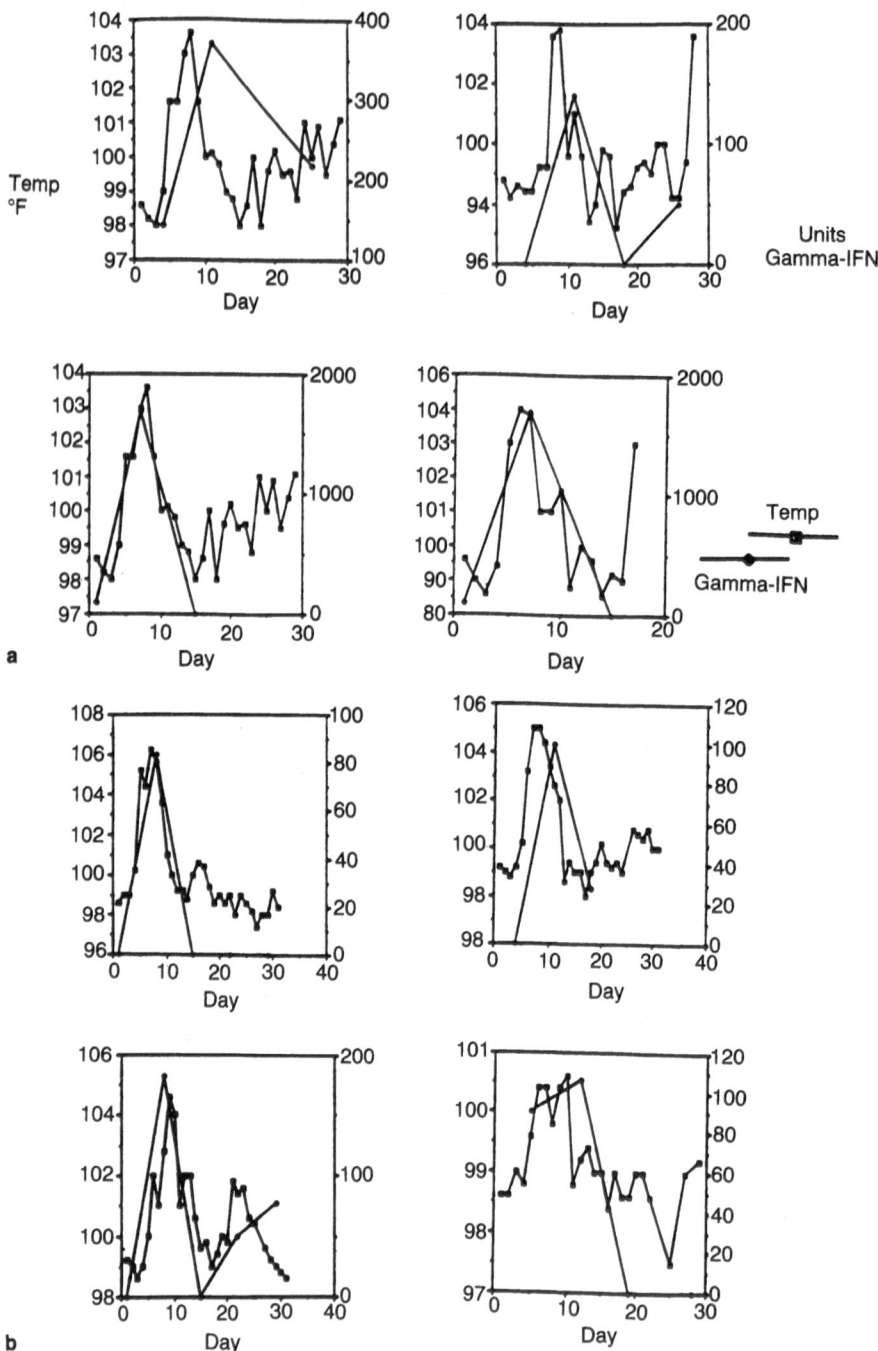

Fig. 1. Correlation of fever and serum gamma interferon (*Gamma-IFN* **a**) levels. **b** X axis: time post BMT; *squares*, temperature; *diamonds*, gamma interferon

This intricate relationship can also be interpreted as infections being the result of GVHD. Damage of the target organs of acute GVHD will again lead to severe compromise of the physical defense barriers with resulting diffuse dermatitis, denudation of the gastrointestinal mucosa, and lymphocytic bronchitis. Hence, bacterial infections, often with resistant bacterial organisms and opportunistic fungi caused by the profound immunosuppression and prolonged antibiotic therapy, are frequently encountered. Moreover, the lymphoid organs are an important target for GVHD, compounding the devastating effect on an already severely impaired immune system. The combination of radiotherapy and chemotherapy, used to condition the recipient, has effectively destroyed the host's own immune system. B cell function of host origin therefore has ceased and serum immunoglobulin levels have declined to less than 50% by 3 weeks after transplantation. Although B cell function of donor origin can be appreciated as early as 1 month after transplantation and T helper function for B cell production of immunoglobulins has started to return, normal immunoglobulin levels are not reached until at least 4 months post-transplant.

Even more devastated than the B cell is the impaired cellular immune function. After total body irradiation, host T cells have promptly disappeared, and for up to 2 months the only T cell immunity present is that of donor T lymphocytes in the donor marrow inoculum that have adoptively transferred some immunity of donor type. Even this adoptively transferred immunity declines during the first 2 months and a very severe defect, in particular of helper T cell immunity, is present primarily due to an inhibition of interleukin 2 production as the central immune defect. Cytotoxic effector function is equally impaired, possibly due to the difficulties of a new immune system that has to reorient itself in a new setting of MHC restriction. This complexity of the immune biology after marrow grafting is further compounded by the development of nonspecific suppressor cells of donor origin with T cell phenotype which nonspecifically suppress the proliferative function of T cells against a variety of mitogens and antigens, and might contribute to the global immune deficiency that is at its peak at 2–3 months after marrow grafting (Atkinson 1990; Witherspoon et al. 1984; Lum et al. 1989; Keever et al. 1989). This severe global immune defect, worsened by the presence of acute GVHD and its therapy with immunosuppressants, might be the prime cause for development of the two most important opportunistic infections, interstitial pneumonia and hemorrhagic gastroenteritis.

Interstitial pneumonia, a complication which used to have an incidence between 30% and 48% and a mortality of greater than 60%, is associated at least in half of the cases with cytomegalovirus (CMV). Risk factors, such as the presence of serum positivity to CMV before transplantation, the transfusion of blood products from CMV-seropositive donors, acute GVHD, and a radiation dose to the lungs exceeding 600 rad, together with some prognostic factors, such as the ability to generate a CMV-specific lymphocytotoxic response, or the ability to mount a humoral antibody response to CMV, have suggested a number of strategies which indeed seem to have reduced the overall incidence to 20% or less in most transplant programs. These efforts center on early detection of CMV disease, particularly with the help of bronchoalveolar lavage, the use of CMV-seronegative blood products, the early use of ganciclovir, and the prophylactic administration of high-titered antisera to CMV. These efforts have resulted in our own patient population in the prevention of CMV pneumonia in CMV-seronegative recipients, and in a reduction in the incidence of CMV interstitial pneumonia to less than 30% in CMV-seropositive patients.

The outlook for the other major complication in this phase, hemorrhagic gastroenteritis, is by far not as optimistic. This severe, progressive hemorrhagic gastroenteritis, which can occur even in the absence of acute GVHD, has an incidence of almost 30% with a mortality approaching 60%. Several prospective studies have incriminated viruses that are prevalent in the community, such as rotavirus and adenovirus, transmitted likely through an exogenous route, as well as CMV, usually a reactivation of an endogenous virus. This likely infectious syndrome further compromises the gastrointestinal tract which has already been severely impaired by the preparative therapy as well as GVHD, where the mucosa is damaged, where the Peyer's patches and other gut-associated lymphoid tissues have been destroyed, and where IgA- and IgM-producing plasma cells in the lamina propria have entirely disappeared. Attempts to counteract this progressive gastrointestinal syndrome with its relentless mucosal destruction by employing strict isolation techniques, better prophylaxis of GVHD, aggressive administration of systemic immunoglobulins, and even the application of immunoglobulins through the oral route, have not shown convincing results (Fegan et al. 1990; Beschorner et al. 1981; Copelan et al. 1988).

As with interstitial pneumonia, the course of the patient with hemorrhagic gastroenteritis is often complicated by superinfections with resistant bacterial organisms or, in particular, by superinfections with fungal organisms. Unfortunately, infections caused by *Aspergillus* species are often encountered, usually leading to the demise of the patient. The necessary administration of amphotericin B in high doses requires the reduction of immunosuppressive therapy with cyclosporine to prevent complete renal failure and necessitates the institution of adrenal steroids to counterbalance acute GVHD. Given the profound immunodeficiency, compounded by the use of adrenal steroids, the therapy of invasive aspergillosis is often futile. New therapeutic strategies to combat this devastating infection, such as the institution of macrophage colony-stimulating factor, new antifungal agents such as imidazoles and new amphotericin formulations, e.g., liposomal amphotericin B, will be required. Most importantly, however, rational strategies need to be sought to rapidly accelerate immunocompetence and tolerance without increasing the potential for acute GVHD (Tutschka 1985, 1988; Burakoff et al. 1990).

References

Atkinson K (1990) Reconstruction of the haemopoietic and immune systems after marrow transplantation. Bone Marrow Transplant 5:209–226

Bearman SI, Appelbaum FR, Buckner CD, Petersen FB, Fisher LD, Clift RA, Thomas ED (1988) Regimen-related toxicity in patients undergoing bone marrow transplantation. J Clin Oncol 6:1562–1568

Beschorner WE, Yardley JH, Tutschka PJ et al. (1981) Deficiency of intestinal immunity with graft versus host disease in humans. J Infect Dis 144:38–46

Bostrom L, Ringden O, Gratama JW et al. (1990) A role of herpes virus serology for the development of acute graft versus host disease. Bone Marrow Transplant 5:321–326

Burakoff SJ, Deeg HT, Ferrara J, Atkinson K (1990) Graft-vs-host disease: immunology, pathophysiology and treatment. Dekker, New York

Copelan EA, Bechtel T, Featheringham NC, Grose MM, Sedmak DD, Kapoor N, Tutschka PJ (1988) Oral administration of IgG in marrow transplant recipients. Drug Intell Clin Pharm 22:912

Fegan C, Poynton CA, Whittacker JA (1990) The gut mucosal barrier in bone marrow transplantation. Bone Marrow Transplant 5:373–377

Haller E, Kolb HJ, Moller A et al. (1990) Increased levels of tumor necrosis factor alpha precede major complications of bone marrow transplantation. Blood 75:1011–1016

Keever CA, Small TN, Flomenberg N et al. (1989) Immune reconstitution following bone marrow transplantation: comparison of recipients of T-cell depleted marrow with recipients of conventional marrow grafts. Blood 73:1340–1350

Lum LG, Seigneuret MC, Orcuff-Thordarson N et al. (1989) The regulation of immunoglobulin synthesis after HLA-identical bone marrow transplantation: VI. Differential rates of maturation of distinct functional groups within lymphoid subpopulations in patients after human marrow grafting. Blood 65:1422–1433

Meyers JD (1986) Infection in bone marrow transplant recipients. Am J Med 81:27–38

Meyers JD, Atkinson K (1983) Infection in bone marrow transplantation. Clin Hematol 12:791–810

Pizzo PA (1985) Empiric therapy and prevention of infection in the immunocompromised host. In: Mandell GL, Douglas RG Jr, Bennett JE (eds) Principles and practice of infectious diseases, 2nd edn. Wiley, New York, pp 1680–1688

Pollard M, Chang CF, Srivasfava KK (1976) The role of microflora in development of graft versus host disease. Transplant Proc 8:533–536

Rossie KM, Sheridan JF, Barthhold SW, Tutschka PJ (1988) Graft versus host disease and sialodacryoadenitis viral infection in bone marrow transplanted rates. Transplantation 45:1012–1016

Rubin RH (1988) Empiric antibacterial therapy in granulocytopenia induced by cancer chemotherapy. Ann Intern Med 108:143–141

Storb R, Prentice RL, Buckner CD et al. (1983) Graft versus host disease and survival in patients with aplastic anemia treated by marrow graft from HLA-identical siblings: beneficial effect of a protective environment. N Engl J Med 308:302–307

Sullivan KM, Kopecky KJ, Jocom J et al. (1990) Immunomodulatory and antimicrobial efficacy of intravenous immunoglobulin in bone marrow. N Engl J Med 323:705–712

Thomas ED (1983) Marrow transplantation for malignant disease. J Clin Oncol 1:517–531

Tutschka PJ (1985) Graft-versus-host disease in experimental and clinical bone marrow transplantation. Plasma Ther Transfus Technol 6:257–274

Tutschka PJ (1987) Complications of bone marrow transplantation. Am J Med Sci 294:86–90

Tutschka PJ (1988) Infections and immunodeficiency in bone marrow transplantation. Pediatr Infect Dis J 7:S24–S29

Tutschka PJ, Kapoor N, Copelan EA (1989) A non-infectious, steroid responsive febrile syndrome in the very early post-transplant phase after allogeneic marrow grafting. Exp Hematol 17:192

Wasserman R, August CS, Plotkin SA (1988) Viral infections in pediatric bone marrow transplant patients. Pediatr Infect Dis J 7:109–115

Winston DJ, Ho WG, Champlin RE (1984) Infectious complications of bone marrow transplantation. Exp Hematol 12:205–215

Witherspoon RP, Matthews D, Storb R et al. (1984) Recovery of in view cellular immunity after human marrow grafting. Influence of time post grafting and acute graft versus host disease. Transplantation 37:145–150

Young LS (1984) An overview of infection in bone marrow transplant recipients. Clin Hematol 13:661–679

Further Reading

Tutschka PJ (1988) Infections and immunodeficiency in bone marrow transplantation. Pediatr Infect Dis J 7:S24–S29
    This is a rather concise yet comprehensive review of infections in bone marrow transplantation as they relate to the underlying immunobiology and pathophysiology of allogeneic bone marrow transplantation.
Tutschka PJ (1985) Graft-versus-host disease in experimental and clinical bone marrow transplantation. Plasma Ther Transfus Technol 6:257–274
    This is a rather comprehensive review of the immunobiology of GVHD, in particular, as it relates to preclinical animal systems as a model for human GVHD. The general concepts expressed in this review article have held up to date.
Burakoff SJ, Deeg HJ, Ferrar J, Atkinson K (1990) Graft-vs-host disease: immunology, pathophysiology and treatment. Hematology, volume 12. Dekker, New York
    This is a well-edited and comprehensive book about all aspects of GVHD containing a wealth of knowledge by recognized experts in the field. Chapter 28 discusses infections in patients with GVHD, corresponding to Tutschka (1988). Chapter 16 is a rather comprehensive overview of the clinical spectrum and pathophysiology of human GVHD, corresponding to Tutschka (1985). Chapter 13 discusses the contribution of tumor necrosis factor alpha to the pathophysiology of the GVHD lesions. This reading corresponds to Bianco et al. (1991).
Bianco JA, Appelbaum FR, Nemunaitis J, Almgren J, Andrews F, Kettner P, Shields A, Singer JW (1991) Phase I–II trial of pentoxifylline for the prevention of transplant-related toxicities following bone marrow transplantation. Blood 78:1205–1211
    In 1989, Tutschka et al. presented a clinical syndrome occurring early after bone marrow transplantation that was likely due to the release of a cascade of cytokines. This interesting paper by Bianco et al. reports about the beneficial effect of a TNF alpha antagonist, pentoxifylline, in counteracting a number of complications germane to bone marrow transplantation, such as mucositis, hepatic veno-occlusive disease, renal insufficiency, and significantly also GVHD of clinical grade II or greater. This paper is further proof that cytokines play an important role in the pathogenesis of post-transplant complications and, in particular, acute GVHD.

V. Infections Related to Humoral Immune Deficiency Vascular Access/Transfusions

Late Bacterial Infections in Humoral Immune Deficiency

P.J. Tutschka

Bone Marrow Transplantation Program, Hematology/Oncology Division, Department of Medicine, Room L-3092, University Health Center, 263 Farmington Avenue, Farmington, CT 06030, USA

Between 2 and 3 months after allogeneic marrow transplantation, once past the hurdles of acute GVHD, opportunistic viral infections, and fungal and bacterial superinfections, the cellular immune system is slowly progressing toward full immunocompetence, a process that will not be completed until close to 2 years after transplantation when finally delayed-type hypersensitivity response is normalized. Equally, T helper function for B cell production of immunoglobulins starts to return, normal immunoglobulin levels being reached not before 4 months after transplantation (Atkinson 1990b; Lum 1987). This state of relative calm can be interrupted by an important complication of allogeneic bone marrow transplantation, chronic graft-versus-host disease which, as more and more patients survive the early post-transplant complications, is becoming an ever-increasing problem (Atkinson 1990a). This syndrome, a chronic, severe and often relentlessly progressing complication, now affects more than half of the transplanted patients and is associated with a number of distinct immunobiological features. Clinically chronic GVHD resembles autoimmune diseases and most often includes a Sjögren's syndrome with xerophthalmia and xerostomia, poikiloderma and cutaneous sclerosis, and hepatic dysfunction with features of cholestasis. Apart from T cell dysfunction with poor response to alloantigens and mitogens, a central feature is the presence of primitive, prethymic T cells that are both CD5- and CD8-negative and resemble natural suppressor cells. Indeed, these cells not only have nonspecific T cell suppressor function that further impairs cellular immune responses, but also autocytotoxic potential. The targets of these killer cells are donor cells that express class 2 antigens, in particular dendritic cells such as Langerhans cells, Kupffer cells, and type 2 pneumocytes. Animal models indicate that the central defect in this disordered immunity syndrome is an impaired

Recent Results in Cancer Research, Vol. 132
© Springer-Verlag Berlin · Heidelberg 1993

thymus which can either not further process these prethymic T cells or not effectively delete them, giving rise to a true autoimmune disease of donor against donor cells (Tutschka 1986, 1987).

The mainstay of therapy for this progressive disease has been a combination of azathioprine and prednisone, agents that will not only further impair the immunocompetence of the patient, but also reduce the cellularity of the bone marrow which is already compromised by the effect of suppressor cells against hematopoietic stem cell elements.

The most common infectious complications seen with this disease are infections primarily with Gram-positive encapsulated organisms such as *Streptococcus pneumoniae* (Atkinson et al. 1979; Sullivan et al. 1981). Several factors might contribute to the high susceptibility of the patient to this infection. The impairment of mucous production as part of the Sjögren's syndrome certainly reduces the barrier function of the sinopulmonary mucosa. The reduction of phagocytic function, worsened by the administration of adrenal steroids and augmented by decrease in opsonizing antibody production, might prevent the proper elimination of encapsulated organisms. Lastly, in patients with severe chronic GVHD, an impairment of spleen function has been described, further compromising the opsonizing ability of the defense system (Al-Eid et al. 1983). This hyposplenism has been regarded as the major reason for the development of fulminant and highly fatal sepsis syndromes associated with *S. pneumoniae*, which can kill the afflicted patient within hours after clinical presentation.

Although associated with chronic GVHD, these life-threatening infectious complications can clearly occur in the absence of any clinically evident chronic GVHD. Since infection by encapsulated organisms occurs commonly in individuals with low levels of serum immunoglobulin associated with primary and acquired immunodeficiency syndromes, such an association was felt possible with bone marrow transplant patients (Sheridan et al. 1990). While many patients with isolated immunoglobulin A (IgA) deficiency do not appear to have an increased risk of infection, patients with a concomitant deficiency in the IgG subclasses, in particular IgG2 or both IgG2 and IgG4, commonly develop a recurrent pattern of severe upper and lower respiratory tract infections caused mainly by *S. pneumoniae* and *Hemophilus influenzae*. In a retrospective analysis (Table 1) we studied nine patients who developed pneumococcal infections at 6 months or longer post-transplant and compared them to 16 patients without pneumococcal infections during a similar time frame. Infection was associated with low levels or the absence of detectable serum IgG2 and IgG4. At the time of infection four of seven patients evaluated had undetectable IgG2, while five of seven had undetectable levels of IgG4. After infection none of the eight patients evaluated had detectable levels of IgG2 and only two of eight had detectable levels of IgG4. In contrast, all 16 patients without pneumococcal infection had IgG2 levels of 102 mg/dl or greater, and IgG4 levels of 20 mg/dl or greater (Table 2). This study confirmed the existence of a long-lasting IgG subclass

Table 1. Patient diagnosis, infections and serum Ig levels. (From Sheridan et al. 1990)

Patient no.	Age (years)	Sex	Diagnosis	GVHD		Infections		Post-transplant (months)	Serum Ig (mg/dl)		
				Acute	Chronic				IgG	IgA	IgM
1	20	M	AML	–	–	Pneumonia	St pn	13	ND	ND	ND
2	21	M	AML	–	–	Pneumonia	St pn	10	2420	80	740
						Sinusitis					
						Otitis media					
3	33	M	AML	–	–	Pneumonia	St pn	7	ND	ND	ND
						Sinusitis					
4	27	F	AML	–	–	Pneumonia	St pn	7	1430	15	380
						Pneumonia	St pn	14			
						Pneumonia	H influ	35			
5	23	F	AML	–	+	Pneumonia	St pn	8	1400	25	100
						Pneumonia	H influ	11			
6	20	F	AML	–	+	Pneumonia	St pn	7	155	50	115
						Septicemia	St pn	10			
						Pneumonia	H influ	11			
7	19	F	CML	–	+	Pneumonia	St pn	13	805	65	360
8	35	M	CML	–	+	Sinusitis	St pn	6	660	10	65
						Pneumonia	St pn	23			
9	38	F	CML	–	+	Pneumonia	St pn	7	330	15	25

Normal Ig concentrations (mg/dl, range): IgG, 600–1200; IgA, 150–350; IgM, 75–150.
CML, chronic myelogenous leukemia; AML, acute myelogenous leukemia; St pn, Streptococcus pneumoniae; H influ, Hemophilus influenzae; ND, not done.

Table 2. Serum IgG subclass levels from infected and noninfected BMT patients. From Sheridan et al. (1990)

Patient group	Serum sample	Time from BMT (Median)	(Range)	(n)	IgG subclass level (mg/dl)[a]							
					IgG1 (Mean)	(Range)	IgG2 (Mean)	(Range)	IgG3 (Mean)	(Range)	IgG4 (Mean)	(Range)
Noninfected	Pre-BMT	-2	-7-12	16	997	852-1165	126	111-144	115	80-166	22	16-32
Infected	Pre-BMT	-3	-10--1	6	877	372-2065	94[b]	54-165	62	40-96	25	11-55
Noninfected	Sample 1	96	62-97	16	950	685-1318	134	119-151	97	75-124	26	19-35
Infected	Before infection	113	75-244	8	1330	1033-1713	93[b]	59-148	32	17-59	10	6-17
Noninfected	Sample 2	204	108-368	14	862	650-1142	119	106-133	106	80-140	17	11-27
Infected	During infection	228	188-399	7	1258	630-2512	77[b]	51-114	50	19-131	5[b]	3-11
Noninfected	Sample 3	560	393-768	11	909	682-1212	101	96-107	97	70-133	15[b]	10-25
Infected	Postinfection	388	277-594	8	1103	563-2162	<50[b,c]		56	30-106	4[b]	3-6

[a] Geometric mean titers (95% confidence intervals).
[b] $p < 0.01$ by Fisher's exact test.
[c] None of the infected patients had detectable levels of IgG2 antibody.

deficiency after transplantation which seemed to contribute to the susceptibility to pneumococcal infection.

More than one mechanism for subclass deficiency may exist in patients who develop bacterial infections. One group of patients had a pre-existing deficiency of IgG2 before transplantation, and the deficiency was not corrected in the year after bone marrow transplant, suggesting that the underlying disorder or previous therapy was responsible for the deficiency. A second group of patients was making detectable levels of IgG2 before bone marrow transplantation and before infection, but ceased to make it after resolution of the infection. In these individuals, bone marrow allograft did not replenish the ability of the host to make Ig of the IgG2 and IgG4 subclasses. Speculation as to the mechanisms operative in the development of this subclass deficiency includes a lack of sufficient T cell help for IgG2/IgG4 production as a consequence of the disordered reconstitution of T cell subsets, and a long-lasting deficit of functional T cell precursors. The group of patients deficient for IgG2 and IgG4 appeared to be at risk for development of respiratory infections caused by *pneumococci*, a premise supported by the clinical observation of second and third episodes of infections by encapsulated bacteria in patients who remained IgG2 and IgG4 deficient. Attempts to prevent these often serious infections have utilized trimethoprim-sulfamethoxozole (TMP-SMX) prophylaxis, hoping to not only prevent *Pneumocystis carinii* infections, but also streptococcal pneumonias and sepsis during the susceptible time periods. Unfortunately, the strains of streptococci encountered frequently were resistant to TMP-SMX. Therefore, it is advisable to use other prophylactic measures such as low-dose daily amoxicillin, which appears sufficient. Another approach is the continuous administration of immunoglobulins until the time that the subclass deficiency has repaired itself. Preliminary trials with intravenous immunoglobulin (IVIG) in children with selective IgG2 deficiency have suggested clinical effectiveness, as have recent studies which demonstrated that Ig infusions after marrow transplantation, which restore sufficient levels of at least IgG2 subclasses, may reduce the frequency of all forms of serious infections.

Unfortunately, infections with encapsulated organisms are not the only threat to patients with chronic GVHD. Preliminary data indicate that in chronic GVHD there is not only a humoral and cellular immune deficiency, but white cell function may also be seriously disturbed. Opsonization and phagocytosis are impaired, as are antibody-dependent cell-mediated cytotoxicity (ADCC), directed macrophage migration and chemotaxis, as well as respiratory burst activity and cyclocytic function of granulocytes. These functional impairments are certainly worsened by the therapy with adrenal steroids and compounded by azathioprine and the associated reduction in marrow cellularity, leading often to neutropenia. Although infections with Gram-negative organisms do occur, the more common and more devastating ones are infections with filamentous fungi. This is particularly true for fungal infections with *Aspergillus* species which are virtually impossible to eradicate in this clinical setting.

Attempts to combat these infectious complications follow two directions. One is the possible use of hematopoietic growth factors, in particular granulocyte–macrophage colony-stimulating factor which would not only increase the cellularity of neutrophils, but likely also increase their functionality. The other utilizes phototherapy. It could be shown that both the putative target cells, the dendritic cells, as well as the putative aggressor cells, the prethymic autocytotoxic T cells, are susceptible to ultraviolet light destruction. Phototherapy utilizing psoralens and ultraviolet A has been effective even in patients with advanced and refractory chronic GVHD, permitting the reduction and eventual discontinuation of the adrenal steroids (Hymes et al. 1990). Such therapies are now being used earlier in the course of the disease, raising the hope that the infectious complications associated with chronic GVHD can be more easily counteracted.

References

Al-Eid MA, Tutschka PJ, Wagner HN et al. (1983) Functional asplesia in patients with chronic graft-versus-host disease: course communication. J Nucl Med 24:1123–1126

Atkinson K (1990a) Chronic graft-versus-host disease. Bone Marrow Transplant 5:69–82

Atkinson K (1990b) Reconstruction of the haemopoietic and immune systems after marrow transplantation. Bone Marrow Transplant 5:209–226

Atkinson K, Storb R, Prentice RL et al. (1979) Analysis of late infections in 89 long-term survivors of bone marrow transplantation. Blood 53:720–731

Hymes SR, Morison WO, Farmer ER et al. (1985) Methoxsalen and ultraviolet A radiation in treatment of chronic cutaneous graft-versus-host reaction. J Am Acad Dermatol 12:30–37

Lum LG (1987) The kinetics of immune reconstitution after human bone marrow transplantation. Blood 69:369

Sheridan JF, Tutschka PJ, Sedmak DD, Copelan EA (1990) Immunoglobulin G subclass deficiency and pneumococcal infection after allogeneic bone marrow transplantation. Blood 75:1583–1588

Sullivan KM, Shulman HM, Storb R et al. (1981) Chronic graft-versus-host disease in 52 patients: adverse natural course and successful treatment with combination immunosuppression. Blood 57:267

Tutschka PJ (1986) Mechanism of chronic GVHD. In: Gale RP, Champlin R (eds) Progress in bone marrow transplantation. UCLA symposia on molecular and cellular biology. Liss, New York, p 457

Tutschka PJ (1987) The role of the thymus in regulating tolerance to self and non-self. Transplant Proc XIX:486–489

Further Reading

Atkinson K (1990a) Chronic graft-versus-host disease. Bone Marrow Transplant 5:69–82

This paper is a concise yet comprehensive review of the clinical entity chronic GVHD with sufficient information about pathophysiology, immunobiology, and therapy of this complex disorder.

Atkinson K (1990b) Reconstruction of the hematopoietic and immune systems after marrow transplantation. Bone Marrow Transplant 5:209–226
This is a very thorough and comprehensive review article about the re-establishment of the immune system, which is concisely written and gives an excellent background of this complex field of immunobiology. There is an exhaustive reference list of 209 articles which covers the topic comprehensively.

Lum LG (1987) The kinetics of immune reconstitution after human bone marrow transplantation. Blood 69:369
This article complements the review article by Atkinson (1990b) and focuses more on the modulating effects of GVHD on the immune reconstitution. Special emphasis is placed on humoral immune recovery and the influence of chronic GVHD on the long-term humoral immune response.

Sheridan JF, Tutschka PJ, Sedmak DD, Copelan EA (1990) Immunoglobulin G subclass deficiency and pneumococcal infection after allogeneic bone marrow transplantation. Blood 75:1583–1588
This paper describes the infections with encapsulated bacterial organisms that occur late in bone marrow transplantation and, in particular, in the presence of chronic GVHD. The focus of this paper is the correlation of these late-occurring bacterial infections with immunoglobulin subclass deficiency states.

Sullivan KM, Shulman HM, Storb R et al. (1981) Chronic graft-versus-host disease in 52 patients: adverse natural course and successful treatment with combination immunosuppression. Blood 57:267
This article describes in detail the clinical manifestations of chronic GVHD and represents the classical paper that defines the syndrome.

Tutschka PJ (1986) Mechanism of chronic GVHD. In: Gale RP, Champlin R (eds) Progress in bone marrow transplantation. UCLA symposia on molecular and cellular biology. Liss, New York, p 457
This paper reviews the pathophysiology of chronic GVHD not only in the clinical situation but, in particular, in the preclinical animal model that mimics human disease. The etiologic contribution of prethymic, autocytotoxic effector T cells, the importance of the thymic defect, and the concept of chronic GVHD as a true autoimmune disease rather than an alloimmune phenomenon are detailed.

Hepatitis B and C: Influence of Immunosuppression

G.L. Davis

Section of Hepatobiliary Diseases, Division of Gastroenterology, Hepatology and Nutrition, J-214, JHMHC, University of Florida, Gainesville, 32610-0214, USA

The differential diagnosis of acute liver disease occurring in the patient with neoplastic disease treated with either chemotherapy or transplantation is extensive (Table 1). Recurrence of primary disease, drug-induced liver disease, vascular disease including veno-occlusive disease, Budd-Chiari syndrome, infarction, graft-versus-host disease, and infection may all occur. The major infectious causes of liver disease include hepatitis B, hepatitis C, cytomegalovirus, and hepatosplenic candidiasis. Additionally, multiple types of hepatic injury may coexist, thereby potentiating the extent of liver cell injury and increasing the severity of clinical illness.

Diagnosis is based on clinical assessment, history of risk factors, time of onset, culture and serologic testing, and liver biopsy. For instance, hepatic veno-occlusive disease is usually associated with abdominal pain and onset of ascites within a few weeks of chemotherapy or bone marrow transplantation. Hepatosplenic candidiasis is characterized by a rising serum alkaline phosphatase and low-density lesions in liver and spleen on computerized tomography scanning. However, diagnosis is difficult in most patients. Clinical history and easily available tests such as serum liver tests and radiologic studies are insensitive and provide only circumstantial evidence to support the diagnoses. Serologic tests are also insensitive. The ability of immunocompromised patients to develop a significant primary antibody response to poorly immunogenic viral antigens is reduced or delayed so that antibody levels may be below levels of detectibility or may disappear with follow up. Finally, direct confirmation of the diagnosis by percutaneous liver biopsy is usually not possible because of thrombocytopenia. Although transvenous biopsy may be more safely accomplished, the technique is more tedious and specimens are frequently inadequate.

This discussion will concentrate on hepatitis virus infections, specifically hepatitis B and C (formerly non-A, non-B hepatitis), in this group of patients. Hepatitis A and E do not occur more frequently and do not cause chronic disease. Hepatitis D (delta agent) infection occurs only in hepatitis

Recent Results in Cancer Research, Vol. 132
© Springer-Verlag Berlin · Heidelberg 1993

Table 1. Liver diseases in immunosuppressed patients

Oncology	Primary or metastatic malignancy	
	Drug-induced hepatotoxicity	
	Vascular:	Hepatic veno-occlusive disease
		Hepatic vein thrombosis
		Hepatic infarction
	Infection:	Hepatitis viruses (A, B, C, D)
		Cytomegalovirus
		Epstein-Barr virus
		Hepatosplenic candidiasis
		Other fungal, viral, and
		bacterial infections
Transplant	Graft-versus-host disease	
	(bone marrow transplant)	
	Rejection (liver transplant)	
	Drug-induced hepatotoxicity	
	Vascular:	(see above)
	Infection:	(see above)

B-infected individuals and is rare in the United States, especially in individuals without a history of intravenous drug use.

Hepatitis B

Hepatitis B is a 42-nm partially double-stranded DNA virus of the hepadnavirus group (Seeff 1990). Characteristics of the virus and disease resulting from hepatitis B infection are reviewed in Table 2. The most common routes of viral transmission are perinatal from an infected mother, sexual through either homo- or heterosexual intercourse, and via shared intravenous drug use paraphernalia. Healthcare workers and frequently hospitalized patients are at risk via needlesticks and exposure to contaminated bodily secretions. Transmission of hepatitis B by blood transfusion is now rare, since donors have been screened for HBsAg since 1972 and anti-HBc since 1986. The risk of acquiring hepatitis B from blood transfusion is estimated to be less than 0.05% (<1 in 2000). The few remaining cases probably result from donors who are incubating infection. About 30%–40% of cases of acute hepatitis B infection have no identifiable risk factor. The incubation period of infection ranges from 30 to 120 days. Acute illness is usually anicteric and minimally symptomatic (Seeff 1990).

Chronic infection develops after acute infection in 2%–5% of immunocompetent adults, 20%–30% of children, and 90%–100% of neonates (Hoofnagle et al. 1981). Since eradication of hepatitis B virus (HBV) is felt to be accomplished by the host cellular immune response to viral antigens expressed on the hepatocyte, it is not surprising that chronic infection is more common in immunocompromised patients (Wands et al. 1974).

Table 2. Characteristics of HBV infection

Double-stranded DNA virus of hepadnavirus family	
Mode of infection	Percutaneous/parenteral
	Sexual
	Perinatal
	Unknown (40%)
Chronicity	Neonates (>90%)
	Children (20%–30%)
	Adults (2%–5%)
	Immunosuppressed adults
	(20%–60%)
Injury	Immune mediated
Course	Three phases of activity

The course of chronic infection is variable and is related to the immune status of the patient, duration of infection, and virus load. In general, hepatitis B is an immune-mediated disease, i.e., the virus is not directly cytopathic and liver cell injury results from host cellular immune response to expression of nucleocapsid antigen on hepatocyte membranes (Ferrari et al. 1988). Typically, the disease has three phases which relate to the levels of viral replication and the presence of liver disease (Fig. 1) (Davis 1991a). The early high replicative phase is characterized by serologic markers of viral replication (HBeAg, HBV-DNA by unamplified techniques), infectivity, and, in most cases, abnormal liver tests and liver disease. Progressive liver injury occurs in this stage of infection. Approximately 7%–10% of immuno-competent patients in the first phase spontaneously lose serologic markers of viral replication each year (Seeff 1990; Hoofnagle et al. 1981). Evolution into the second or low replicative phase is characterized by return of liver tests to normal, reduction of hepatic inflammation, and loss of risk of progressive liver injury (Hoofnagle et al. 1981). However, HBV-DNA is still detectable in liver tissue and in serum by polymerase chain reaction (PCR). This explains the occurrence of spontaneous reactivation in up to 30% of patients within the first few months after losing serum HBV-DNA (Davis et al. 1989). The third phase of infection is convalescence which is characterized by loss of HBsAg and HBV-DNA (PCR) and development of anti-HBs (Korenman et al. 1991). It is unusual for patients to spontaneously enter this third stage (~2% per year).

The course of infection is distinctly different in immunocompromised patients. Immunosuppression (either endogenous or iatrogenic) is associated with diminution of immune-mediated cytolysis (Davis 1989). Thus, serum alanine aminotransferase (ALT) levels commonly fall and liver histology may initially improve. However, the HBV load increases, often drama-tically. This is felt to be due to the loss of immune-mediated control of replication and, when patients are treated with corticosteroids, direct

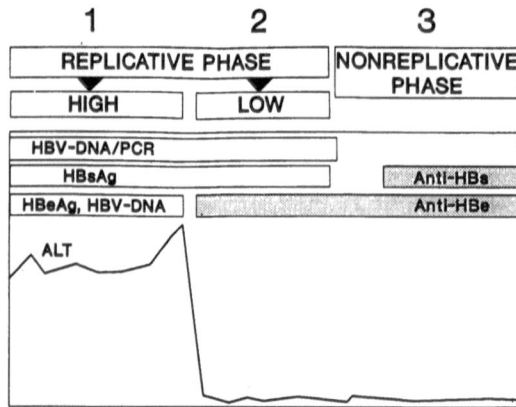

Fig. 1. Phases of HBV infection

Table 3. Influence of antiviral and immunomodulatory agents on hepatitis infections

	Immune-mediated injury (e.g., HBV)		Cytopathic injury (e.g., HCV)	
	ALT	DNA	ALT	RNA
Immunosuppression	↓	↑	–	–
Immunostimulation	↑	↕	–	–
Antiviral	–	↓	↓	↓

induction of replication through enhancing elements in the HBV genome (Davis 1989; Tur-Kaspa et al. 1986). Thus, *acute* immune suppression with cytotoxic agents, corticosteroids, or other immunosuppressants results in increased HBV replication, reduced host immune response to the virus, and lowered serum ALT levels (Table 3). In patients who have previously been in the second (low replication) phase of infection, immune suppression frequently results in return of serum HBV-DNA (reactivation) (Dusheiko et al. 1983). Withdrawal of immunosuppressive agents is associated with a return of immunocompetence against viral antigens and may result in acute hepatitis and even hepatic failure (20%) (Fig. 2) (Davis 1989; Hoofnagle et al. 1986; Pinto et al. 1990). *Chronic* immunosuppression results in a different course. Again, HBV replication typically increases and patients who previously had no detectable serum HBV-DNA will often reactivate (Dusheiko et al. 1983). Although serum ALT levels and histologic evidence of hepatitis are lacking early in the course, these may become abnormal with time. It is now believed that huge viral loads, such as those seen in immuno-suppressed transplant recipients, may be directly cytopathic to the liver cell.

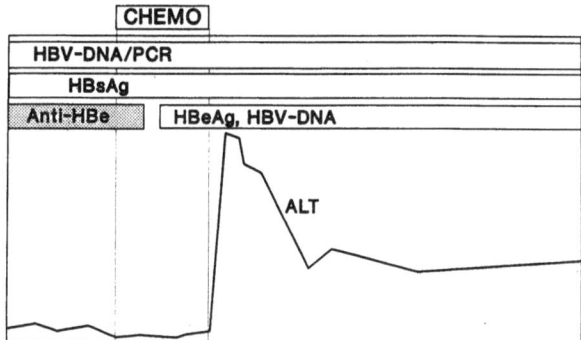

Fig. 2. Reactivation of chronic hepatitis B after chemotherapy withdrawal

Indeed, a particular form of aggressive liver disease (fibrosing cholestatic hepatitis) has recently been described in such patients (Davies et al. 1991). This is particularly prevalent in hepatitis B-infected liver transplant recipients and accounts for the poor long-term survival in this group of patients. Interestingly, the detrimental effect on survival appears to be less in recipients of marrow or nonhepatic solid organ transplants.

Treatment of HBV infection in immunosuppressed patients is difficult and the results are disappointing (Davis 1989). As discussed above, eradication of HBV is felt to be mediated through immune clearance of the virus. Alpha interferon, the only agent of proven therapeutic efficacy in this disease, is felt to have its effect through reduction of HBV load *and* stimulation of the cellular immune response against the virus (Perrillo et al. 1991). Unfortunately, most immunosuppressed patients do not appear to be capable of mounting an adequate cellular immune response. In addition, currently available antiviral agents, including alpha interferons, do not appear to be capable of significantly reducing viral load in these patients. Thus, therapeutic options are currently extremely limited (Davis 1989).

Hepatitis C

Hepatitis C virus (HCV) is a single-stranded RNA virus similar, but not identical, to the flavi- and pestiviridae (Davis 1991b). The agent is responsible for most of what was previously called non-A, non-B hepatitis. The characteristics of the virus and the disease resulting from infection with it are reviewed in Table 4. As with hepatitis B, 40% of patients with hepatitis C have no identifiable risk factor (Davis 1991b). Recognized routes of transmission are primarily parenteral. Forty percent of patients have a history of intravenous drug use. Transfusion was a major cause of infection in the past but now accounts for only about 5% of acute cases (Davis 1991).

Table 4. Characteristics of HCV infection

Single-stranded RNA virus similar to flavi-/pestiviruses	
Mode of infection	Percutaneous/parenteral
	Sexual (probable, but uncommon)
	Perinatal (probable, but uncommon)
	Unknown (40%)
Chronicity	Immunocompetent (30%–70%)
	Immunosuppressed (30%–90%)
Injury	Directly cytopathic
	Other modes of injury unknown
Course	Insidiously progressive
	Spontaneous resolution unusual

This reduction in transfusion-related hepatitis is due to improvement in donor screening, elimination of commercial donors for routine blood donation, institution of testing for surrogate markers of hepatitis C infection in 1986, and use of anti-HCV beginning in May 1990. However, hepatitis C is still the most common infection transmitted by transfusion with a risk per recipient of 1.7%–3.0% (one in 30–60). The incubation period of the HCV is 2–12 weeks with the majority of cases occurring 6–8 weeks after exposure (Dienstag 1983).

The major liability of acute hepatitis C infection is the propensity to progress to chronicity in 50%–60% of cases (Davis 1991b; Dienstag 1983). The natural history of chronic hepatitis C is incompletely characterized, but appears to be insidiously progressive in most patients. Cirrhosis develops in at least 20% of cases during short-term follow up and probably half of patients over the course of disease (Davis 1991b; Dienstag 1983). However, cirrhosis is clinically inapparent in the majority of these patients and hepatic failure develops in only about a quarter of cirrhotic patients (Dienstag 1983). Like hepatitis B, hepatitis C is associated with the development of hepatocellular carcinoma (Davis 1991b). Unlike hepatitis B, HCV is thought to be directly cytopathic to the hepatocyte. Whether other mechanisms of hepatic injury, e.g., immune-mediated, act as well is not yet known.

Chronic hepatitis C is common in oncology, hematology, and transplant patients (Davis 1989). Indeed, more than a third of solid organ transplant recipients have chronic serum ALT elevations that are felt to be secondary to this infection (Davies et al. 1991). The course of the disease in the immunosuppressed patient appears to be aggressive. Non-A, non-B hepatitis (diagnosed prior to hepatitis C serologic testing) is the major cause of death in renal transplant recipients more than 5 years from transplant (Reinke et al. 1987). Hepatitis C has been shown to be particularly aggressive in acquired immunodeficiency syndrome (AIDS) patients (Martin et al. 1989). Although common, the infection has not yet been shown to be a major factor influencing survival in infected liver and heart transplant patients. In fact, the course of hepatitis C in these patients remains difficult to document since serologic tests for HCV are unreliable in immunosuppressed patients. Considerable work needs to be done to document the course of disease in these patients.

Recombinant interferon alfa-2b was recently licensed for treatment of chronic hepatitis C. Interferon controls disease activity (normalizes serum ALT levels and reduces hepatic inflammation) in 40%–50% of patients (Davis et al. 1989). It is felt that interferon acts by a direct antiviral effect to suppress HCV. Indeed, serum HCV-RNA becomes undetectable in responding patients (Brillanti et al. 1991). However, interferon does not appear to eradicate infection in many patients. Indeed, 50%–80% of patients demonstrate return of serum HCV-RNA and relapse of serum ALT after discontinuation of treatment (Davis et al. 1989; Brillanti et al. 1991). These patients require further therapy, often with long-term maintenance.

Interferon treatment of HCV should be used with extreme caution in immunosuppressed transplant recipients. In fact, the licensing for the drug specifically excludes transplant recipients from treatment consideration. The rationale for this recommendation is that interferon is a potent immuno-stimulant which increases HLA display and activates a number of arms of the immune response process (Davis 1989). Not surprisingly, it has been reported to result in graft rejection (Weimar et al. 1985). Trials are underway to document the extent of these effects and the limits of drug safety in transplant recipients.

References

Brillanti S, Garson JA, Tuke PW et al. (1991) Effect of alpha-interferon therapy on hepatitis C viraemia in community-acquired chronic non-A, non-B hepatitis: a quantitative polymerase chain reaction study. J Med Virol 34:136–141

Davies SE, Portmann BC, O'Grady JG et al. (1991) Hepatic histological findings after transplantation for chronic hepatitis B virus infection, including a unique pattern of fibrosing cholestatic hepatitis. Hepatology 13:150–157

Davis GL (1989) Interferon treatment of viral hepatitis in immunocompromised patients. Semin Liver Dis 9:267–272

Davis GL (1991a) Chronic hepatitis. In: Kaplowitz N (ed) Liver and biliary diseases. Williams and Wilkins, Baltimore

Davis GL (1991b) Hepatitis C virus. In: Mandell GL, Douglas RG, Bennett JE (eds) Principles and practice of infectious diseases. Churchill Livingstone, New York, pp 3–11

Davis GL, Hoofnagle JH, Waggoner JG (1984) Spontaneous reactivation of chronic hepatitis B virus infection. Gastroenterology 86:230–235

Davis GL, Balart LA, Schiff ER et al. (1989) Treatment of chronic hepatitis C with recombinant alfa interferon: a multicenter randomized controlled trial. N Engl J Med 321:1501–1506

Dienstag JL (1983) Non-A, non-B hepatitis: I. Recognition, epidemiology, and clinical features. Gastroenterology 85:439–462

Dusheiko G, Song E, Bowyer S et al. (1983) Natural history of hepatitis B virus infection in renal transplant recipients – a fifteen year follow-up. Hepatology 3:330–336

Ferrari C, Penna A, DegliAntoni A, Fiaccardori F (1988) Cellular immune response to hepatitis B virus antigens: an overview. J Hepatol 7:21–33

Hoofnagle JH, Dusheiko GM, Seeff LB et al. (1981) Seroconversion from hepatitis Be antigen to antibody in chronic type B hepatitis. Ann Intern Med 94:744–748

Hoofnagle JH, Davis GL, Hanson RG et al. (1986) A short course of prednisolone in chronic type B hepatitis: report of a randomized double-blind placebo-controlled trial. Ann Intern Med 104:12–16

Korenman J, Baker B, Waggoner J et al. (1991) Long-term remission of chronic hepatitis B after alpha-interferon therapy. Ann Intern Med 114:629–634

Martin P, DiBisceglie AM, Kassianides C (1989) Rapidly progressive non-A, non-B hepatitis in patients with human immunodeficiency virus infection. Gastroenterology 97:1559–1561

Perrillo RP, Schiff ER, Davis GL et al. (1991) A randomized, controlled study of interferon alfa, alone and following prednisone withdrawal, in the treatment of chronic hepatitis B. N Engl J Med 323:295–301

Pinto PC, Hu E, Bernstein-Singer M, Pinter-Brown L, Govindarajan S (1990) Acute hepatic injury after withdrawal of immunosuppressive chemotherapy in patients with hepatitis B. Cancer 65:878–884

Reinke P, David H, Scholz D (1987) The significance of liver changes as the cause of death in kidney transplant patients: an analysis of 689 autopsy cases. Zentralbl Allg Pathol 133:447–452

Seeff LB (1990) Diagnosis, therapy, and prognosis of viral hepatitis. In: Zakim D, Boyer TD (eds) Hepatology: a textbook of liver disease, 2nd edn. Saunders, Philadelphia, pp 958–1025

Tur-Kaspa R, Burk RD, Shaul Y, Shafritz DA (1986) Hepatitis B virus contains a glucocorticoid responsive element. Proc Natl Acad Sci USA 83:1627–1631

Wands JR, Walker JA, Davis TT et al. (1974) Hepatitis B in an oncology unit. N Engl J Med 29:1371–1375

Weimar W, Kramer P, Bijnen AB et al. (1985) The incidence of cytomegalo- and herpes simplex virus infections in renal allograft recipients treated with high-dose recombinant leukocyte interferon: a controlled study. Scand J Urol Nephrol 92[Suppl]:37–39

Further Reading

Davis GL (1989) Interferon treatment of viral hepatitis in immunocompromised patients. Semin Liver Dis 9:267–272
    Review of the natural history and treatment of viral hepatitis in immunocompromised patients.

Davis GL, Balart LA, Schiff ER et al. (1989) Treatment of chronic hepatitis C with recombinant alfa interferon: a multicenter randomized controlled trial. N Engl J Med 321:1501–1506
    Report of large multicenter study which documented effectiveness of treatment of chronic non-A, non-B hepatitis (hepatitis C) with recombinant interferon alfa2b.

Pinto PC, Hu E, Bernstein-Singer M, Pinter-Brown L, Govindarajan S (1990) Acute hepatic injury after withdrawal of immunosuppressive chemotherapy in patients with hepatitis B. Cancer 65:878–884
    Report of cases and discussion of post-chemotherapy liver failure due to activation of hepatitis B.

Emergence of Gram-Positive Infections: Relationship to Indwelling Catheters and Management During Chemotherapy-Induced Aplasia

J.E. Karp[1] and J.D. Dick[2]

[1] The National Cancer Institute, Bethesda, MD 20892, USA
[2] Johns Hopkins Oncology Center and Department of Laboratory Medicine, The Johns Hopkins Medical Institutions, Baltimore, MD 21205, USA

The empiric use of broad-spectrum antibacterial antibiotics for first fever in the granulocytopenic patient has had a major impact in lowering mortality from overwhelming infection caused by aerobic Gram-negative bacteria (Schimpff et al. 1971; Hathorn et al. 1987; Klastersky 1989; Karp et al. 1990). Despite this decrease in early infectious death, there has been an increased prevalence of Gram-positive (GP) infections in this same population which, while less life-threatening than their Gram-negative counterparts, can result in significant morbidity. Several factors are likely responsible for the emerging prominence of GP infections in this clinical setting (Table 1). In particular, the use of indwelling, multiport central venous catheters (CVC) as a routine adjunct to optimize venous access during lengthy aplasia has accentuated the problems of GP infection (Lowder et al. 1982; Lokich et al. 1985; Dickinson and Bisno 1989). Both initial catheter placement and long-term catheterization are accompanied by skin barrier invasion. The mechanical interruption of barrier integrity predisposes to local infection at exit and/or tunnel sites, thrombophlebitis, and sepsis from colonization along the entire catheter tract by common skin organisms including coagulase-negative staphylococci and *Corynebacterium jeikeium*. These bacteria are often resistant to beta lactam antibiotics and other antibiotics commonly used in empiric regiments for treatment of first infectious fever during aplasia (Karp et al. 1986; Anaissie et al. 1988a; Shenep et al. 1988). They are susceptible, however, to vancomycin, a cell wall-acting glycopeptide antibiotic with efficacy against both beta lactam-susceptible and resistant staphylococci and corynebacteria.

The frequency of local and disseminated GP infections in these compromised hosts has led to a number of trials evaluating the therapeutic role of empirically administered vancomycin during deep aplasia. In prospective clinical trials at centers where GP infections have been particularly prevalent (Karp et al. 1986; Shenep et al. 1988), empiric vancomycin therapy begun at the time of first infectious fever has resulted in prompt fever resolution,

Table 1. Increased incidence of Gram-positive infectious complications during induced granulocytopenia

1. Improved intervention against specific tumor-related complications (leukostasis, coagulopathy, tumor lysis)
2. Effective empiric antibacterial coverage of potentially life-threatening Gram-negative infections at the time of first infectious fever
3. Increased use of indwelling catheters, leading to increased skin barrier breakdown
4. Increased use of parenteral hyperalimentation
5. Development of beta lactam antibiotic resistance by Gram-positive organisms

rapid clearance of local and/or disseminated GP infections, and prevention of late-onset GP infections in acute leukemia patients with indwelling venous catheters and chemotherapy-induced granulocytopenia. Antibiotic susceptibility testing of GP pathogens demonstrates uniform susceptibility to vancomycin in vitro, with the large majority being susceptible at minimal inhibitory drug concentration of $1-2\,\mu g/ml$. However, in centers where GP infections have been less prevalent, the role for early empiric vancomycin has been less clear. While vancomycin has been effective in treating established infection, these latter trials suggest that the drug can be added selectively and nonempirically (Hathorn et al. 1987; Rubin et al. 1988).

Pharmacologic, microbiologic, and perhaps physiologic factors suggest that the current dose schedule of vancomycin could be modified without sacrificing efficacy in this patient population. In traditional dosing schedules of vancomycin, the intravenous administration of 500 mg every 6 h to patients with normal renal function affords peak serum drug concentrations of $20-40\,\mu g/ml$ and 6-h trough concentrations of at least $10\,\mu g/ml$. These findings are consistent with pharmacokinetic studies demonstrating a $T_{1/2}$ of 6 h in normal subjects with a predominant renal route for excretion of active drug. Secondly, the antibiotic susceptibility profiles for most GP pathogens, as noted previously, suggest that lower peak and trough serum drug levels should still provide full therapeutic coverage for GP infections and thorough protection against breakthrough infection. Finally, the patient with profound marrow aplasia lacks both granulocytes and platelets and is unable to form abscesses or loculations, thus theoretically permitting more efficient drug penetration into infected sites.

On the basis of the above considerations, we compared the clinical pharmacology and efficacy of empirically instituted vancomycin given intravenously in a reduced total dose and schedule (low-dose vancomycin, LDV; 500 mg every 12 h) with vancomycin given in standard dosage (SDV, 500 mg every 6 h) in 94 adult acute leukemia patients undergoing 143 courses of antileukemic therapy-induced profound marrow aplasia (granulocytes <100/ mm^3) lasting a median of 32 days (range 16–75). In this study, LDV or SDV was instituted for first infectious fever in combination with gentamicin (2 mg/kg every 6 h) and ticarcillin (45 mg/kg every 4 h). Pharmacologically,

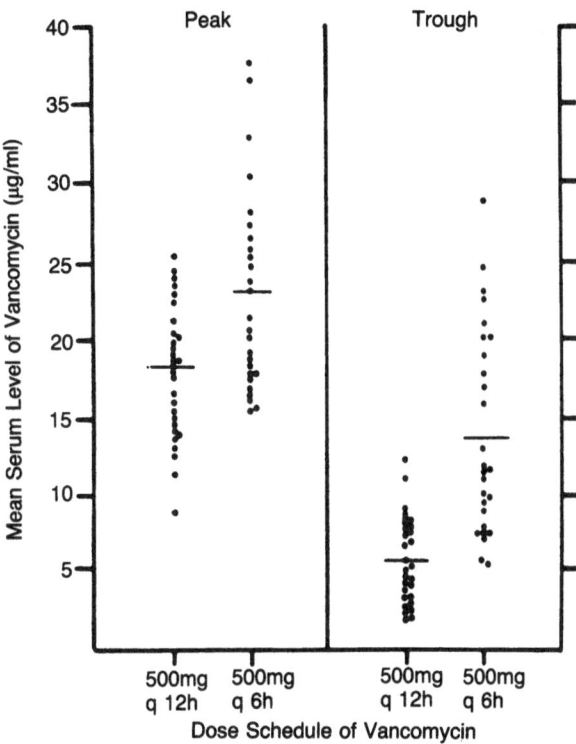

Fig. 1. Mean individual peak and trough serum vancomycin levels obtained twice weekly throughout granulocytopenia from 29 LDV and 27 SDV patients undergoing the prospective randomized trial. Mean peak serum drug levels were 17.9 µg/ml (range 8.7–25.2) for individual LDV patients and 23.1 µg/ml (range 15.3–37.4) for individual SDV patients ($p < 0.0007$). Mean trough serum drug levels were 5.7 µg/ml (range 1.8–12.1) for LDV and 13.8 µg/ml (range 5.4–28.7) for SDV patients ($p < 10^6$)

the individual and mean peak serum levels obtained 1 h post-drug infusion were at least 10 µg/ml for both dose schedules. Mean trough levels were at least 2.0 µg/ml in all but two patients receiving LDV and in all patients receiving SDV. Peak and trough serum drug levels in all individuals were closely and directly correlated for both dose schedules (LDV, $r = 0.82$, $p < 10^6$; SDV, $r = 0.94$, $p < 10^6$) (Fig. 1).

The clinical effects of LDV equalled those of SDV begun at the time of first infectious fever and continued throughout aplasia until granulocyte counts recovered to more than 500/mm³. In both groups, the occurrence of first fever systemic and local GP infection was similar (approximately 30%; Table 2). In all patients with sepsis, both LDV and SDV effected rapid (<24 h) clearance of bacteremia and the time to response of first fever, independent of documented infection, was similar in both groups (defer-

Table 2. Incidence of Gram-positive infections using empiric standard versus low-dose vancomycin

Time	Empiric LDV ($n = 71$)						Empiric SDV ($n = 72$)					
	Sepsis[a]		Local		Total		Sepsis		Local		Total	
	(n)	(%)	(n)	(%)	(n)	(%)	(n)	(%)	(n)	(%)	(n)	(%)
First infectious fever	18	25	4	5.6	22	31	17	24	6	8.3	23	31.9
Breakthrough fever	3	4.2	1	1.4	4	5.6	0	0	2	2.8	2	2.8

[a] ≥Positive blood cultures.

vescence within a mean 3 days). Importantly, late-onset GP infections were uncommon events in both groups, occurring in four of 71 (6%) LDV patients and two of 72 (3%) SDV patients. All three episodes of late-onset GP sepsis occurred in LDV patients, however (Table 2). Nonetheless, this trial demonstrated the feasibility and efficacy of using LDV throughout prolonged aplasia without incurring significant breakthrough GP infections or predisposing to the development of colonization or superinfection with vancomycin-resistant GP organisms.

Still, the striking incidence of GP infections in association with first infectious fever in aplasia – consistently 25%–30% over a 4-year period of close observation during antibiotic clinical trials (1983–1986) – led us to evaluate the role of LDV given prophylactically following CVC placement, prior to antileukemic therapy, and throughout aplasia in suppressing the occurrence of early as well as late GP complications during profound marrow aplasia. The adult leukemia patient population undergoing 281 consecutive treatment episodes and their relevant clinical features are delineated in Table 3. The prevention of early GP infection by prophylactic use of LDV is depicted in Table 4. Prophylactic LDV had a major impact on early infection, reducing GP infection from 31% when vancomycin was begun empirically for first infectious fever to 5% when vancomycin was instituted at the time of CVC placement ($\chi^2 = 53.3$, $p < 10^6$). Thus, prophylactic vancomycin prevented 80% of all early GP infections. The remaining 20% occurred prior to or within 48 h of prophylactic LDV institution. The spectrum of GP organisms causing early infections remained similar to the spectrum detected during previous study periods. In addition, there was been no change during the years 1986–1990 throughout which vancomycin prophylaxis was routinely implemented.

As in the preceding trial of empirically administered vancomycin, breakthrough sepsis and/or local GP infections were detected in only 16 (6%) of the 281 prophylactic LDV courses. Similarly, the predominant organisms

Table 3. Prophylactic low-dose vancomycin in leukemia patient population (1986–1990)

Type of leukemia (treatment episode)	Episodes (n)	Duration of Aplasia (days) (Median)	(Range)	Age (years) (Median)	(Range)
Acute myelogenous	236	32	17–65	55	18–76
Induction	101				
Remission	66				
Relapse	69				
Acute lymphocytic	45	28	15–50	35	18–71
Induction	26				
Remission	6				
Relapse	13				

Table 4. Incidence of Gram-positive infections during induced granulocytopenia using prophylactic low-dose vancomycin

Infecting organism	Initial presentation[a]			Breakthrough		
	Sepsis[b]	Local	Total	Sepsis	Local	Total
Staphylococcus spp. (coagulase-negative)	10	0	10	10	2	12
Staphylococcus aureus	1	3	4	0	1	1
Corynectacterium spp.	1	0	1	0	1	1
Streptococcus viridans	1	1	2	1	1	2
Enterococcus spp.	0	0	0	0	2	2
Total isolates			17 from 14/281 (5%) patients			18 from 16/281 (6%) patients

[a] At time of admission, prior to institution of prophylactic LDV and chemotherapy.
[b] ≥2 Positive blood cultures.

were beta lactam-resistant, coagulase-negative staphylococci. There was no emergence of vancomycin resistance or shift to other causative GP bacteria (Table 5). All GP isolates had vancomycin minimal inhibitory concentrations (MIC) of four or less. Bacteremias and local infections occurred with equal frequency. All 281 patients had multiport CVC inserted before beginning antileukemic therapy and vancomycin was begun as soon as proper placement was confirmed. Mean length of catheter life was 35 days (median 34, range 1–74). CVCs were removed and replaced during chemotherapy-induced aplasia only for mechanical or infectious complications. Mechanical complications, manifested primarily by thrombosis, occurred early in four (1.4%) patients on mean day 2.7 of placement, without evidence for con-

Table 5. Gram-positive bacteria causing infections during prophylactic low-dose vancomycin (1986–1990)

Organism	(n)	(%)
Staphylococcus spp. (coagulase-negative)	22	63
Staphylococcus aureus	5	14
Streptococcus viridans group	4	11
Enterococcus spp.	2	6
Corynebacterium spp.	2	6
Total isolates	35 Strains from 30/281 (11%) patients	

Table 6. Multiport central venous catheter complications during prophylactic low-dose vancomycin (1986–1990)

	Thrombosis	Infection
Incidence (n)	4/281	7/281
(%)	1.4	2.5
Day of placement (Mean)	2.7	25
(Median)	3	22
(Range)	1–6	6–59

Mean catheter life = 35 days (median = 34; range = 1–74).

comitant GP infection. In contrast, CVC GP infection occurred in seven (2.5%) patients late in the chemotherapy course on mean day 25 of placement (Table 6). Of note, the incidence of GP infections did not increase during serial courses of intensive antileukemic therapy. During initial induction therapy of newly diagnosed acute leukemia, GP infections occurred early (prior to or within 48 h of beginning prophylactic LDV) in eight of 127 patients (6.3%) and late in seven patients (5.5%). Similarly, in 154 subsequent chemotherapy cycles, GP infections occurred early in six (3.8%) and late in seven patients (4.5%). Thus, during the 4-year period of continuous prophylactic LDV usage, there was no increase in GP infections during repeated courses of therapy and no evidence for resistance development or shift in causative organisms for individual patients, as well as for the whole group of adults with acute leukemia. Figure 2 summarizes our experience with GP sepsis in the granulocytopenic adult leukemia patient and the effect of vancomycin utilization in various dose schedules on the treatment and prevention of GP infection during profound bone marrow aplasia.

A recent prospective, randomized trial in patients undergoing bone marrow transplantation (BMT) (Attal 1991) substantiates these findings by

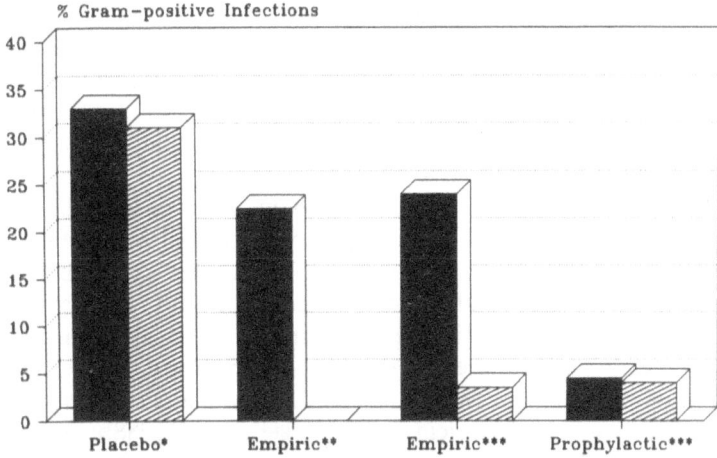

Fig. 2. The effects of vancomycin administered empirically (first infectious fever) and prophylactically on Gram-positive infections during antileukemia therapy-induced granulocytopenia. *Solid columns*, Gram-positive infection causing first fever; *hatched columns*, Gram-positive infection causing late-onset fever; *, no vancomycin; **, vancomycin 500 mg every 6 h; ***, vancomycin 500 mg every 12 h

demonstrating that prophylactically administered vancomycin prevents the majority of early GP infections and, as a consequence, delays the onset of first infectious fever. In both BMT (Attal et al. 1991) and antileukemic chemotherapy settings (Karp et al. 1986; Shenep et al. 1988), continuation of vancomycin throughout profound granulocytopenia successfully suppresses late-onset GP infections without evidence for development of clinically significant vancomycin resistance to date. As a result of delaying the onset of first fever and decreasing total numbers of febrile days, total antibiotic usage (and the attendant total costs of care) may in some cases decrease.

Yet, indwelling catheters are not the sole source of local and disseminated GP infections in this compromised patient population. Chemotherapy-induced cytotoxicity to skin and oropharyngeal mucosal barriers, in addition to skin invasion and granulocytopenia, is a significant factor in development of first fever GP infections. The dissemination of GP organisms from any of these potential sites of barrier breakdown can be suppressed by effective prophylactic therapy directed against GP pathogens. The role for anti-GP prophylaxis is supported by recent studies in patients receiving immunotherapy who are compromised by lymphocyte dysfunction and perhaps by the induction of certain tissue-active cytokines, rather than by absence of granulocytes (Bock et al. 1990). The recent recognition of overwhelming infections caused by *Streptococcus mitis* in association with therapy-induced oropharyngeal mucositis lends further credence to a prophylactic approach, particularly in patients predisposed to this potentially fatal complication (Karp et al. 1990; Weisman et al. 1990). Recently, concerns have been raised that quinolone prophylaxis against gastrointestinally based Gram-negative infections could possibly predispose to colonization and subsequent infection by GP organisms, particularly *S. mitis* (Winston et al. 1987; Karp et al. 1990). However, this potential complication can be averted by prophylaxis directed against GP pathogens throughout the period of maximal mucosal and hematopoietic toxicities.

An emerging problem is that of colonization of indwelling catheters and subsequent local and systemic infection by fungal pathogens (Lowder et al. 1982; Klastersky 1989; Karp et al. 1991). This problem has emerged as consequence of several factors including lengthy aplasias, prolonged use of broad-spectrum antibacterial antibiotics and hyperalimentation. Many of these organisms are either non-albicans yeast (for example, *Candida parapsilosis*) or filamentous fungi (for example, *Fusarium* spp.) which are refractory to amphotericin B (Anaissie et al. 1988b; Merz et al. 1988; Karp et al. 1991). While aggressive antifungal approaches have proven to be successful therapeutically, strategies to prevent these fungal infections remain to be elucidated.

In summary, the empiric use of vancomycin, with concomitant broad-spectrum anti-Gram-negative antibiotics, is effective in treating early GP infections and preventing the emergence of late-onset GP infections in patients undergoing intensive antileukemic therapy attended by prolonged granulocytopenia. Further, the prophylactic use of LDV has proven successful in preventing 80% of early GP infections. The use of vancomycin either prophylactically or therapeutically for GP infections contributes to the length of indwelling catheter life in the deeply aplastic host. It is likely that the suppression of local catheter or surrounding tissue colonization and infection by GP pathogens prevents the occurrence and/or propogation of infection-related thrombophlebitis. In addition, the absence of granulocytes and the inability to sequester pathogens in a formed abscess may actually facilitate the eradication of any local foci of infection, since organisms are not protected from antibiotic penetration. Thus, in adults with acute leukemia and indwelling CVC, the use of prophylactic LDV (500 mg every 12 h) can suppress systemic and local GP infections both early and late during profound chemotherapy-induced bone marrow aplasia, without development of vancomycin resistance despite continued long-term use in these compromised hosts.

References

Anaissie EL, Fainstein V, Bodey GP et al. (1988a) Randomized trial of beta-lactam regimens in the febrile neutropenic cancer patients. Am J Med 84:581–589

Anaissie EL, Kantarjian H, Ro J et al. (1988b) The emerging role of Fusarium infections in patients with cancer. Medicine (Baltimore) 67:77–83

Attal M, Schlaifer D, Rubie H et al. (1991) Prevention of Gram-positive infections after bone marrow transplantation by systemic vancomycin: a prospective, randomized trial. J Clin Oncol 9:865–870

Bock SN, Lee RE, Fisher B et al. (1990) A prospective randomized trail evaluating prophylactic antibiotics to prevent triple-lumen catheter-related sepsis in patients treated with immunotherapy. J Clin Oncol 8:161–169

Dickinson GM, Bisno AL (1989) Infections associated with indwelling devices: concepts of pathogenesis; infections associated with intravascular devices. Antimicrob Agents Chemother 33:597–601

Hathorn JW, Rubin M, Pizzo PA (1987) Empirical antibiotic therapy in the febrile neutropenic cancer patient: clinical efficacy and impact of monotherapy. Antimicrob Agents Chemother 31:971–977

Karp JE, Dick JD, Angelopulos C et al. (1986) Empiric use of vancomycin during prolonged treatment-induced granulocytopenia: a randomized, double-blind, placebo-controlled clinical trial in patients with acute leukemia. Am J Med 81:237–242

Karp JE, Merz WG, Dick JD et al. (1990) Management of infectious complications of acute leukemia and antileukemia therapy. Oncology 4:45–53

Karp JE, Merz WG, Charache P (1991) An evaluation of the response to empiric amphotericin B during antileukemic therapy-induced granulocytopenia. Rev Infect Dis 13:592–599

Klastersky J (1989) Empiric treatment of infection during granulocytopenia: a comprehensive approach. Infection 17:59–64

Lokich JJ, Bothe A Jr, Benotti et al. (1985) Complications and management of implanted venous access catheters. J Clin Oncol 3:710–717

Lowder JN, Lazarus HM, Herzig RH et al. (1982) Bacteremias and fungemias in oncologic patients with central venous catheters: changing spectrum of infection. Arch Intern Med 142:1456–1459

Merz WG, Karp JE, Hoagland M et al. (1988) Diagnosis and successful treatment of fusariosis in the compromised host. J Infect Dis 158:1046–1055

Rubin M, Hathorn JW, Marshall D et al. (1988) Gram-positive infections and the use of vancomycin in 550 episodes of fever and neutropenia. Ann Intern Med 108:30–35

Schimpff SC, Satterlee W, Young VM et al. (1971) Empiric therapy with carbenicillin and gentamicin for febrile patients with cancer and granulocytopenia. N Engl J Med 284:1061–1065

Shenep J, Hughes WT, Robertson PJ et al. (1988) Vancomycin, ticarcillin and amikacin compared with ticarcillin-clavulanate and amikacin in the empirical treatment of febrile, neutropenic children with cancer. N Engl J Med 319:1053–105

Weisman SJ, Scoopo FJ, Johnson GM et al. (1990) Septicemia in pediatric oncology patients: the significance of viridans streptococcal infections. J Clin Oncol 8:453–459

Winston DJ, Ho WG, Karp JE et al. (1987) Norfloxacin for prevention of bacterial infections in granulocytopenic patients. Am J Med 82:40–46

VI. New Pathogens/Resistance/Drug Delivery

New Pathogens in the Immunocompromised Host

S.H. Zinner

Brown University Division of Infectious Diseases, Roger Williams Medical Center, Rhode Island Hospital Providence, RI 02129, USA

As more patients receive ever-increasing and more potent chemotherapy for cancer and more potent immunosuppressive agents for bone marrow and other transplantations we are likely to encounter increasing numbers of opportunistic infections and also new types of infecting organisms. Even in the past decade several changes have occurred in the distribution of organisms causing bacteremia in neutropenic patients.

The importance of an intact immune system in the prevention of serious infection is emphasized by the human immunodeficiency virus (HIV) epidemic. Clearly, the acquired immunodeficiency syndrome (AIDS) epidemic has allowed the emergence of serious pathogenic organisms which either were unknown or were previously thought to be commensals. This paper will review the current trends in infections in neutropenic patients caused by bacteria and other organisms and also will highlight some of the organisms newly recognized as pathogens in patients with AIDS and other altered immune states.

Trends in Bacterial Pathogens in the Febrile Neutropenic Patient

To most oncologists, the neutropenic patient remains the most common "immunosuppressed" patient in their practice. Patients with hematologic malignancies are often rendered profoundly neutropenic for several weeks as a result of their chemotherapy and increasingly as patients with solid tumors receive intensive cancer chemotherapy with or without bone marrow transplantation. All these patients may be granulocytopenic for several days or weeks.

Fever is very common in granulocytopenic patients and several studies have estimated that approximately 60% of these fevers are associated with microbiologically documented infections (including bacteremia) and clinically

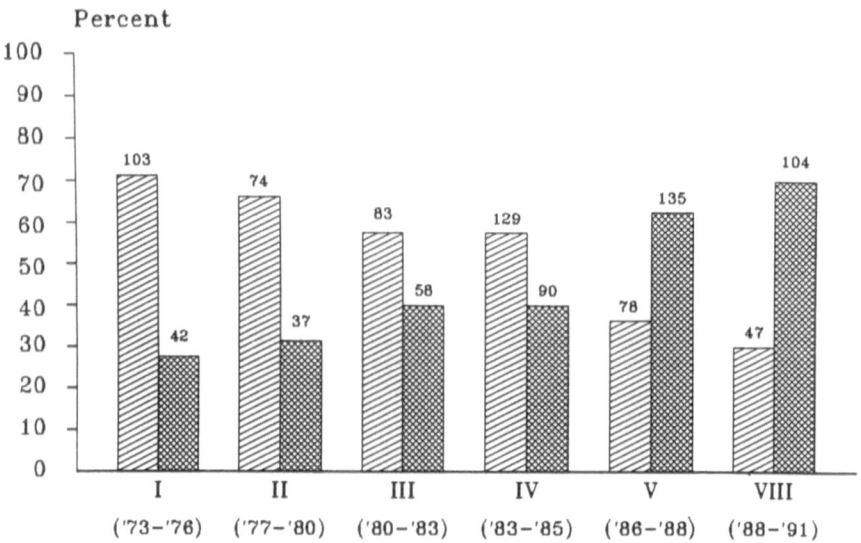

Fig. 1. Trends in single organism bacteremia (EORTC—IATCG). *Hatched columns*, Gram-negative bacteria; *crossed hatched columns*, Gram-positive bacteria

documented infections. This high frequency of presumptive infection in febrile neutropenic patients has justified the empirical approach to therapy.

A decade ago, Gram-negative rod bacteremia was the most frequent and lethal infection in neutropenic patients with cancer. *Escherichia coli, Klebsiella* species, and *Pseudomonas aeruginosa* were the most common organisms and overall Gram-negative rods were responsible for more than two thirds of the bacteremic episodes in these patients. More recently, Gram-positive cocci have emerged as important agents of bacteremia in neutropenic patients. Possibly because of the mucositis associated with intensive chemotherapy, the increasing use of Hickman or Broviac intravascular catheters and/or the increasing use of quinolone antibiotics as prophylactic agents, Gram-positive cocci now are responsible for most episodes of bacteremia in neutropenic patients (EORTC International Antimicrobial Therapy Cooperative Group and National Cancer Institute of Canada – Clinical Trials Group 1991).

The International Antimicrobial Therapy Cooperative Group (IATCG) of the European Organization for Research and Treatment of Cancer has been studying infections in neutropenic patients with cancer for the past 20 years. As seen in Fig. 1, although the overall incidence of blood stream infections has not changed dramatically, there has been a major shift in the distribution of Gram-negative versus Gram-positive organisms. For example, in the first EORTC-IATCG trial in 1973–1976, Gram-negative rods accounted for 71% of the bacteremic isolates and Gram-positive cocci for 29%. In the eighth therapeutic trial, completed in early 1991, Gram-negative rods were responsible for bacteremia in 47 of 151 patients (31%), whereas Gram-positive cocci were responsible in 104 patients or 69%

Moreover, 1 decade ago, most Gram-positive isolates were either *Staphylococcus aureus* or *Staphylococcus epidermidis*. In the past few years other Gram-positive cocci including viridans streptococci, *Staphylococcus mitis*, *Streptococcus pyogenes*, *Streptococcus pneumoniae*, and *Enterococcus* species have emerged as major bacteremic pathogens. As seen in Table 1, viridans streptococci and coagulase-negative staphylococci accounted for 70% of the 134 single-organism bacteremias caused by Gram-positive organisms in a recent IATCG Trial (EORTC International Antimicrobial Therapy Cooperative Group and National Cancer Institute of Canada – Clinical Trials Group 1991). Also, several neutropenic febrile patients with viridans streptococcal bacteremia reportedly have developed bacterial endocarditis even in the face of thrombocytopenia.

Although bacteremias caused by Gram-positive cocci are clearly increasing in this population, the mortality associated with these organisms remains low, and empiric therapy directed specifically at Gram-positive bacteria is not recommended by all investigators unless there is a special incidence of breakthrough bacteremia or resistant organisms in a given institution.

New Pathogenic Organisms in Neutropenic and Other Immunocompromised Patients

Bacteria

In the past 5–10 years several other bacteria have emerged as causes of infection in neutropenic and non-neutropenic patients with cancer. Several Gram-negative bacteria can be included here such as *Legionella pneumophila* and other *Legionella* species, *Xanthomonas maltophilia*, *Pseudomonas putrefaciens*, and *Leptotrichia buccalis*.

Xanthomonas maltophilia (previously *Pseudomonas maltophilia*) is increasing as a cause of nosocomial infections in neutropenic patients (Khardori et al. 1990). This organism has been associated with nosocomial infections and, in particular, may emanate from water sources. Strains of *X. maltophilia* are generally resistant to imipenem and othe beta lactam agents as well as the aminoglycosides. Trimethoprim sulfamethoxazole and some of the new fluoroquinolones may be effective clinically.

Pseudomonas putrefaciens (possible new name: *Alteromonas putrefaciens*) is an oxidase-positive, non-glucose-fermenting flagellated Gram-negative rod which produces H_2S on triple sugar iron agar. It can be found in "tainted" butter, sewage, dairy products, spoiled meats, oysters, etc. Initially *P. putrefaciens* was thought to be a cause of chronic otitis media. However, more recently it has been identified as a cause of cutaneous ulcers, cellulitis, and septicemia. This organism is susceptible to most second- and third-

Table 1. Single organism bacteremic isolates in the fifth IATCG therapeutic trial (747 patients). (From EORTC Group 1991)

Organism	Number isolated	
	(n)	(%)
Streptococcus species	57	
Viridans group		44
Group D		5[b]
S. pneumoniae		4
Other streptococci		4
Coagulase-negative staphylococci	49	
Staphylococcus aureus	20	
Corynebacterium spp.	5	
Other organisms[a]	3	
Total Gram-positive organisms	134	64
Total Gram-negative organisms	77	36

[a] Includes Listeria monocytogenes, Bacillus cereus, Propionibacterium acnes.
[b] Includes Enterococcus faecium (n = 4), Enterococcus faecalis (n = 1).

generation cephalosporins, ureidopenicillins, aminoglycosides, imipenem, and the fluoroquinolones. This organism was recently described as a cause of fulminant septicemia in a neutropenic patient and in a patient with metastatic carcinoma (Kim et al. 1989).

Leptotrichia buccalis is an anaerobic Gram-negative rod normally present in the oral flora. This organism recently has been described as a cause of bacteremia in patients with advanced malignancies and especially those who have oral mucosal ulceration or inflammation. Weinberger et al. (1991) described four patients with *L. buccalis* septicemia and reviewed the literature of six other patients. New infections have been caused in patients with leukemia and solid tumors, especially those with mucositis or esophageal or colon lesions. This organism is resistant to the aminoglycosides, vancomycin, fluoroquinolones, and erythromycin but is susceptible to penicillins, clindamycin, cephalosporins, metronidazole, and tetracycline.

Legionella pneumophila and *Legionella micdadei* are well recognized causes of pneumonia and they also may disseminate to other organs in bone marrow transplant recipients and other immunocompromised patients. *L. micdadei* is a cause of nosocomial infection in immunocompromised patients with serious chronic diseases. Risk factors associated with pneumonia caused by *L. micdadei* and *L. pneumophila* include corticosteroid use, prolonged hospitalization, renal transplantation, and, as recently described, bone marrow transplantation (Schwebke et al. 1990). *Legionella* pneumonia presents with abrupt onset of fever and cough, which may be associated with pleuritic pain. *L. micdadei* and *L. pneumophila* infections may present with similar chest X-ray findings but pulmonary nodules which expand rapidly are seen with the former organism. Useful antibiotics against the Legionellae include erythromycin, trimethoprim-sulfamethoxazole with or without rifampin, the fluoroquinolones, and the new azalide-macrolide drugs.

Gram-positive bacteria continue to be major bacteremic pathogens in neutropenic patients. *Leuconostoc* species used to be considered as non-pathogens. These Streptococcaceae would appear in the laboratory as vancomycin-resistant viridans streptococci. They may be relatively fastidious and slow growing and they must be distinguished in the laboratory from enterococci and lactobacilli. They are reported to cause bacteremia, leukocytosis, fever, and abdominal pain in a wide spectrum of underlying diseases (Handwerger et al. 1990). One case of purulent meningitis in a normal host has been reported. *Leuconostoc* species may cause intravenous catheter-associated infections, some of which may be cured with simple removal of the catheter. Colitis and gastroenteritis also have been described.

Leuconostoc species are highly resistant to vancomycin and teichoplanin but they may be susceptible to daptomycin. These organisms are moderately susceptible to penicillins and early cephalosporins and are sensitive to aminoglycosides and clindamycin. Variable or intermediate susceptibility has been demonstrated with trimethoprim and second- and third-generation cephalosporins.

Rhodococcus equi (formally known as *Corynebacterium equi*) is a well-known veterinary pathogen but has been described only recently as a cause of infections in humans. *R. equi* is a non-motile pleomorphic Gram-positive organism. This organism is characteristically acid fast when grown on Löwenstein-Jensen medium but may be non-acid fast when grown on blood agar plates. It is nonhemolytic and grows in conventional blood culture, TSB media, and in thioglycolate broth. This organism has been reported to cause suppurative pneumonitis with abscesses, effusion, or empyema (Harvey and Sunstrum 1991). Subcutaneous abscesses and brain abscesses have been reported.

Rhodococcus equi is usually resistant to penicillin and first-generation cephalosporins. It is susceptible to chloramphenicol, erythromycin, vancomycin, and aminoglycosides. Clindamycin, rifampin, sulfamethoxazole, and ampicillin are reported to have in vitro activity (Harvey and Sunstrum 1991). The use of intracellularly active antibiotics has been suggested. Therapy should be continued until cultures are negative and the patient's signs and symptoms of infection have resolved.

Although not necessarily a new pathogen, *Enterococcus* species (*E. fecalis* and *E. faecium*) are becoming more dangerous in neutropenic patients because of their multiple antibiotic resistance. Recently, strains of beta lactamase-producing enterococci as well as those resistant to vancomycin and high concentrations of aminoglycoside have been described with increasing frequency.

Corynebacterium jeikeium or *Corynebacterium* group JK causes nosocomial infection in patients with cancer and other immunocompromised states. It can colonize various body sites especially skin and soft tissue; it may be cultured from the axilla and the rectum. The risk of colonization is probably associated with prior antibiotic use, especially of third-generation cephalosporins. Group JK corynebacteria cause bacteremia especially in neutropenic patients with lymphoma usually in the presence of vascular catheters (Young et al. 1981). *C. jeikeium* also may cause endocarditis, peritonitis, prosthetic joint infections, and other infections associated with indwelling devices. Vancomycin is the treatment of choice along with removal of intravenous devices.

Fungi

Anaissie et al. (1989) recently called attention to a broadening spectrum of fungal pathogens which cause infections in neutropenic and other cancer patients. These agents include: *Trichosporon beigelii, Pseudallescheria boydii, Fusarium* species, *Saccharomyces cerevisiae, Torulopsis pintolopesii, Drechslera* species, *Rhodotorula rubra, Curvularia* species, and *Geotrichum* species. Most of these organisms have plant or soil sources and caused skin lesions, soft tissue infections, and sinusitis as well as fungemia in a series of 44 patients with cancer. In this series, which included 30 patients with leukemia and 14 with other malignancies, profound neutropenia with less than 100 granulocytes per milliliter was present in 34. Twenty-four of these patients had disseminated fungal infections and eight had fungemia.

Trichosporon beigelii was the most-frequently isolated fungal infection in this series. *T. beigelii* is related to the organism that causes white piedra, a common infection of hair shafts. It has been described as an important cause of pneumonia, nodular purpuric necrotic skin lesions, hepatitis, glomerulonephritis, and fungal emboli. Multiple organ involvement with vascular invasion similar to that with *Mucor* and *Aspergillus* species may occur, as may endocarditis and endophthalmitis. *T. beigelii* may crossreact with cryptococcal antigens and this may cause some diagnostic confusion.

In the Anaissie et al. series (1989) *Fusarium* species were the cause of infection in four neutropenic patients with cancer who presented with pneumonia, fungemia, or disseminated disease. The nasal sinuses were believed to be the sites of entry of these *Fusarium* infections. The authors also point out the concurrent nature of infections with other fungi as well as bacteria in these severely immunosuppressed patients.

The other species listed above were responsible for infections in one or two patients each. The authors stress the importance of the isolation of these fungi on culture as well as on histological appearance. Since these organisms can be quite ubiquitous in nature, a positive culture with histological documentation may be needed to diagnose these infections. It is important to identify the organisms as their antifungal susceptibilities differ somewhat. Since the organisms may look similar in tissue sections culture is necessary to confirm the organisms' identity. Several strains including *P. boydii* and *Trichosporon* species may be resistant to amphotericin B but most of the other organisms remain susceptible. *Trichosporon, P. boydii; Curvularia, Geotrichum,* and *Drechslera* species may be susceptible to the imidazoles and therapy has been successful in non-neutropenic infected patients.

Anaissie et al. (1989) also describe infections due to *Pichia farinosa* as a cause of fungemia in a patient with an abdominal teratoma. This organism was thought not to cause infection in humans.

Hansenula anomala, another organism rarely causing human infections, has been described as a cause of catheter-related fungemia in leukemic patients (Haron et al. 1988). This organism is also known to cause pneumonia and fungemia (usually vascular catheter associated) in low-birthweight babies in neonatal intensive care units. Amphotericin B remains the drug of choice.

Blastoschizomyces capitatus is a yeast-like fungus previously named *Trichosporon capitatum* or *Geotrichum capitatum*. *B. capitatus* has been described recently to cause infections in immunocompromised patients. Martino et al. (1990) reported 20 patients with leukemia or other malignancies who were infected or colonized with *B. capitatus*. The organism was isolated from blood, sputum, lung tissue, liver, spleen, kidney, brain, skin, myocardium, endocardium, the oropharynx, and the gastrointestinal tract. It was associated with focal hepatitis, pulmonary infiltrates, and fungemia in patients with persistent fever. Response to therapy with amphotericin B was dependent upon remission of the underlying disease.

Phialophora parasitica, a plant fungus, is a rare cause of chronic subcutaneous abscesses or septic arthritis in diabetic patients and immunocompromised individuals. Recurrent systemic infection in an elderly patient initially presented as a draining sinus on the chest and ultimately with invasive infection in the aorta, hip, vertebra, and other bone sites. Amphotericin B and terbinafine were tried without success in this patient (Wong et al. 1989). *Exophiala pisciphila* recently has been reported as a cause of a localized ulcerating pustule in a patient who had previously received a liver transplant and was receiving high-dose corticosteroids for organ rejection. This organism is a well-known fish pathogen and presumably entered while this patient was walking barefoot (Sughayer et al. 1991).

The fungal class of Zygomycetes includes the organisms of mucormycosis and infections caused by *Absidia, Rhizopus,* and *Cunninghamella* species. These well-known but relatively uncommon pathogens may disseminate in patients with leukemia, lymphoma, and other malignancies as well as in patients with chronic renal disease, and gastrointestinal and liver disease. Acute neutropenia, splenectomy and diabetes also may predispose to these infections. Patients with chronic renal insufficiency treated with deferoxamine may be at particular risk of zygomycoses. An excellent review of disseminated zygomycosis has been reported recently (Ingram et al. 1989).

Others

Other novel pathogens that have been described recently include the achloric alga *Prototheca wickerhamii*. One report describes a Hickman catheter-related algemia due to this organism in a young patient with Hodgkin's lymphoma. Protothecosis has also been described in association with other malignancies, diabetes mellitus, ambulatory peritoneal dialysis, use of corticosteroids, and in renal transplants (Heney et al. 1991).

New Pathogens in Patients with AIDS; Potential Pathogens in Other Immunocompromised Hosts

The epidemic of infection with human immunodeficiency virus has allowed the emergence of several new organisms which were previously unknown or unappreciated as agents of human disease. Many of these microorganisms have serious implications for patients with other immunocompromising diseases. Although not new pathogens, *Pneumocystis carinii* and *Cryptococcus neoformans* have become much more prevalent and have appeared in new forms with new organ distributions.

Cryptosporidia are among the most frequent causes of self-limited diarrhea in children but they were not well recognized prior to the AIDS epidemic. These protozoa cause serious secretory diarrhea in HIV-infected persons.

A new Gram-negative organism has been isolated from the blood in several immunocompromised and immunocompetent patients with sepsis (Slater et al. 1990). This organism is known as *Rochalimaea henseli* and it resembles *Rochalimaea quintana*. It was isolated in blood cultures using the RBC-lysis-centrifugation method. Fever and bacteremia resolved after therapy with erythromycin, ceftazidime or tetracycline. This organism is also susceptible in vitro to aztreonam, trimethoprim-sulfamethoxazole, aminoglycosides, chloramphenicol, rifampin, and fluoroquinolones.

R. henseli has been elegantly isolated as the causal organism of bacillary angiomatosis and peliosis hepatis, rare conditions seen in AIDS patients (Relman et al. 1990). Bacillary angiomatosis is a proliferative vascular lesion found on the skin and in visceral organs. Peliosis hepatis is recognized by blood-filled cystic spaces in the liver and it may also occur in the spleen. The organism can be detected histopathologically with the Warthin-Starry stain and may respond clinically to erythromycin, tetracycline, and antituberculous agents. The cat scratch bacillus, possibly related to this organism, also can cause disseminated visceral infection in patients with AIDS.

Rhodococcus equi, a Gram-positive bacillus previously known as *Coryne-bacterium equi* and a known veterinary pathogen, has been reported to cause cavitary pneumonitis in patients with AIDS and may cause bacteremia or pelvic abscess. It may also cause pulmonary infection in other immuno-compromised patients.

Still other newly recognized organisms in patients with AIDS and other immunocompromising conditions include the protozoal microsporidia *Encephalitozoon cuniculi*, *Encephalitozoon hellem*, and *Nosema* species which may cause keratoconjunctivitis and widespread infection in many tissues (Didier et al. 1991). *Blastocystis hominis* may be a pathogen in patients with AIDS and in other immunocompromised patients (Garavelli and Libanore 1990).

Respiratory viruses such as adenovirus may cause serious hepatic infection in patients with AIDS. A recent paper described three patients and reviewed 16 others with disseminated adenovirus infection due to common serotypes (Krilov et al. 1990). Fatal fulminant hepatitis associated with fever, coagulo-pathy, evidence of respiratory infection, and gastrointestinal hemorrhage was described. Treatment remains elusive but ribavirin, thymic hormone, and immune serum globulin might prove useful.

References

Anaissie E, Bodey GP, Kantarjian H, Ro J, Vartivarian SE et al. (1989) New spectrum of fungal infections in patients with cancer. Rev Infect Dis 11:369–378

Didier ES, Didier PJ, Friedberg DN, Stenson SM, Orenstein JM et al. (1991) Isolation and characterization of a new human microsporidian, Encephalitozoon hellem from three AIDS patients with keratoconjunctivitis. J Infect Dis 163:617–621

EORTC International Antimicrobial Therapy Cooperative Group and the National Cancer Institute of Canada – Clinical Trials Group (1991) Vancomycin added to empirical combination antibiotic therapy for fever in granulocytopenic cancer patients. J Infect Dis 163:951–958

Garavelli PL Libanore M (1990) *Blastocystis* in immunodeficiency diseases. Rev Infect Dis 12:158

Handwerger S, Horowitz H, Coburn K, Kolokathis A, Wormser GP (1990) Infection due to *Leuconostoc* species:six cases and review. Rev Infect Dis 12:602–610

Haron E, Anaissie E, Dumphy F, McCredie K, Fainstein V (1988) *Hansenula anomala* fungemia. Rev Infect Dis 10:1182–1186

Harvey RL, Sunstrum JC (1991) *Rhodococcus equi* infection in patients with and without human immunodeficiency virus infection. Rev Infect Dis 13:139–145

Heney C, Greeff M, Davis V (1991) Hickman catheter-related prototheca1 algaemia in an immunocompromised child. J Infect Dis 163:930–931

Ingram CW, Sennesh J, Cooper JN, Perfect JR (1989) Disseminated zygomycosis: report of four cases and review. Rev Infect Dis 11:741–754

Khardori N, Elting L, Wong E, Schable B, Bodey GP (1990) Nosocomial infections due to *Xanthomonas maltophilia* (*Pseudomonas maltophilia*) in patients with cancer. Rev Infect Dis 12:997–1003

Kim JH, Cooper RA, Welty-Wolf KE, Harrell LJ, Zwadyk P, Klotman ME (1989) *Pseudomonas putrefaciens* bacteremia. Rev Infect Dis 11:97–104

Krilov LR, Rubin LG, Frogel M, Gloster E, Ni K, Kaplan M, Lipson SM (1990) Disseminated adenovirus infection with hepatic necrosis in patients with human immunodeficiency virus infection and other immunodeficiency states. Rev Infect Dis 12:303–307

Martino P, Venditti M, Micozzi A, Morace G, Polonelli L et al. (1990) *Blastoschizomyces capitatus*:an emerging cause of invasive fungal disease in leukemia patients. Rev Infect Dis 12:570–582

Relman DA, Loutit JS, Schmidt TM, Falkow S, Tompkins LS (1990) The agent of bacillary angiomatosis:an approach to the identification of uncultured pathogens. N Engl J Med 323:1573–1580

Schwebke JR, Hackman R, Bowden R (1990) Pneumonia due to *Legionella micdadei* in bone marrow transplant recipients. Rev Infect Dis 12:824–828

Slater LN, Welch DF, Hensel D, Coody DW (1990) A newly recognized fastidious Gram-negative pathogen as a cause of fever and bacteremia. N Engl J Med 323:1587–1593

Sughayer M, DeGirolami PC, Khettry U, Korzeniowski D, Grumney A et al. (1991) Human infection caused by *Exophiala psiciphila*:case report and review. Rev Infect Dis 13:379–382

Weinberger M, Wu T, Rubin M, Gill VJ, Pizzo PA (1991) *Leptotrichia buccalis* bacteremia in patients with cancer:report of four cases and review. Rev Infect Dis 13:201–206

Wong PK, Ching WTW, Kwon-Chung KJ, Meyer RD (1989) Disseminated *Phialophora parasitica* infection in humans:case report and review. Rev Infect Dis 11:770–775

Young VM, Meyers WF, Moody MR et al. (1981) The emergence of coryneform bacteria as a cause of nosocomial infections in compromised hosts. Am J Med 70:646–650.

Further Reading

Anaissie E, Bodey GP, Kantarjian H, Ro J, Vartivarian SE et al. (1989) New spectrum of fungal infections in patients with cancer. Rev Infect Dis 11:369–378

Khardori N, Elting L, Wong E, Schable B, Bodey GP (1990) Nosocomial infections due to Xanthomonas maltophilia (Pseudomonas maltophilia) in patients with cancer. Rev Infect Dis 12:997–1003

Slater LN, Welch DF, Hensel D, Coody DW (1990) A newly recognized fastidious Gram-negative pathogen as a cause of fever and bacteremia. N Engl J Med 323:1587–1593

Resistant Bacterial Infections

G.A. Jacoby

Infectious Disease Unit, Massachusetts General Hospital, Boston, MA 02114, USA

Bacterial resistance is only one of the factors to consider in selecting a regimen for empiric therapy in the immunocompromised patient with fever, but it may become a more important consideration because of recent developments on the part of our bacterial adversaries (Jacoby and Archer 1991). Presently susceptibility or resistance is largely predictable even though a sizable fraction of infections are due to bacteria acquired in the hospital where antibiotic resistance has a selective advantage. At most institutions 90% or more of *Pseudomonas aeruginosa* and enteric Gram-negative organisms are reliably susceptible to aminoglycosides like amikacin, gentamicin, and tobramycin or to β-lactams like aztreonam, ceftazidime, and imipenem. Virtually 100% susceptibility can be anticipated for *Pneumocystis carinii* to sulfamethoxazole and trimethoprim, for *Legionella pneumophila* to erythromycin, and for staphylococci to vancomycin. What are emerging, but not yet prevalent, are new mechanisms for resistance to aminoglycosides, β-lactams, quinolones, and vancomycin. Time will tell how important these resistance mechanisms will become clinically.

Among the aminoglycosides, the lowest incidence of resistance can still be claimed by amikacin which was designed to be a poor substrate for many of the modifying enzymes that attack gentamicin, kanamycin, or tobramycin. As detailed in Table 1 enzymatic mechanisms for amikacin resistance have appeared in a variety of Gram-positive and Gram-negative organisms. Furthermore, *P. aeruginosa* broadly resistant by a general defect in aminoglycoside permeability have been isolated from patients treated with amikacin (Maloney et al. 1989). Fortunately, despite this potential for resistance, the frequency of amikacin resistance remains low at most institutions, even when it has been made the aminoglycoside of choice (Moody et al. 1982).

Bacteria demonstrate even greater versatility in β-lactam resistance. In some organisms, such as methicillin-resistant staphylococci, an altered or substitute target is responsible for resistance. In others loss or alteration of

Table 1. Mechanisms for amikacin resistance. (Modified from Jacoby and Archer 1991)

Mechanism	Aminoglycosides affected	Species involved
Impermeability	Amikacin, gentamicin kanamycin, netilmicin, tobramycin	*Pseudomonas aeruginosa*
Phosphorylation APH(3′)-VI and others	Amikacin, kanamycin	*Acinetobacter* spp., *Escherichia coli, Klebsiella pneumoniae, Proteus* spp., *Providencia* spp., *P. aeruginosa, Serratia marcescens*
Acetylation AAC(3)-V	Amikacin, gentamicin, kanamycin, netilmicin, tobramycin	*Citrobacter freundii, Enterobacter cloacae, E. coli*
AAC(6′)-IV	Amikacin, kanamycin, netilmicin, tobramycin	*Citrobacter* spp., *E. cloacae, E. coli, K. pneumoniae, P. aeruginosa, S. marcescens*
AAC(6′)-APH(2″)	Amikacin, gentamicin, kanamycin, netilmicin, tobramycin	*Staphylococcus aureus, Staphylococcus epidermidis Enterococcus faecalis Enterococcus faecium*
Nucleotidylation ANT(4′)	Amikacin, kanamycin, tobramycin	*E. coli, K. pneumoniae, P. aeruginosa*
ANT(4′,4″)	Amikacin[a], kanamycin, tobramycin	*C. freundii, E. faecium, S. marcescens S. aureus, S. epidermidis*

[a] ANT(4′,4″) confers amikacin resistance in Gram-positive organisms; however, Gram-negative isolates with this activity are kanamycin and tobramycin resistant but amikacin sensitive.
Aminoglycoside-modifying enzyme abbreviations: APH(3′), 3′-O-phosphotransferase; AAC(3), 3-N-acetyltransferase; AAC(3), 3-N-acetyltransferase; AAC(6′), 6′-N-acetyltransferase; AAC(6′)-APH(2″), bifunctional 6′-N-acetyltransferase, 2″-O-phosphotransferase; ANT(4′), 4′-O-nucleotidyltransferase; ANT(4′,4″), 4′,4″-O-nucleotidyltransferase.

an outer membrane porin protein contributes to resistance by removing a channel for β-lactam entry into the cell. The major mechanism for β-lactam resistance, however, is enzymatic destruction mediated by β-lactamase. The gene for this enzyme may be located on the bacterial chromosome or

Table 2. Characteristics of broad-spectrum resistance to β-lactam antibiotics. (From Jacoby and Medeiros 1991)

Mechanism	Clinical isolates	β-Lactams affected	β-Lactams not affected[a]
Common plasmid-mediated β-lactamases	Many Gram-negative organisms	Ampicillin azlocillin, carbenicillin, cefamandole, cephalothin, mezlocillin, piperacillin, ticarcillin	Cefotetan, cefoxitin, oxyimino-cephalosporins, carbapenems, monobactams
Plasmid-mediated extended-spectrum β-lactamase in TEM or SHV families	K. pneumoniae, E. coli, C. freundii, S. marcescens, E. cloacae	Above plus aztreonam, cefotaxime, ceftazidime, ceftizoxime, ceftriaxone, cefuroxime	Cefmetazole, cefotetan, cefoxitin, imipenem
Constitutive production of chromosomal β-lactamase	E. cloacae, C. freundii, P. aeruginosa, S. marcescens	Above plus cefmetazole, cefotetan, cefoxitin	Imipenem
Plasmid-mediated extended-spectrum β-lactamase related to AmpC	K. pneumoniae E. coli	Above	Imipenem
Carbapenem hydrolyzing chromosomal β-lactamases	X. maltophilia B. fragilis, S. marcescens, E. cloacae	Imipenem	Variable
Plasmid-mediated β-lactamase conferring carbapenem resistance	P. aeruginosa	Above	Aztreonam, piperacillin

[a] Investigational drugs have not been included.

on a plasmid. Often the plasmid is transmissible thus facilitating spread of β-lactam resistance. Table 2 describes the characteristics of β-lactamase-mediated resistance. Many Gram-negative pathogens of concern in the immunocompromised patient produce one or more of the common plasmid-mediated β-lactamases such as TEM-1, TEM-2, SHV-1, or in *P. aeruginosa* PSE-1. These enzymes provide resistance to ampicillin, cephalothin, and also more specialized penicillins like carbenicillin, ticarcillin, and the ureido compounds azlocillin, mezlocillin, and piperacillin; but they are not able to deal with oxyiminocephalosporins like cefotaxime, ceftazidime, or ceftriaxone, with cephamycins like cefotetan or cefoxitin, with a carbapenem such as imipenem, or with a monobactam like aztreonam.

Bacteria have recently met this challenge by modifying TEM-1, TEM-2, and SHV-1 to produce enzymes of broader specificity that can attack oxyimino-β-lactams (Philippon et al. 1989; Jacoby and Medeiros 1991). The extended-spectrum β-lactamases were first recognized in Europe but have now been reported from a number of centers in the United States. These enzymes differ from their progenitors by one, two, or three amino acid substitutions that alter the configuration around the active site of the enzyme, thus increasing its affinity for broad-spectrum β-lactam antibiotics. For some reason, broad-spectrum β-lactamases are particularly likely to be found in *Klebsiella pneumoniae*, but because they are carried on plasmids, they can spread to other Gram-negative pathogens. The mutations that broaden the spectrum of the β-lactamase often weaken its absolute activity (Jacoby and Carreras 1990). Consequently the level of broad-spectrum resistance may be low, so low that the clinical laboratory can miss its presence, especially if some automated susceptibility testing methods are used. This could be important at heavily infected sites because β-lactamase-mediated resistance shows a marked inoculum effect, and an organism that tested susceptible at low inoculum in the laboratory could prove highly resistant at high inoculum in the patient. Weak extended-spectrum enzymes are probably more prevalent than is currently appreciated. An additional reason to recognize such β-lactamases is that other mutations can augment resistance further. For example, another mutation in the β-lactamase gene could augment resistance to a higher level, or a mutation decreasing outer membrane permeability to β-lactams could permit even a weak β-lactamase to work more effectively by allowing substrate to be delivered to it more slowly.

Strains making this kind of extended-spectrum β-lactamase remain susceptible to cephamycins and carbapenems. Some are also susceptible in vitro to treatment with a β-lactam and a β-lactamase inhibitor such as clavulanic acid, sulbactam, or tazobactam; but there is little clinical experience with such combination therapy, and its benefit has not been impressive in animal model infections (Caron et al. 1990). Cephamycins also have the drawback that some initially susceptible Gram-negative bacilli can become resistant to them by enhanced production of a chromosomal β-lactamase. *Enterobacter* species, *Serratia* species, indole-positive *Proteus* species, *Citrobacter freundii*, *P. aeruginosa*, and a few other organisms have an inducible system for β-lactamase production and can undergo single-step mutations to constitutive, high-level enzyme formation. Even though the AmpC chromosomal β-lactamase hydrolyzes broad-spectrum cephalosporins poorly, if enough of the enzyme is made, resistance to aztreonam, cefotaxime, cefoxitin, cefotetan, ceftazidime, and other β-lactams results. The development of resistance is estimated to occur in 5%–19% of patients with *Enterobacter* bacteremia treated with broad-spectrum β-lactams and consequently has led to recommendations against their use in serious *Enterobacter* infections (Chow et al.

1991). A new concern is that an AmpC-like β-lactamase gene has appeared on plasmids in clinical isolates of *K. pneumoniae* and *E. coli* that are resistant to oxyimino-β-lactams and to cephamycins (Papanicolaou et al. 1990). Such "second-generation" plasmid-mediated extended-spectrum β-lactamases are still rare, but if they become more common in organisms likely to infect immunocompromised patients, recommendations for empiric antibiotic coverage will need to be altered.

The one β-lactam effective against all the β-lactamase-producing strains mentioned thus far is imipenem. Unfortunately, bacteria are prepared to deal with it, too, although imipenem resistance is still rare. *P. aeruginosa* can rather readily become imipenem resistant by loss of an outer-membrane protein that provides a channel for imipenem entry (Quinn et al. 1986), and *Enterobacter aerogenes* can occasionally do the same thing as well. A few reports have appeared of imipenem resistance attributed to an altered penicillin-binding protein. There are also a few organisms with chromosomal β-lactamases that can attack carbapenems including virtually all strains of *Xanthomonas* (formerly *Pseudomonas*) *maltophilia*, which is being increasingly recognized as an important nosocomial pathogen in immunocompromised patients with cancer (Khardori et al. 1990). A plasmid-mediated β-lactamase that can hydrolyze imipenem has been reported in a single isolate of *P. aeruginosa* from Japan (Watanabe et al. 1991). This metalo-β-lactamase also conferred resistance to carbenicillin, cefoperazone, and ceftazidime, but not to aztreonam or piperacillin. Whether this enzyme, which could be termed a "third-generation" β lactamase, will spread to organisms other than *P. aeruginosa* or appear in countries other than Japan remains to be seen.

At long last, reports of bacterial resistance to vancomycin have begun to appear. Table 3 lists Gram-positive organisms that are either naturally vancomycin resistant or have recently acquired this property. Organisms like

Table 3. Vancomycin-resistant Gram-positive pathogens[a]

Organism	MIC (μg/ml)	Mechanism
Enterococcus faecalis	256–1000	Plasmid-mediated *vanA*
Enterococcus faecium	64–1000	Plasmid-mediated *vanA*
Enterococcus faecium	64	Chromosomal *vanB*
Enterococcus casseliflavus	16	Chromosomal *vanC*
Enterococcus gallinarum	16	Chromosomal *vanC*
Erysipelothrix spp.	25	Not yet known
Lactobacillus spp.	>256	Not yet known
Leuconostoc spp.	>1000	Not yet known
Pediococcus spp.	>1000	Not yet known
Staphylococcus haemolyticus	8–16	Not yet known

[a] Susceptible organisms have MICs of 5 μg/ml or less.

Leuconostoc spp. or *Pediococcus* spp. uniformly show high-level vancomycin resistance. *Leuconostoc* spp. are potential pathogens in cancer patients (Handwerger et al. 1990), but of greater concern in this immunocompromised population are coagulase-negative *Staphylococcus haemolyticus*, some of which demonstrate low-level vancomycin resistance, and enterococci. Transmissible plasmids have been found in both *Enterococcus faecalis* and *Enterococcus faecium* that encode inducible vancomycin resistance by a mechanism that involves alteration in the terminal D-Ala-D-Ala residues of the peptidoglycan stem peptide where vancomycin binds to block cell wall synthesis (Bugg et al. 1991). Vancomycin-resistant enterococci are beginning to appear in medical centers in the United States. Furthermore, some plasmids found in enterococci can transfer to *Staphylococcus aureus* and, although the particular plasmids that carry VanA seem not able to do so, the concern is that in time high-level vancomycin resistance might appear in methicillin-resistant *S. aureus*, leaving very few options for treatment.

Resistance is also a problem with prophylactic regimens to prevent infection during neutropenia relying on trimethoprim sulfamethoxazole or one of the fluoroquinolones. Resistance to trimethoprim is spreading (Huovinen 1987), and as norfloxacin, ciprofloxacin, and ofloxacin have come into increasing use, quinolone resistance has increased particularly in organisms like *P. aeruginosa* and *S. aureus*. This resistance results from mutations in the DNA gyrase target for quinolone action and also from alteration in drug accumulation (Wolfson and Hooper 1989). Mutations that diminish quinolone uptake may also confer cross-resistance to β-lactams, chloramphenicol, tetracycline, and other antimicrobial agents so that the danger of selecting multiresistant strains by prophylactic use of quinolones should be recognized.

Predicting what bacteria will do in the future is always hazardous. For the present the reassuring message is that available antibiotics are still broadly enough effective that resistance is rarely the cause of treatment failure. However, vigilance is always advisable, local problem pathogens and resistance patterns need to be taken into account, and monotherapy should be recognized as carrying more of a risk from resistant organisms than empiric use of several agents.

References

Bugg TDH, Dutka-Malen S, Arthur M, Courvalin P, Walsh CT (1991) Identification of vancomycin resistance protein VanA as a D-alanine: D-alanine ligase of altered substrate specificity. Biochemistry 30:2017–2021

Caron F, Gutmann L, Bure A, Pangon B, Vallois J-M, Pechinot A, Carbon C (1990) Ceftriaxone-sulbactam combination in rabbit endocarditis caused by a strain of *Klebsiella pneumoniae* producing extended-broad-spectrum TEM-3 β-lactamase. Antimicrob Agents Chemother 34:2070–2074

Handwerger S, Horowitz H, Coburn K, Kolokathis A, Wormser GP (1990) Infection due to *Leuconostoc* species: six cases and review. Rev Invect Dis 12:602–610

Huovinen P (1987) Trimethoprim resistance. Antimicrob Agents Chemother 31:1451–1456

Jacoby GA, Archer GL (1991) New mechanisms of bacterial resistance to antimicrobial agents. N Engl J Med 324:601–612

Jacoby GA, Carreras I (1990) Activities of β-lactam antibiotics against *Escherichia coli* strains producing extended-spectrum β-lactamases. Antimicrob Agents Chemother 34:858–862

Jacoby GA, Medeiros AA (1991) More extended-spectrum β-lactamases. Antimicrob Agents Chemother 35:1697–1704

Khardori N, Elting L, Wong E, Schable B, Bodey GP (1990) Nosocomial infections due to *Xanthomonas maltophilia* (*Pseudomonas maltophilia*) in patients with cancer. Rev Infect Dis 12:997–1003

Maloney J, Rimland D, Stephens DS, Terry P, Whitney AM (1989) Analysis of amikacin-resistant *Pseudomonas aeruginosa* developing in patients receiving amikacin. Arch Intern Med 149:630–634

Moody MM, De Jongh CA, Schimpff SC, Tillman GL (1982) Long-term amikacin use. Effects on aminoglycoside susceptibility patterns of Gram-negative bacilli. JAMA 248:1199–1202

Papanicolaou GA, Medeiros AA, Jacoby GA (1990) Novel plasmid-mediated β-lactamase (MIR-1) conferring resistance to oxyimino- and α-methoxy β-lactams in clinical isolates of *Klebsiella pneumoniae*. Antimicrob Agents Chemother 34:2200–2209

Philippon A, Labia R, Jacoby G (1989) Extended-spectrum β-lactamases. Antimicrob Agents Chemother 33:1131–1136

Quinn JP, Dudek EJ, DiVincenzo CA, Lucks DA, Lerner SA (1986) Emergence of resistance to imipenem during therapy for *Pseudomonas aeruginosa* infections. J Infect Dis 154:289–294

Watanabe M, Iyobe S, Inoue M, Mitsuhashi S (1991) Transferable imipenem resistance in *Pseudomonas aeruginosa*. Antimicrob Agents Chemother 35:147–151

Wolfson JS, Hooper DC (1989) Fluoroquinolone antimicrobial agents. Clin Microbiol Rev 2:378–424

Further Reading

Bryan LE (ed) (1989) Microbial resistance to drugs. Springer, Berlin Heidelberg New York (Handbook of experimental pharmacology, vol 91)

A collection of authoritative reviews on all aspects of resistance to antimicrobial agents.

Jacoby GA, Archer GL (1991) New mechanisms of bacterial resistance to antimicrobial agents. N Engl J Med 324:601–612

A review of current issues in antimicrobial resistance.

VII. Clinical Trials: Perspectives

Organization of Clinical Trials: Problems, Controversies, Definitions, and Methodology Related to Infections in Neutropenic Patients

R. Feld

University of Toronto, Department of Medicine, Princess Margaret Hospital, 500 Sherbourne Street, Toronto, ON M4X 1K9, Canada

Introduction

This subject is a rather complicated one since there is very little literature specifically addressing it. In this short review I plan to state my own views while taking into account the Immunocompromised Host Society review article published in 1990 in the *Journal of Infectious Diseases* and the report by Pater and Weir in the *Journal of Clinical Oncology* in March 1986 dealing with a critical survey of 21 randomized trials on the therapy of febrile neutropenic patients reviewed by these authors. The third paper of significance is one by Elliott and Pater published in 1988 in *Clinical Investigative Medicine* dealing with the effect of different measures of outcome on the results of these kinds of studies. Although other literature may be pertinent, I believe these papers address the issues best. Therapeutic approaches in these patients were well summarized in a recent Infectious Diseases Society of America consensus paper (Hughes et al. 1990).

Organization of Clinical Trials

The two major types of clinical trials that can be carried out in febrile neutropenic patients are the *phase II exploratory trial* with a new regimen or the *large phase III randomized controlled trial* comparing a new treatment regimen to an accepted standard regimen looking for evidence of progress either in efficacy, toxicity, or improved cost effectiveness.

Phase II Trials

The standard *phase II trial* often includes approximately 50–75 patients because of the large number of patients *without* documented infection. This

Recent Results in Cancer Research, Vol. 132
© Springer-Verlag Berlin · Heidelberg 1993

can be used to ensure that a new regimen is reasonably safe and that its efficacy is sufficient to consider for comparison with a more standard regimen. The use of confidence intervals for response may be useful for the latter. If one does this by defining well all the endpoints that one is seeking, especially infection response, then these trials are relatively simple and create no major controversy.

Randomized Phase III Trials

There are two major approaches to such trials, that is, the *single-institution* versus the *multi-institution* trial. In addition, the trial can be an *open-labelled* trial or a *double-blind* trial. The latter is most commonly carried out in single centres.

Single-Institution Studies. These have some significant *advantages* over multi-institution trials. These include: (a) a more homogeneous patient population; (b) there is often more uniform response criteria evaluated by a limited number of trained investigators; (c) double-blind studies are much easier to carry out in individual institutions and it is easy to carefully audit individual cases and studies because all the data are available in the one centre. However, there are at least two *disadvantages* to these studies: (a) it is usually difficult to accrue the number of patients required to achieve the power to answer the question posed. Even in a very large and busy centre it may take in excess of 3–4 years to accrue the required patient numbers. This may frustrate the individual investigator(s) who might at that point prefer to go on to other more interesting regimens that might become available. This might then lead to the early discontinuation of a trial that does not reach its objectives of accrual (the worst of all possibilities); (b) because of the specialized homogeneous populations studied in single institutions, results from such a study may not be applicable to populations in other centres. Even the organisms that colonize the patients and subsequently cause infection may be quite different from one institution to another.

Multicentre Trials. The *advantages* of multi-institutional trials are: (a) the potential for large numbers of patients to be entered on trials, making it feasible to complete large trials in relatively short periods of time; (b) because of the large numbers of potential patients, there is a high likelihood of adequate numbers and adequate power to obtain the endpoints desired in the study; (c) the variety of patients in different centres allows the results of these trials to be potentially applicable in most centres despite variations in patient populations and microbial flora; (d) the larger numbers may also allow for subset analysis which might otherwise not be possible. The *disadvantages* of multi-institutional studies are: (a) heterogeneity of patients and investigators *may* result in lower-quality data – very complex trials may be exceedingly difficult to carry out because of problems in individual centres, for example, doing double-blind trials; (b) in multi-institutional trials, some centre(s) will enter the majority of patients while a large number of other centres will enter the minority – the limited experience of those centres enrolling relatively few patients may result in lower-quality data and usually there is not a requirement for a minimum number of patients to be entered for an individual centre's data to be included in the analyses.

Other Issues Related to the Design of Clinical Trials for Infections in Febrile Neutropenic Patients. A number of factors may influence eventual conclusions from clinical trials in this patient population. These include: (a) *stratification factors* such as the type of underlying malignancy (acute leukemia and bone marrow transplants versus solid tumours), pediatric versus adult patients, state of the malignancy (remission or relapse or even multiple relapses), type of bone marrow transplantation (autologous versus allogeneic), presence or absence of indwelling venous catheters, and the use or absence of prophylactic oral systemic antibiotics. The degree and duration of neutropenia as well as the type and site of infections are also very important but often these cannot be stratified ahead of time, since they are not known until after the fact. Any or all of these as well as the institution entering patients (usually part of the stratification) might influence the outcome in patients on such trials and, therefore, ideally should be stratified prior to randomization. The majority of trials are stratified primarily by acute leukemia and bone marrow transplants versus solid tumours, and by institution. Usually either pediatric or adult patients are included in the trial rather than both. The other factors may only be considered post-randomization. This, of course, can lead to serious misinterpretations of the trial. *All patients approached for study entry should be recorded and any reasons for exclusion should be noted.* Both febrile episodes and febrile patients can be analyzed, assuming one accepts the hypothesis that one can re-enter patients on the protocol. Statisticians are very unhappy with this approach but it is fairly commonly done by clinicians who usually insist on at least a 7-day period of time from a prior episode of neutropenia before entering patients again. Many people use even longer time intervals between study entries.

All patients on such trials should be followed daily. In multi-institutional studies, an independent review board should evaluate cases retrospectively to ensure that they meet the trial's eligibility criteria and where necessary an appropriate committee should be available to monitor prospectively for any unexpected toxicity or very poor clinical efficacy which may lead to an early discontinuation of the study (Immunocompromised Host Consensus Panel 1990).

Definitions on Trials of Empirical Antibiotic Therapy in
Febrile Neutropenic Patients

The main definitions required include: infection at specific sites, infections caused by specific organisms and unexplained fever (FUO) as well as definitions of response and other potential endpoints.

Definitions of specific infections are quite simple as is unexplained fever (Immunocompromised Host Society Consensus Panel 1990). However, the definitions of response to therapy and other endpoints are much more difficult. Multiple ways of defining response have been used in the literature and they can clearly influence the eventual interpretation of the study. Elliott and Pater (1988) looked at this issue in two cross-Canada trials of febrile, neutropenic patients. Their *first definition* for response required complete resolution of all signs and symptoms of infection and the patient had to remain afebrile for 4 days following discontinuation of study antibiotics. There was an intermediate category of temporary improvement in which there was a decrease in the temperature of at least 1.7°C and improvement at the site of infection. A *second definition* required that all superinfections and subsequent infections be considered failures while a *third definition* required that failures only be patients dying from their infection. Using these various definitions the authors were able to show very major differences in response rates based on the response definition used. In addition, of course, patients had to be stratified by important prognostic factors for the final analysis before the results using each definition could be compared. This study showed that the definitions of response had a substantial influence not only on the response rates but on the magnitude of the differences in response rates between groups. Patients with acute leukemia or bone marrow transplantation who have long-term severe neutropenia, superinfection and subsequent infections have frequent problems requiring further modifications of antimicrobial therapy, and any definition which fails to take this into account may underestimate the benefits of certain empiric antibiotic treatments. Since all antibiotic regimens presently available are quite successful, survival as the major endpoint of response may over-exaggerate the benefits of treatment and will not usually allow demonstrable differences between empiric regiments, making it exceedingly difficult to show that one treatment is more effective than another. Therefore, this approach may be too insensitive for this purpose although it may pick up toxicity.

The most frequently used response criteria are those of the EORTC International Antimicrobial Therapy Cooperative Group (1991) and those developed by Dr. Phillip Pizzo et al. (1986) at the National Cancer institute. The major difference between the criteria for response in these two systems is that in the EORTC antimicrobial group system, most types of modifications will be called failures virtually whenever they occur in the course of treatment. This may result in an overly low response rate. Pizzo et al.'s approach is to consider all patients who do not succumb to their infection as having responded with or without antimicrobial modification (very high response rates). Because of this major difference in response definitions, the various trials presented in the literature may be extremely difficult to compare.

This difficulty led to the convening of an international consensus conference by the Immunocompromised Host Society (IHS) to try to better define various aspects of trials in febrile neutropenic patients, much of which has been alluded to in this review, and, in particular, to come up with a new definition for response. The results of the conference are described in the previously mentioned paper (Immunocompromised Host Society Consensus Panel 1990). It recommends that all modifications be stated regardless of the method of evaluation. In addition, modifications when an organism is not identified are not considered failures but, instead, are called non-responses if a new antibacterial has been added. In microbiologically and clinically documented infections the new definitions include a category called "initial response but regimen modified". This means that there was in fact an initial response from the initial empiric antibacterials but other agents, that is, antifungals, antivirals or antiparasitics, were required and these then do not make the initial antibiotic regimen a failure since other antibacterials were not required. Unfortunately, this new classification of response has yet to be tested in clinical trials.

Definitions of response become even more of a problem when one looks at endpoints for trials testing treatment with antifungals and antivirals in febrile neutropenic patients. These are often used empirically, particularly antifungals such as amphotericin B or perhaps fluconazole, in patients who have failed initial antibiotic regimens. The efficacy of such approaches is extremely difficult to evaluate especially when no pathogen is isolated. Usually the patient becomes afebrile which may be a useful endpoint; however, this certainly could be influenced by an increase in the neutrophil count in the patients being studied. Those whose neutrophils are recovering will likely have their fever drop whether or not the empiric antifungal has had an effect. The use of the number of documented fungal infections as an endpoint is extremely difficult to use since isolation of such pathogens is so rare, therefore differences will be extremely difficult to identify. Usually antibacterials are continued on both arms of such trials making them even more dificult to interpret. The use of empiric antivirals, especially in bone marrow transplant patients, is at least as difficult to interpret, with similar problems to antifungals.

Another area of major difficulty is interpretation of trials involving *antimicrobial prophylaxis*. About 50% of patients worldwide with acute leukemia or undergoing bone marrow transplantation are treated with prophylactic oral antibiotics, the main agents used being cotrimoxizole or quinolones (norfloxacin, ciprofloxacin, ofloxacin and others). It would appear that the quinolones reduce the frequency of Gram-negative bacteremia more so than cotrimoxizole but have less effect on the Gram-positive pathogens. They seem to have little effect on the frequency of febrile episodes no matter what pathogens are identified. Numerous recent studies employ quinolones plus additional anti-Gram-positive coverage to try to reduce the febrile episodes and bacteremias even further. Studies testing such hypotheses are extremely difficult to carry out as the endpoints usually relate to the frequency of febrile episodes, the duration of antibiotic therapy, the types of infections seen, etc. Similar problems arise with studies using prophylactic colony stimulating factors (CSF) such as granulocyte CSF or granulocyte–macrophage CSF. The use of these agents affects the duration of neutropenia, and therefore theoretically, should reduce the frequency and severity of infectious complications. This has, in fact, been shown in solid tumours, especially small cell lung cancer, but these agents have not been compared to prophylactic oral systemic antibiotics.

In addition to being extremely difficult studies to carry out in their own right, prophylactic antibiotics, by affecting the gastrointestinal flora of the patients when they become febrile neutropenics, may influence the types of pathogens seen in these patients and, therefore, probably influence the outcome of empiric regimens used to treat such patients. For example, if no antibiotic prophylaxis is used, there is probably more likelihood of isolation of Gram-negative pathogens and therefore excellent Gram-negative antibiotic coverage is required. On the other hand, when one uses a prophylactic antibiotic, particularly quinolones, one often selects out Gram-positive pathogens. Therefore, a high failure rate may be seen on an empiric antibiotic regimen in patients who have received these agents if adequate Gram-positive coverage was not included; this can create difficulties in response evaluations.

Another endpoint of such trials that has only rarely been used in this group of patients is *cost effectiveness*. Obviously in the situation where multiple empiric antibiotic regimens may be successful, those that are the least costly, either for the individual or the health care system, are preferable. In these evaluations, the number of injections per day and, therefore, nursing help, pharmacy costs, etc. must be considered as well as the drug costs. Further trials involving such endpoints are essential for this group of patients. Of course, if efficacy differences exist, then it becomes much more difficult to be as concerned about the costs. However, the majority of empiric antibiotic regimens achieve similar efficacy based on recent studies and even monotherapy, particularly with certain third-generation cephalosporins or carbapenems, are at least as efficacious as antibiotic combinations. Therefore, with minimal differences in efficacy, cost comparisons can become very important.

Conclusions

This brief review has dealt with some of the problems and controversies surrounding the design, analysis and reporting of clinical trials on empiric antibiotic management of the febrile neutropenic patient. Much more work needs to be done in this area so that we can more appropriately recommend the best and most cost-effective therapy for our patients.

References

Elliott CR, Pater JL (1988) The effect of different measures of outcome on the results of studies of empiric antibiotic therapy in febrile neutropenic patients. Clin Invest Med 11:327–330

EORTC International Antimicrobial Therapy Cooperative Group and National Cancer Institute of Canada – Clinical Trials Group (1991) Vancomycin added to empirical combination antibiotic therapy for fever in granulocytopenic cancer patients. J Infect Dis 163:951–958

Hughes WT, Armstrong D, Bodey GP, Feld R, Mandell GL, Meyers JD, Pizzo PA, Schimpff SC, Shenep JL, Wade JC, Young L, Yow MJ (1990) Guidelines for the use of antimicrobial agents in neutropenic patients with unexplained fever. J Infect Dis 161:381–396

Immunocompromised Host Society Consensus Panel (1990) The design, analysis and reporting of clinical trials on the empirical antibiotic management of the neutropenic patient. J Infect Dis 161:397–401

Pater JL, Wier L (1986) Reporting the results of randomized trials of empiric antibiotics in febrile neutropenic patients – a critical survey. J Clin Oncol 4:346–352

Pizzo PA, Hathorn JW, Hiemenz J, Browne M, Commers J, Cotton D, Gress J, Longo D, Marshall D, McKnight J, Rubin M, Skelton J, Thaler M, Wesley R (1986) A randomized trial comparing ceftazidime alone with combination antibiotic therapy in cancer patients with fever and neutropenia. N Engl J Med 315:552–558

Further Reading

A critical paper pointing out that the definitions of response can heavily influence the interpretation of results in such studies.

Hughes WT, Armstrong D, Bodey GP, Feld R, Mandell GL, Meyers JD, Pizzo PA, Schimpff SC, Shenep JL, Wade JC, Young L, Yow MJ (1990) Guidelines for the use of antimicrobial agents in neutropenic patients with unexplained fever. J Infect Dis 161:381–396

A description of the recommendations of an expert North American panel consisting of fellows of the Infectious Diseases Society of America on how best to use antimicrobial agents in febrile neutropenic patients.

Immunocompromised Host Society Consensus Panel (1990) The design, analysis and reporting of clinical trials on the empirical antibiotic management of the neutropenic patient. J Infect Dis 161:397–401

The description of the recommendations for carrying out clinical trials on empiric antibiotic management of neutropenic patients based on a consensus meeting of international experts held in 1989.

Pater JL, Wier L (1986) Reporting the results of randomized trials of empiric
antibiotics in febrile neutropenic patients – a critical survey. J Clin Oncol 4:346–352
A retrospective review of 21 randomized trials on empiric antibiotics in febrile
neutropenic patients pointing out the reporting problems in different studies.

Organization of Clinical Trials: Problems, Controversies, Definitions, Methodology

R.L. Comis

Fox Chase Cancer Center, 7701 Burholme Avenue, Philadelphia, PA 19111, USA

In internal medicine, there are two disciplies in which patients are treated with curative intent – infectious disease and medical oncology. Systemic drug therapy is the cornerstone of curative treatment in both disciplines. In both areas there has been an explosion in the number of agents employed, a broadening of the types of agents available, as well as an increase in the spectrum of activity *and* toxicity associated with their use. With the widespread use of cytotoxic agents, treatment algorithms were required to deal with the intense, often sustained iatrogenic induction of granulocytopenia integral to the appropriate therapy of a variety of cancers. All of these historic developments have led to a welding of the activities of the infectious disease and medical oncology subspecialist.

This paper will try to put this topic into perspective and illustrate some of the issues that impact on oncology as well as on infectious diseases approaching this issue from the viewpoint of a medical oncologist. Those of us in medical oncology are very proud of the fact that the development of this field has had tremendous impact on internal medicine overall. There are two areas in particular where there has been a tremendous impact: one is in clinical trials study design (oncologists have been working on this for 25–30 years) and the second is in supportive care.

First, consider some of the convergences of infectious diseases and medical oncology as subspecialities of internal medicine. The history of these two fields were steeped in nihilism. I, in fact, as well as many others, entered oncology through the influence of a man named Dr. Kenneth B. Olson who was Director of Oncology at the Albany Medical Center, Albany, New York. A victim of tuberculosis, he ran the Saranac Lake Sanitarium. He lived through the era when tuberculosis was a hopelessly incurable disease. Participating in the personal and general curative advance in the fight of tuberculosis, he decided to enter oncology, a field in which the same nihilistic attitude prevailed.

Drug development has been the key to progress in the treatment of infectious diseases and cancer. Pharmacology is the basis of both fields, so the understanding of drugs and drug delivery is extremely important. The real convergence of these two fields is in the treatment of the immuno-suppressed host. Twenty-five years ago, when a patient was granulocytopenic and septic, the therapeutic armamentarium included only a few drugs. House officers were taught how difficult and treacherous this setting was. But now, trainees, in the average situation, are able to take care of such patients routinely. This transition is a remarkable outgrowth of the interaction between medical oncology and infectious disease.

What are the divergences? Although both specialties treat with curative intent, curative therapy is more generally available in infectious diseases than in cancer. In infectious diseases, there is a wide spectrum of curative agents; in medical oncology, the spectrum is narrower. The therapeutic index is much better with the drugs used to treat infection and much less with the drugs that treat cancer. An area in which divergence exists now, but in which convergence is developing is in the response to the immunologic challenge of these diseases. In infectious diseases there is a clearly unique immunologic challenge. The immunologic challenge in cancer has yet to be precisely defined and exploited. The hope is that the mechanisms operational in infectious diseases may be understood and exploited in the treatment of cancer. For instance, we all know that when we have a granulocytopenic patient who has a persistent fever spike, we are waiting, and waiting, and waiting until the monocytes return and herald granulocyte recovery. With appropriate hematopoietic growth factors can we accelerate this recovery? Another divergence has been the treatment of acute versus chronic diseases in our respective specialties. Today, with the treatment of acquired immuno-deficiency syndrome (AIDS), another convergence is developing. Once, infectious disease specialists were involved with us primarily in the acute management of infectious disease. This is now in the process of changing as more chronic diseases, such as AIDS, fungal and parasitic diseases become more prevalent in our patients.

The principles of drug development have been very precisely established in the oncology setting, probably more so than in any other pharmacologically based discipline. This precision was required by the generally narrow therapeutic index associated with most cytotoxic agents and the rather elusive native efficacy of the drugs employed. By general definition, phase I studies: are designed to establish the maximally tolerated dose (MTD) of a given agent; phase II studies are designed to determine an acceptable level of efficacy in a variety of disease specific, good risk settings; and phase III trials, employing a concurrently randomized control group, are designed to establish the role of the new therapy in the therapeutic armamentarium within a given disease state.

Although there are certain distinctions, these three purposes are integral to the proper evaluation of new antibiotics, as well as new anticancer drugs, and precision in the questions asked, endpoints and analysis should be commensurately rigorous.

To discuss the distinctions first, it must be admitted that the target dose sought it phase I studies of antibiotics and anticancer drugs are inherently different. In the case of the anticancer drug, the MTD is sought because there are considerable animal data (and albeit fewer human data) to suggest a steep dose–response curve. No reliable in vitro models are available to establish a specific drug concentration or biologically effective dose as a target. With myelotoxicity being a common endpoint of cytotoxic therapy, its attainment has become an end, for better or worse, of defining the MTD.

In medical oncology we tend to enter heterogeneous groups of patients into phase I studies: patients who were previously treated with different diseases and levels of performance status. In infectious disease, normal subjects are often used; there is a targeted drug concentration sought which represents the biologically effective dose anticipated for phase II trials. Phase II evaluations of anticancer agents are performed at a fraction of the established MTD, rather than at a specific dose which could lead to a serum concentration which might be associated with clinical benefit. Superimposing these unknowns upon the heterogeneity of the patient populations treated, it is a wonder that any cancer drugs have the power to pass the positivity test. In this regard, efficacy testing of antibiotics has a decided edge in excluding a false negative, if not in establishing a true positive. Another distinction in phase II trials relates to the magnitude of the penumbra in defining "activity" where many effective antibiotics already exist, as compared to the clear edge defined by an active new agent in the setting of totally ineffective therapy (e.g., interleukin 2 in renal cell cancer).

The proper design, execution and analysis embodied in the phase III trial represents a point of convergence for all clinical research trials. In this setting, a new treatment modality is given the acid test of: stratification, to balance prognostic variables; randomization, to eliminate investigator bias; delineation of evaluation and response criteria, to establish consistency; programmed interim analysis schedules, to deter the natural inclination of the physician–scientist to deliver the best conceivable therapy at the earliest possible point; and final analysis, at which point predetermined accrual goals assure a defined alpha and beta error relating to outcome. Although, this is the norm in oncologic research, oftentimes antibiotics enter general usage without this vigorous supportive data. Pater and Weir (1986) have extensively analyzed the deficiencies often encountered in randomized trials of empiric antibiotic trials performed in febrile granulocytopenic patients. It is possible that the urgency associated with this life-threatening situation sometimes deters the proper design or execution of such studies. On the other hand, such a patient can be treated on a properly designed clinical trial as well as, if not better than, in a less controlled setting. The framework of a clinical trial demands attention to detail, the presence of a stable clinical research team, standardization of entry and evaluation criteria, crisp definition of endpoint, and a controlled prospective plan of action which relates to outcome. Superimposed upon this individual protection is the general good which can arise from a properly designed trial, where the overall outcome can enhance the therapeutic approach for future patients.

A recent treatise eloquently described the tension between the inclinations and responsibilities of treating physicians versus the physician–scientists, favoring the former (Hellman and Hellman 1991). An accompanying article challenged the value of uncontrolled observations as the foundation for medical practice (Passamani 1991). The current climate in the nation as it relates to the so-called health-care industry will increasingly demand hard data to justify the increasing costs of sophisticated, new approaches to sustain the life of severely ill individuals. Such data can only be obtained within the framework of a properly designed and executed clinical trial.

Recent communications from the Infectious Disease Society of America have addressed guidelines for the use of antibiotics in the febrile, granulocytopenic patient and specific criteria for the proper design of clinical research studies relating to antibiotic therapy in this setting. Once again, the convergence of both disciplines was represented by the constitution of the committees, with representation from both the Infectious Disease and Medical Oncology communities (Hughes et al. 1990; Pizzo et al. 1990). Such interaction will undoubtedly strengthen both disciplines, in which well-designed clinical trials become the norm, rather than the exception in describing future approaches for the patients served.

References

Hellman S, Hellman DS (1991) (Sounding Board) Problems of randomized clinical trial. N Engl J Med 324:1585–1589

Hughes WT, Armstrong D, Bodey GP, Feld R, Mandell GL, Meyers JD et al. (1990) Guidelines for the use of antimicrobial agents in neutropenic patients with unexplained fever. J Infect Dis 161:381–396

Passamani E (1991) (Sounding Board) Clinical trials – are they ethical? N Engl J Med 324:1589–1592

Pater JL, Weir C (1986) Reporting the results of randomized trials of empiric antibiotics in febrile neutropenic patients – a critical survey. J Clin Oncol 4:346–352

Pizzo PA, Armstrong D, Bodey G et al. (1990) The design, analysis, and reporting of clinical trials on the empirical antibiotic management of the neutropenic patient (From the Immunocompromised Host Society: Report of a consensus panel). J Infect Dis 161:397–401

Case Presentation with Answers to Questions

S.C. Schimpff

University of Maryland School of Medicine, 22 South Greene Street,
Baltimore, MD 21201, USA

The Case Presentation offered at the beginning of the text is repeated here
along with a brief discussion of the correct answer. The reader will note that
the 23 experts at The Greenbrier Conference were frequently not unanimous in
their opinion. Obviously, there remains much to be learned as to the
management of these patients.

Case Presentation

A 33-year-old previously healthy male is found to have acute myelocytic
(monocytic) leukemia. He is treated with cytotoxic combination chemotherapy, and a complete remission is achieved following a stormy course.
He goes home for 2 months and then is readmitted for bone marrow
transplantation. The donor is to be his HLA-identical sister. In advance
preparation, he has a Hickman catheter placed into his venous system.

Three days before the transplantation, he receives total body irradiation
and 3 consecutive days of high-dose cyclophosphamide. The bone marrow
material is infused intravenously without incident. Within 4 days, he has no
circulating granulocytes, and his platelets are being supported by every-
other-day platelet transfusions.

On day 9 following transplantation, without concurrent symptomatology,
he develops a fever of 102°F with a shaking chill. Complete history and
physical examination are unremarkable. Chest X-ray is negative, and urinalysis is negative.

1. In the absence of any other detectable historical, physical, or X-ray
   finding should this patient be treated empirically with broad-spectrum
   antibiotic(s)?
   A. Yes
   B. No

Recent Results in Cancer Research, Vol. 132
© Springer-Verlag Berlin · Heidelberg 1993

The individual who develops an infection while neutropenic has a very poor inflammatory response so that the four cardinal signs pointing to a site of infection (swelling, redness, warmth, and pain) may be absent, but fever will be present because interleukin 1 IL-1, IL-6, and tumor necrosis factor (TNF) (endogenous pyrogens) are produced by monocytes and macrophages. The finding of new fever in a patient with <500 granulocytes/μl is associated with infection in at least 60% of cases of which about 20% will be bacteremias. Therefore, prompt initiation of empiric antibiotic therapy is indicated. (See the chapter by Bustamante.)

2. Assuming the decision was to begin a combination of antibiotics, which one of the following combinations would not be appropriate?
   A. Cephalothin plus gentamicin
   B. Ceftazidime plus gentamicin
   C. Imipenem plus gentamicin
   D. Piperacillin plus gentamicin

   The least appropriate combination of those suggested is cephalothin plus gentamicin, because cephalothin, unlike the other beta lactams/carbapenem noted here, is not effective against *Pseudomonas aeruginosa*. Although *P. aeruginosa* is susceptible to gentamicin in vitro, an aminoglycoside alone in the profoundly neutropenic patient is often not effective against Gram-negative bacilli, especially *P. aeruginosa*.

3. The hospital microbiology laboratory reports that approximately 20% of Gram-negative rod isolates in recent months have been resistant to gentamicin. In that situation, which one of the following would be an appropriate aminoglycoside to utilize?
   A. Gentamicin
   B. Tobramycin
   C. Netilmicin
   D. Amikacin

   When Gram-negative bacilli are resistant to gentamicin, they are often also resistant to tobramycin and netilmicin but not amikacin. The correct answer therefore is amikacin.

4. Under what circumstances would a "double beta lactam" combination (e.g., piperacillin plus ceftazidime) be utilized?
   A. Never
   B. Patient with pre-existing renal dysfunction
   C. Patient with aminoglycoside ototoxicity
   D. Hospital with high incidence of gentamicin resistance

   Double beta lactam combinations have enjoyed increased popularity since the advent of the extended spectrum penicillins which are effective against *P. aeruginosa*, *Klebsiella* and *Escherichia coli* and the third-generation cephalosporins which are likewise effective against these three Gram-negative bacilli. Although many clinicians who prefer to use combination therapy would consider a beta lactam plus aminoglycoside combination as their first choice, the double beta lactam combination approach has been considered for patients with pre-existing renal dysfunction and for patients who have developed ototoxity from repeated uses of aminoglycosides. Gentamicin resistance per se would probably not be an indication to use a double beta lactam as one could use amikacin in most cases where there is resistance to gentamicin. It needs to be noted that there is concern that the use of double beta lactam regimens will lead to more rapid development of resistance than with the use of a beta lactam/aminoglycoside combination. Finally, since some clinicians would use monotherapy, they would see no need for the use of a double beta lactam combination. (See the chapter by Vogelzang and Flaherty.)

5. Which of the following (choose one or more) have an adequate spectrum of coverage when using monotherapy as an initial empiric regimen?
   A. Piperacillin
   B. Ticarcillin plus clavulanate
   C. Imipenem
   D. Ceftazidime

   Ceftazidime and imipenem are the two agents with a broad spectrum of activity which have been used extensively in trials of monotherapy in the neutropenic patient. The addition of clavulanate to ticarcillin gives it a very broad spectrum; however, there are few clinical data on its use as monotherapy. Piperacillin's broad spectrum does not include most strains of *Staphylococcus aureus*; it has not been considered for monotherapy in clinical trials. (See the chapter by Pizzo.)

6. Monotherapy is appropriate initial therapy when the initial granulocyte count is (choose one or more):
   A. 0–99/μl
   B. 100–499/μl
   C. 500–999/μl
   D. ≥1000/μl

   There is a difference of opinion among experts in the field as regards the answer to this question. Most would find monotherapy appropriate therapy in the setting of at least some circulating granulocytes. Although experts would use monotherapy even for patients with profound, persistent granulocytopenia, i.e., essentially an aplastic marrow as is seen during the first few weeks after bone marrow transplantation, others would use a combination regimen is this setting. To date, the number of patients with Gram-negative rod bacteremia and <100 PMN/μl treated with monotherapy and reported in the literature are too few to reach a definite conclusion one way or the other.

7. Some institutions have noted a particularly high frequency of *Staphylococcus epidermidis*, streptococcal species bacteremias and a near absence of Gram-negative rod infections among their patients who

develop fever during neutropenia. Given that setting, which of the following might be appropriate regimens for empiric therapy in the febrile neutropenic cancer patient? (Choose one or more.)

A. Piperacillin plus gentamicin plus vancomycin
B. Piperacillin plus vancomycin
C. Ceftazidime plus vancomycin
D. Imipenem plus vancomycin
E. Vancomycin

In the setting suggested here, one would add vancomycin to whatever regimen one was otherwise comfortable with, which would include adequate coverage for Gram-negative bacilli, albeit occurring infrequently. In this situation, the broad spectrum of ceftazidime or imipenem in addition to vancomycin should be sufficient; the combination of piperacillin plus gentamicin in addition to vancomycin, while certainly adequate therapy, would seem to be excessive compared to the two regimens just mentioned. Only a few of the experts at this meeting were satisfied with using piperacillin alone in combination with vancomycin. (See the chapter by Karp and Dick, and Shenep.)

8. The changing epidemiology of infections in neutropenic patients continues. Which Gram-positive cocci are most likely to cause bacteremia in this patient?

A. *Staphylococcus aureus*
B. *Staphylococcus epidermidis*
C. Viridans streptococci
D. *Streptococcus pneumoniae*

Twenty years ago, *S. aureus* was a fairly frequent cause of infection in the setting of neutropenia; this organism is still a cause of infection but in much less frequency than in years gone by. *S. epidermidis* and various streptococci, especially the viridans streptococci have become common causes of infection in recent years. *S. pneumoniae* remains a relatively uncommon cause of infection in the setting of neutropenia.

9. Repeat history and examination on a daily basis demonstrate a site of infection 48 h after initial fever documentation. Which of the following are the five most likely sites for infection in this patient?

A. Acute exacerbation of chronic periodontitis
B. Sinusitis
C. Pharyngitis
D. Otitis media
E. Pneumonitis
F. Esophagitis
G. Perianal lesion
H. Urinary tract infection
I. Prostatitis
J. Hickman catheter exit site infection
K. Hickman catheter tunnel infection

L. Hickman catheter-related bacteremia

The most common sites of infection in the neutropenic patient relate to some form of damage to an anatomic barrier such as chemotherapy- or radiation therapy-induced mucosal damage along the alimentary canal, damage to the cells along the tracheobronchial tree, or infections associated with damage to the integument, such as an indwelling vascular catheter. Thus, from this list, the most common sites of infection are pharyngitis, pneumonitis, perianal lesions, and Hickman catheter exit site infections. In addition, pre-existing chronic peri- odontitis, present in most adult individuals, can be frequently exacer- bated into an acute infection during granulocytopenia. Sinusitis seems to occur in individuals who have a past history of recurrent episodes of sinusitis. Otitis media is rare unless there is an added predisposing factor, such as lymphomatous obstruction of the eustachian tube. Esophagitis tends not to occur early during neutropenia but rather a few weeks later if neutropenia persists. Urinary tract infections should not occur unless the patient has some additional predisposing factors, such as an indwelling catheter. Prostatitis, likewise, should not occur except in someone who has exacerbation of a chronic condition. Deep-seated Hickman catheter tunnel infections and catheter-related bacteremias, in particular those caused by Gram-negative bacteria or fungi, both very serious infections, are not only uncommon but are rarely the site of infection early during the patient's neutropenic episode.

10. Blood cultures drawn when fever first began are reported negative. However, which of the following organisms are likely causes of bacteremia (fungemia) in patients such as this one? (Choose one or more.)

A. *Pseudomonas aeruginosa*
B. *Xanthomonas (Pseudomonas) maltophilia*
C. *Escherichia coli*
D. *Enterobacter cloacae*
E. *Staphylococcus epidermidis*
F. *Clostridium difficile*
G. *Candida albicans*
H. *Streptococcus mitis*

The question asks which are the likely causes of bacteremia, and, although there is variation from institution to institution, the correct answers would be *P. aeruginosa*, *E. coli*, *S. epidermidis*, and *S. mitis*. *S. mitis* has recently had a resurgence as a particularly virulent pathogen and seems to be associated with highly intensive therapies that cause marked oropharyngeal and/or esophageal mucositis (for example, bone marrow transplant preparative regimens). *X. maltophilia* has been noted to occur in neutropenic patients recently but is certainly not a frequent cause of infection or bacteremia, nor is *E. cloacae*. *C. difficile* is seen frequently among these patients as a cause of enterocolitis; but these infections occur later after the patient has received antibiotics. *C. albicans*, likewise, is the most common cause of fungal infection in these patients but is uncommon as an infecting agent early in the clinical course, especially before the patient has received broad-spectrum antibiotics.

11. What novel bacteria are emerging as agents of bacteremia in neutropenic patients?

   A. *Corynebacterium jikeium*
   B. *Leuconostoc* species
   C. *Xanthomonas maltophilia*
   D. *Pseudomonas putrefaciens*
   E. *Leptotrichia buccalis*
   F. *Rhodococcus equi*

   It is still true that the granulocytopenic patient tends to become infected with a relatively limited number of organisms, most notably three Gram-negative bacilli (*E. coli*, *K. pneumoniae*, and *P. aeruginosa*), three types of Gram-positive cocci (*S. epidermidis*, *Streptococcus* species, and *S. aureus*), and, if the patient has received broad-spectrum antibiotics and remains neutropenic, then one is likely to see infections with two yeasts (*C. albicans* and *C. tropicalis*) and two fungi (*A. flavus* and *A. fumigatus*). However, reports in the recent literature have noted each of the organisms listed in this question. (See the chapter by Zinner.)

12. Fever resolves over a 3-day period as do symptoms and signs of perianal cellulitis (recognized the day after fever occurred) by day 5. How long should the empiric antibiotic regimen be continued? (Choose one.)

   A. Discontinue when fever/symptoms and signs resolve
   B. For a total course of 7–10 days
   C. Until resolution of granulocytopenia

   The experts at this symposium did not think that it was sufficient to treat for only 5 days in a patient with a documented serious infection and no circulating granulocytes. About half thought that a total course of 7–10 days was sufficient, whereas the other half felt that it was more appropriate to continue antibiotics until granulocytopenia resolved. Given that the patient's granulocyte count is expected to return toward normal approximately 3 weeks after transplantation, there may be little difference in the two approaches. However, in a different patient with an expectation of continued profound granulocytopenia, the difference in approach could become marked.

13. If fever had persisted, but the signs and symptoms of local infection had resolved, which course of action would be appropriate? (Assume daily repeat examinations are negative, chest X-rays every 2–3 days are unrevealing, and the empiric regimen was a beta lactam or carbapenem plus gentamicin.) (Choose one or more.)

   A. Add amphotericin B (i.v.)
   B. Add acyclovir (i.v.)

C. Replace gentamicin with amikacin
D. Add vancomycin
E. Replace beta lactam/carbapenem with a different class (e.g., substitute carbapenem for cephalosporin or vice versa)
F. Removal of indwelling catheter

In many ways, this is the most difficult question in the entire group in that it asks the clinician to consider the possibility of fungal infection, viral infection, such as herpes simplex, the presence of a gentamicin-resistant Gram-negative rod, the possibility of *Staphylococcus epidermidis* which would respond only to vancomycin in this situation, the possibility that an infecting organism is resistant to the beta lactam or carbapenem, or that there is a catheter-related infection. The point, of course, is that modifications of therapy at this point may well be necessary and that a very organized approach recognizing the most common types of infection in these settings and in one's own individual institution needs to be considered. A critical aspect of the way this question is written is the statement that you have continued to thoroughly evaluate the patient on a daily basis and that these examinations have remained negative, including repeat chest X-rays. Most of the experts at this symposium would have added amphotericin B intravenously at this point in time because of the frequency of fungal infections (candidiasis or aspergillosis) which occur in patients with no circulating granulocytes who are receiving broad-spectrum antibiotic therapy. In many series, response (defervescence) to the empiric institution of amphotericin B for fever that is recurrent or refractory to antibacterial antibiotics occurs in 60%–70% of patients. Given the way the question and commentary are written, we (the editors) would not have added amphotericin B at this relatively early stage in the absence of some identifiable focus. About half the experts at the symposium would have added vancomycin at this point, primarily out of concern for the possibility of a *Staphylococcus epidermidis* infection which had not been recognized. Although very few suggested adding acyclovir, it is important to note that herpes simplex infections occur fairly early following bone marrow transplantation in seropositive individuals; note that no mention was made in the case history of the patient being placed on prophylactic acyclovir. No data were given to suggest that this patient was being treated in an institution with a high frequency of gentamicin resistance, so relatively few individuals suggested a switch to amikacin and, likewise, very few suggested a change in the beta lactam or carbapenem. In our personal opinion, the only answer which one could clearly consider incorrect would be removal of the Hickman catheter. These are vital to patient care and, other than tunnel infections, one can usually treat exit site infections or catheter-related bacteremias with antibiotics, generally vancomycin. (See the chapters by Pizzo; Gallagher; Vogelzang and Flaherty; and Karp and Dick.)

14. Should this patient have been the recipient of granulocyte–macrophage colony-stimulating factor (GM-CSF) to hasten marrow engraftment and return of circulating granulocytes?

   A. Yes

   B. No

   The experts were split on the answer to this question. After the discussions by Drs. Mandell and Peters, there was general agreement that GM- or G-CSF does hasten marrow recovery. (See the chapters by Vollmer and Mandell, and Peters.)

15. Should this patient have been the recipient of granulocyte transfusions?

   A. Yes

   B. No

   Granulocyte transfusions are infrequently utilized in this patient population and generally are reserved for the patient with a Gram-negative rod bacteremia receiving appropriate antimicrobial therapy but who is nevertheless failing to respond.

16. What about other growth factors or growth factor antagonists? (Choose one or more.)

   A. Granulocyte CSF (G-CSF)

   B. Macrophage CSF (M-CSF)

   C. Tumor necrosis factor (TNF)

   D. Anti-TNF compound

   E. Interleukin 1 (IL-1)

   F. IL-6

   G. None of above

   This is a rapidly developing field, but certainly many would consider G-CSF to hasten marrow recovery, and there is now evidence that TNF may be an initiator of GVHD so that anti-TNF substances are being investigated. (See the chapters by Barrett, Tutschka, and Peters.)

17. Are granulocytes that are released "early" due to GM-CSF (or other growth factors) functionally normal?

   A. Yes

   B. No

   The granulocytes which are stimulated by GM-CSF or other growth factors are functionally normal based on in vitro and in vivo testing. (See the chapter by Vollmer and Mandell.)

18. Granulocyte transfusions have fallen from use largely due to limited yields with current technology even following donor priming with corticosteroids. Would the priming of donors with GM-CSF be of potential value in collecting adequate numbers of granulocytes for transfusion?

   A. Yes

   B. No

   The question is stimulating, but the answer is unclear.

19. The patient is treated, as above; however, by day 18, with still no circulating granulocytes, he develops new fever and chest X-ray shows a

left upper lobe pulmonary infiltrate. Bronchoscopy with biopsy is done, and appropriate stains might show which of the following organisms? (Pick the two most likely.)

    A. Gram-negative bacilli

    B. Branching septated hyphae

    C. *Pneumocystis carinii*

    D. *Toxoplasma gondii*

The most likely finding would be branching septated hyphae representing invasive aspergillosis; however, this patient is still at high risk of developing a Gram-negative pneumonia. *P. carinii* causes interstitial pneumonitis in patients with depressed cellular immunity, such as in the bone marrow transplant patient, but this is somewhat early in the course for this infection. Toxoplasma is a very uncommon cause of pneumonia.

20. The biopsy shows branching septated hyphae. You would now treat with (choose all correct answers):

    A. Amphotericin B

    B. Amphotericin B plus rifampin

    C. Fluconazole

    D. Ketoconazole

Amphotericin B remains the "gold standard" for the treatment of aspergillosis in the neutropenic patient. Animal studies have shown that the addition of rifampin to amphotericin B is synergistic, but there are no clinical data in humans to document any added clinical value in this setting. Fluconazole is effective for invasive candidiasis but not invasive aspergillosis. Ketoconazole is not active against *A. flavus* or *fumigatus*.

21. Amphotericin B should be at what dosage? (Choose one best answer)

    A. 0.3 mg/kg per day

    B. 0.6 mg/kg per day

    C. 1.2–1.5 mg/kg per day

    D. 1.2–1.5 mg/kg q.o.d.

The so-called standard dosage of amphotericin B is 0.6 mg/kg per day; however, given the exceedingly poor response rates for aspergillosis in the granulocytopenic state, many increase the dose to 1.2–1.5 mg/kg per day (yet others would give a maximum of 1.0 mg/kg per day). Every-other-day therapy would be reserved for the patient with return of granulocytes, resolving infection, but who needs a long course of therapy.

22. Should amphotericin B be given as a liposomal preparation?

    A. Yes

    B. No

Numerous investigations in recent years have looked at the potential of administering amphotericin B in a liposomal preparation. Although the studies published to date are encouraging, there is yet no definitive answer on efficacy and safety. (See the chapter by Anaissie and Pinczowski.)

23. Assume that the biopsy in Q16 had demonstrated a nonfungal origin for the pulmonary infiltrate and that a few days later the patient developed difficulty swallowing. Esophagoscopy was performed and demonstrated invasive candidiasis. Which of the following would be appropriate therapy? (Choose one or more.)
    A. Amphotericin B
    B. Amphotericin B plus flucytosine
    C. Fluconazole
    D. Nystatin
    E. Ketoconazole
    F. Amphotericin B plus acyclovir

As with aspergillosis, the "standard" for candidiasis remains amphotericin B intravenously. Some would add flucytosine to amphotericin B as the two are known to be synergistic and both effective against *Candida*. Fluconazole has been found to be effective in this setting and could be utilized. Nystatin is only available orally and is not absorbed; this invasive infection requires systemic therapy. Ketoconazole, given orally, is systemically absorbed and might be effective in this setting; however, most believe that amphotericin B or fluconazole would be more appropriate than ketoconazole. Finally, it should be noted that many cases of esophagitis in the neutropenic patient are initiated by herpes simplex and then superinfected by *Candida*; therefore, some of the experts at the symposium would have given the combination of amphotericin B plus acyclovir. For similar reasons, one could utilize fluconazole and acyclovir, thus avoiding the toxicities of amphotericin B. Finally, it is important to note that many would consider using fluconazole prophylactically in these patients to prevent invasive candidiasis. (See the chapter by Anaissie and Pinczowski.)

24. How often is *Candida* esophagitis preceded by herpetic infection? (Choose one.)
    A. Frequently
    B. Occasionally
    C. Rarely

Candida esophagitis is frequently preceded by herpes simplex invasion.

25. Which species of *Candida* is more invasive?
    A. *Candida albicans*
    B. *Candida tropicalis*

C. tropicalis has been found to be more invasive among neutropenic patients than *C. albicans*.

26. Which species of *Candida* is more frequently found to cause infection in this setting?
    A. *Candida albicans*
    B. *Candida tropicalis*

C. albicans colonizes the alimentary canal much more frequently than does *C. tropicalis*, therefore, even though *C. tropicalis* is more invasive, *C. albicans* more frequently causes infection.

27. Which fungi are emerging as new pathogens in the immunocompromised patients with cancer?

   A. *Pseudallescheria boydii*
   B. *Trichosporon* spp.
   C. *Fusarium* spp.
   D. *Drechslera* spp.
   E. *Encephalitozoon cuniculi*

   All of these organisms are now emerging as new pathogens. (See the chapter by Zinner.)

28. This patient was antibody positive for herpes simplex virus at the time of initial admission. Given that such patients have a very high incidence of reactivation of the latent herpes simplex virus, which of the following agents should have been used, beginning on day 0, as prophylaxis?

   A. Ganciclovir
   B. AZT
   C. Acyclovir
   D. Foscarnet

   It is generally agreed that these patients are at exceedingly high risk of herpes simplex infection following bone marrow transplantation and that acyclovir, given orally, will prevent reactivation. (See the chapter by Saral.)

29. Would the same prophylactic approach have been appropriate for this patient when he was receiving his initial remission induction chemotherapy?

   A. Yes
   B. No

   It is not generally appreciated that the patient with acute nonlymphocytic leukemia who receives intensive remission induction chemotherapy, such as a combination of daunorubicin plus cytosine arabinoside, has a very high frequency of developing herpes simplex reactivation infection. As a result, acyclovir prophylaxis is appropriate in seropositive individuals. However, more than 80%–90% of all adults are antibody positive for herpes simplex virus; those who are antibody positive have a strikingly high rate of reactivation during any type of intensive myelosuppressive (and thus mucosa-damaging) therapy.

30. Again, the patient improves, and by day 23, the granulocyte count begins to return toward normal. Antibacterial therapy is given for 14 days and antifungal therapy is planned for 6 weeks. On day 40, new fever develops and chest X-ray now shows bilateral pulmonary infiltrates with an interstitial pattern. Bronchoscopy and biopsy are done again,

avoiding the original area of infiltrate known to be fungal in origin. The findings are most likely which one of the following?

A. *Pseudomonas aeruginosa*
B. Cytomegalovirus (CMV)
C. *Toxoplasma gondii*
D. *Streptococcus pneumoniae*
E. *Aspergillus flavus*
F. *Pneumocystis carinii*
G. Herpes simplex virus
H. Idiopathic IP (regimen-related toxicity)

At this point in time, the patient has return of granulocytes and is therefore much less susceptible to the organisms commonly associated with granulocytopenia, such as *P. aeruginosa*. CMV is the most common recognized cause of interstitial pneumonia, although *P. carinii* can occur, as can idiopathic pneumonitis. Pneumococcal infection is possible but unlikely given the presentation, and, similarly, aspergillosis may still occur in this time frame although this is an unlikely presentation. (See the chapters by Schmidt and Barrett.)

31. The appropriate therapy for this patient would be:

A. Acyclovir
B. Piperacillin plus gentamicin
C. Pyrimethamine plus sulfadiazine
D. Ganciclovir plus immune serum globulin

Given the presumptive diagnosis of CMV pneumonitis, it has been shown that ganciclovir plus immune serum globulin is effective if given early in the course of the infection. (See the chapter by Schmidt.)

32. If this patient has been CMV seronegative prior to bone marrow transplantation and also received his graft from a CMV-negative donor,

A. the patient should have received CMV-negative blood component support exclusively
B. filtered blood component support is equivalent
C. unscreened blood support is adequate

CMV pneumonia or other CMV infection can be avoided in this setting if the patient receives CMV-negative blood component support exclusively.

33. The patient improves and is discharged to home. On day 63, he develops an erythematous painful rash at the level of T4 on the right side. By the next day, a number of vesicles have appeared which are filled with a clear, slightly straw-colored fluid. The diagnosis is herpes zoster caused by the latent varicella zoster virus. The physician prescribes codeine for pain, careful washing with an antiseptic soap, and a skin cream. In addition, this patient should be treated with:

A. Nothing
B. Ganciclovir

C. Acyclovir

D. Adenine arabinoside

Acyclovir, the treatment of choice, is effective against herpes zoster if begun very early in the patient's course. Since many of these patients progress to dissemination and some to death, it is very reasonable to treat these patients early and aggressively with acyclovir intravenously or orally. (See the chapter by Feldman.)

34. About day 70 following transplantation, the patient develops myalgia, abdominal pain, nausea, and malaise. He is afebrile. White blood count and platelet count are normal with no evidence of recurrence of primary disease. Serum ALT is 1330 IU/l, AST is 890 IU/l (nl ALT and AST <40), alkaline phosphatase is 115 IU/l (nl <120), bilirubin is 2.1 mg/dl (1.3 mg/dl direct). Differential diagnosis includes viral hepatitis (A, B, C, D, CMV), drug-induced hepatitis, hepatic recurrence, veno-occlusive disease, and hepatic graft-versus-host disease. Initial serologic evaluation include negative IgG anti-HAV, HBsAg, anti-HBc, and anti-HCV. Blood and urine cultures for CMV are negative. The most effective means of establishing the diagnosis is:

A. CT scan

B. Wedged hepatic venogram

C. Percutaneous liver biopsy

D. Laparoscopic liver biopsy

As stated in the question, the differential diagnosis is broad. Although infection with hepatitis C virus is probably most likely, anti-HCV is not likely to be present this early in the course of infection. If any further diagnostic studies were considered at this time, percutaneous liver biopsy would be most helpful. Laparoscopic biopsy would also be acceptable but would add to the cost and complexity of the evaluation and would not provide any advantage over percutaneous biopsy in this particular situation.

35. The most likely diagnosis is:

A. CMV hepatitis

B. Hepatitis C

C. Veno-occlusive disease

Hepatitis C is very common in multiply transfused and immunosuppressed patients such as the individual under discussion. It is the most likely of the three possibilities to occur this long after transplantation. Veno-occlusive disease usually occurs within the 1st month after transplant. CMV infection should always be considered in immunosuppressed patients, but the degree of elevation of the serum aminotransferase levels makes this diagnosis less likely.

36. The patient is observed. Although the liver tests decline slightly over the next week, the patient becomes jaundiced. A liver biopsy is performed which shows acute hepatitis without viral inclusions. Terminal hepatic

venules are normal (no veno-occlusive disease). The presumptive diagnosis is seronegative hepatitis C (post-transfusion). Appropriate treatment is:

A. Recombinant interferon alfa-2b
B. Ribavirin
C. Decrease immunosuppression
D. Observation

Observation is most appropriate. Although recombinant interferon alfa-2b is effective treatment for *chronic* hepatitis C, preliminary data suggest that it does not prevent development of chronic hepatitis when administered during the acute phase of the disease. Ribavirin has some activity against hepatitis C virus during chronic infection, but it does not appear to be as effective as interferon alfa-2b. Ribavirin has not been studied in acute infections. Finally, hepatitis C virus is directly cytopathic to hepatocytes and does not appear to be effected by immunosuppression. Thus, reduction of immunosuppressive therapy would probably have little, if any, influence on the infection and is not indicated because of the risk of graft-versus-host disease. It is not practical to decrease immunosuppression because of the need to reduce graft-versus-host disease. (See the chapter by Davis.)

37. About day 90 the patient is driving in his car and is obliged to make a sudden stop; his shoulder seat belt strap forcibly restrains him. He notices some discomfort along the Hickman catheter tunnel site for the next week and then begins to have low-grade fever and increased discomfort along the tunnel. Within 2 more days the overlying skin is erythematous and examination demonstrates fluctuance; temperature is now 100.4°F. Gram stain of an aspirate shows Gram-positive cocci. The treatment approach should be (choose one):

A. Vancomycin (i.v.)
B. Nafcillin (i.v.)
C. Cloxacillin (p.o.)
D. Vancomycin plus remove catheter
E. Nafcillin plus remove catheter

There are three types of infections associated with Hickman catheters. The first and most common is an exit site infection and is usually caused by *Staphylococcus epidermidis* or other local skin flora. These infections can be treated with antibiotics, most often vancomycin, without the need to remove the catheter. Bacteremia associated with the catheter is relatively uncommon despite the fact that nearly all catheters after a few weeks will be colonized with *S. epidermidis* well embedded in a glycocalyx matrix. These bacteremias can likewise be treated with intravenous vancomcyin (given through the catheter). These can be successfully treated, in our experience, in most cases. Finally, tunnel infections are serious and life threatening, are usually caused by staphylococci, either *S. aureus* or *S. epidermidis*, and do require removal of the catheter in addition to appropriate therapy which, in this case, would be vancomycin so as to assure coverage for both *S. aureus* and *S. epidermidis*.

38. The patient is well until he calls his physician at 10 p.m. on the evening of the 97th day. He indicates that he has been well except for a minor sore throat for the past day or two. However, 1 h ago, he had the sudden onset of fever to 103°F with very intense shaking chills. He has no other particular symptomatology. His physician had seen him in the office a few days before for routine follow up, and, at that time, he had been in complete remission of leukemia, white blood cell count was normal with a normal differential, and the platelet count was normal. The physical examination was entirely normal. Given the high fever and shaking chills, the patient is instructed to meet his physician in the emergency room immediately. The physician is concerned about the possibility of an overwhelming bacteremia, in its very earliest stages, caused by which (choose the single best answer) of the following organisms?

    A. *Pseudomonas aeruginosa*
    B. *Staphylococcus epidermidis*
    C. *Streptococcus pneumoniae*
    D. *Staphylococcus aureus*

    Not only do these patients have depressed cellular immunity, they also have depressed humoral immunity for a prolonged time. Reduced humoral immunity increases susceptibility to infection by the encapsulated pyogenic cocci, especially *S. pneumoniae*. There is also evidence that these patients develop hyposplenism, probably as a result of chronic graft-versus-host disease. In addition, many patients develop a subclass deficiency of IgG, especially IgG II/IgG IV, apparently as a consequence of disordered reconstitution of T cell subsets and a long-lasting deficit of functional T cell precursors. There is a syndrome among asplenic patients known as overwhelming pneumococcal sepsis syndrome which can progress very quickly, very aggressively, leading to the patient's demise within just a few hours. It is therefore critical to evaluate these patients promptly and begin antibiotic therapy intravenously under hospital observation.

39. Should this patient have received any of the following vaccines following transplantation? (Circle correct choices.)

    A. *Haemophilus influenzae* B
    B. *Streptococcus pneumoniae*
    C. *Neisseria meningitidis*
    D. Varicella zoster
    E. Measles – mumps – rubella

    Given the comments above, one would want to vaccinate with the pneumococcal vaccine and, likewise, the *Haemophilus* and the meningococcal vaccine, recognizing, however, that the patient probably will not develop a strong antibody response and therefore certainly should not be considered no longer at risk for these infections. The varicella zoster viral vaccine would not be given to someone with a prior history of varicella since it presumably will not prevent the development of zoster as reactivation from the prior infection. Generally, one avoids live viral vaccines in individuals with suppressed cellular immunity and hence would not use the measles, mumps, or rubella vaccines but would give the influenza vaccine each fall not only to prevent influenza but also bacterial superinfection.

40. Should this patient have received serum immune globulin (i.v.) prophylactically on a regular basis after transplantation?

    A. Yes

    B. No

There is evidence that immune serum globulin given intravenously helps to prevent some bacterial infections in these patients and, likewise, helps to prevent graft-versus-host disease. (See the chapter by Tutschka.)

41. Should this patient have received trimethoprim sulfamethoxazole (TMP-SMX) as prophylaxis for pneumocystis pneumonia?

    A. Yes

    B. No

Although it would not be inappropriate to use trimethoprim sulfamethoxazole as prophylaxis for Pneumocystis, it should be recalled that pneumocystis pneumonitis is not extremely common in these patients.

42. Would TMP-SMX therapy have prevented this febrile illness?

    A. Yes

    B. No

TMP-SMX has been suggested, but the infecting streptococcal strains are frequently resistant to TMP-SMZ.

43. Should the patient have received prophylaxis with another antibiotic, e.g., amoxacillin?

    A. Yes

    B. No

Opinions differ as to whether the patient at risk for the pneumococcal sepsis syndrome should receive antibiotic prophylaxis. Given all of the other problems the patient is at risk for and the potential for causing overgrowth with other organisms, notably *Candida*, one could argue either way. Amoxacillin has been suggested, but it would appear that the use of repeated doses of intravenous serum globulin may be most useful.

44. On day 120 after bone marrow transplantation on a routine review, he complains of an unusual sensation which he described as "not being able to take a complete breath." Examination of the chest is unremarkable, blood count shows a fall in neutrophils from $2.4 \times 10^9/l$ to $1.3 \times 10^9/l$, the platelet count also fell from 110 to $92 \times 10^9/l$. A chest radiograph

showed no abnormalities, but lung function showed a restrictive–obstructive pattern with a decreased KCO and a prolonged FEV1. He was given a bronchodilator inhaler, and a DEAFF test for CMV was carried out on blood and urine. What possible diagnosis should be considered?

A. CMV pneumonitis
B. Chronic graft-versus-host disease affecting the lungs
C. Pneumocystis pneumonia
D. Bacterial pneumonia
E. *Aspergillus* pneumonia

The two key diagnoses in this setting would be CMV pneumonitis or graft-versus-host disease affecting the lungs. At this late date with normal numbers of granulocytes circulating, bacterial pneumonia or *Aspergillus* pneumonia would not be expected and pneumocystis pneumonia would be uncommon. Although one tends not to think of *Aspergillus* infection so late after marrow transplantation, in fact, it can occur. Apparently, it develops as a result of disturbances of granulocyte function which, in turn, is related to chronic graft-versus-host disease. In these patients with chronic graft-versus-host disease, opsonization and phagocytosis can be impaired as well as respiratory burst function. Gram-negative infections in this setting can occur, but aspergillosis is more common and can be aggressively invasive.

45. Three days later, he reports that the tightness in the chest has improved but he is nevertheless more dyspneic and has developed an unproductive cough. On examination, there are a few scattered crepitations to be heard on auscultation of the chest, and the chest radiograph now shows a widespread diffuse increase in density particularly around the midzones. On further examinations, he is noted to be mildly icteric and has a generalized fine erythema. Liver function results taken 3 days previously show a rise in alkaline phosphatase and raised bilirubin. The DEAFF test for CMV early antigens taken 3 days previously is negative. What would you do next?

A. Bronchoscopy and examination of bronchial washings
B. Open lung biopsy
C. Empiric high-dose intravenous cotrimoxazole
D Repeat DEAFF test
E. Empiric intravenous ceftazidime
F. Empiric intravenous amphotericin B

The correct answer is to do bronchoscopy and examination of bronchial washings as this will usually diagnose CMV infection when it is present and should help to define the presence or absence of graft-versus-host disease. Open lung biopsy should not be necessary in this situation. Given the likely differential diagnosis, one would not prescribe cotrimoxazole for *Pneumocystis carinii* pneumonia, ceftazidime for bacterial pneumonia, or amphotericin B for fungal pneumonia.

46. Bronchial washings were shown to be positive for CMV. How would you treat the patient?
    A. CMV-specific immunoglobulin and ganciclovir
    B. Prednisolone and cyclosporine to treat chronic graft-versus-host disease
    C. Add antibacterial prophylaxis with TMP-SMZ, and antifungal prophylaxis with ketoconazole
    D. Give high-dose intravenous methyl prednisolone to improve lung function

    Specific therapy would include ganciclovir and (CMV serum) high-dose immunoglobulin intravenously. Patients who require ventilatory assistance early on usually have an extremely poor prognosis despite this therapy. Those patients may benefit from high-dose intravenous methylprednisolone.

    Given the unlikely development of either *Pneumocystis* or fungal infections at this time, one would not begin prophylaxis with TMP-SMZ or an antifungal such as ketoconazole.

47. He was admitted to the hospital and treated with ganciclovir and high-dose immunoglobulin. After 3 weeks of treatment, his lung function had improved and the DEAFF test was negative. He is discharged from the hospital. What prophylactic treatment should he continue with and for how long?
    A. Alternate-day prednisolone and cyclosporine
    B. Regular cotrimoxazole
    C. Penicillin daily
    D. Repeated monthly infusions of anti-CMV immunoglobulin

    Patients who successfully complete a treatment course with ganciclovir/ intravenous immunoglobulin should be on a maintenance regimen as long as they require immunosuppressive therapy (as part of their graft-versus-host disease prophylaxis or treatment). The likelihood of re-infection in this setting is high. The length of such maintenance treatment is not standardized, but Tutschka and Schmidt recommend continuing ganciclovir at 5 mg/day five times a week in addition to intravenous immunoglobulin at 500 mg/kg once a week until the patient is off all immunosuppressive drugs.

Subject Index

Springer-Verlag
and the Environment

We at Springer-Verlag firmly believe that an international science publisher has a special obligation to the environment, and our corporate policies consistently reflect this conviction.

We also expect our business partners – paper mills, printers, packaging manufacturers, etc. – to commit themselves to using environmentally friendly materials and production processes.

The paper in this book is made from low- or no-chlorine pulp and is acid free, in conformance with international standards for paper permanency.